2/12

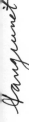

WEYERHAEUSER ENVIRONMENTAL BOOKS

WILLIAM CRONON, EDITOR

Weyerhaeuser Environmental Books explore human relationships
with natural environments in all their variety and complexity. They
seek to cast new light on the ways that natural systems affect human
communities, the ways that people affect the environments of which
they are a part, and the ways that different cultural conceptions of
nature profoundly shape our sense of the world around us. A complete
listing of the books in the series appears at the end of this book.

TOXIC ARCHIPELAGO

A HISTORY OF INDUSTRIAL DISEASE IN JAPAN

BRETT L. WALKER   FOREWORD BY WILLIAM CRONON

UNIVERSITY OF WASHINGTON PRESS   SEATTLE AND LONDON

The Toxic Archipelago: A History of Industrial Disease
in Japan *is published with the assistance of a grant from the
Weyerhaeuser Environmental Books Endowment, established
by the Weyerhaeuser Company Foundation, members of the
Weyerhaeuser family, and Janet and Jack Creighton.*

University of Washington Press
PO Box 50096, Seattle, WA 98145, USA
www.washington.edu/uwpress

Library of Congress Cataloging-in-Publication Data
Walker, Brett L., 1967–
Toxic archipelago: a history of industrial disease in Japan /
Brett L. Walker.
p. cm. —(Wewyerhauser environmental books.)
Includes bibliographical references and index.
ISBN 978-0-295-98954-9 (hardback : alk. paper)
1. Occupational diseases—Japan—History.
2. Human ecology—Japan—History.
3. Japan—Environmental conditions. I. Title
RC963.7.J3W45 2010   616.9'8030952—dc22   2009037663

FOR CLOSE FRIENDS

How delightful it would be to converse intimately
with someone of the same mind, sharing with him
the pleasures of uninhibited conversation on the
amusing and foolish things of this world, but such
friends are hard to find. If you must take care that
your opinions do not differ in the least from those
of the person with whom you are talking, you
might just as well be alone.

—Kenkō, *Tsurezuregusa* (Essays in Idleness)

CONTENTS

FOREWORD: THE PAIN OF A POISONED WORLD

BY WILLIAM CRONON

Among the historical phenomena leading to the rise of modern environmentalism in the second half of the twentieth century, one of the most striking was also one of the least visible: the proliferating presence of toxic compounds in the webs of ecological relationships that sustain life on the planet. What seemed like a new age of toxicity exploded into public view with the atomic bombs dropped on the Japanese cities of Hiroshima and Nagasaki in 1945, followed in turn by countless nuclear tests and the radioactive fallout they generated. As background levels of radiation rose during the 1950s and early 1960s, people around the globe became increasingly concerned that the foods on which they and their children depended were laced with contaminants like Strontium 90 and Cesium 137. In the early years of the Cold War, the "enemy within" symbolized the peril posed by communist agents (and organized criminals) capable of infiltrating and undermining national institutions, but the metaphor gradually extended to include other forms of infiltration and contamination as well. Rachel Carson's *Silent Spring* in 1962 brought those fears into sharp focus. Environmental toxicity was hardly limited to radiation: the intentional use of poisons to control pests, she argued, was having devastating effects as toxins accumulated in the bodies of fish, birds, mammals, and human beings.

Although Carson's intervention might suggest to Americans that concern about toxicity first arose mainly in the United States, in fact this transformation in environmental thinking was world-wide. Japanese concerns about radiation and nuclear weapons made that nation a leader in pointing the way toward a new era. A year before Silent Spring was published, a mysterious wave of birth defects in the United Kingdom and elsewhere was linked to the new drug thalidomide, so that images of newborn babies with missing limbs joined the victims of Hiroshima as sinister icons of the havoc that toxic exposures can wreak. Whereas an earlier era had habitually looked to science and technology for solutions to social and environmental problems, by the 1960s these agents of "progress"—the scare quotes around that word are themselves symptomatic of the new era—seemed as often as not to cause those problems. For a generation growing up in the shadow of the mushroom cloud, the idea that one's own body might harbor the poisonous seeds of future cancers and birth defects became a potent source both of nightmares and political activism. In the history of human fear, the post-Hiroshima age was haunted by new forms of hidden terror that were all the more frightening for lurking so invisibly beneath the bright sunlit surfaces of everyday life.

What was new, though, was less the poisons themselves than the public awareness of their presence. To be sure, radioactive fallout was peculiarly a product of the nuclear age and the widespread use of organic compounds as pesticides were an innovation of modern chemistry. But before DDT was used to control insects, it had precursors, like copper sulphate and lead arsenate, whose biological effects and long-term accumulation in the environment were hardly benign. Factories and mines had been generating toxic by-products world-wide long before World War II, so to really understand the rise of environmental toxicity one has to go much further back in time, to the dawn of the industrial era.

This is what Brett Walker has done in *Toxic Archipelago*, his disturbing new history of industrial disease in Japan. The book's argument is deceptively simple: toxicity was an inevitable outcome of cultural innovations that viewed nature as a resource waiting to be exploited toward useful human ends. The Enlightenment rationality that enabled scientists and engineers to break natural substances and productive processes into their component parts made possible efficiencies and economies of scale that would have been unthinkable to earlier generations. The benefits were obvious: dramatic increases in material outputs of all manner of goods and services, from foods to textiles to machines. The costs were often not so visible, concentrated as they were in the vicinity of individual factories or so diffuse that they could not easily be detected by unaided human senses. Every industrial product, Walker argues, also had by-products, unwanted materials that were inherent to production but undesirable in and of themselves and so were destined for release into environments that seemed capable of diluting or absorbing them without much harm. Or so people thought.

In a series of horrifying case studies, Walker applies his analytical lens to episodes involving different forms of pollution at different moments in the Japanese past: organophosphate pesticide contaminations in agricultural districts; toxic tailings and effluents at the Ashio copper smelter; methylmercury-contaminated shellfish and other marine organisms off the coast of Minamata; asthma-inducing chemicals from the Yokkaichi petroleum refinery; and the all-too-descriptive "it hurts, it hurts disease" caused by toxic waste from the Kamioka lead and zinc mines. Walker's tightly focused narratives of what happened in these places—and his accounts of his own efforts to uncover the toxic legacies of landscapes he has explored himself—enable him to put human faces on events that might otherwise seem abstract and remote, so far from the lived experience of non-Japanese readers that they might be tempted to regard this book as having little relevance to their own lives.

Nothing could be further from the truth, since these vivid stories of contaminated landscapes and grievously injured people and animals point toward two striking moral lessons that could hardly be more relevant to would-be readers of this book no matter where they live. The first is that modernity's promise to liberate humanity from the constraints of nature was a lie, plain and simple. In Walker's words, "transcendence, disengagement, or liberation . . . from nature is a fantasy." The ability of engineers to redesign productive processes so as to maximize desired outputs almost always involved simplifying those processes and turning a blind eye toward the biological contexts within which they took place. To imagine that a reinvented human world could somehow be created in isolation from the rest of nature almost always meant ignoring those parts of nature not immediately relevant to the technological labor being performed in any given place at any given time. From this willful refusal to observe and understand the full range of outputs from a technological system came the toxins that were invisible, mainly because people chose not to see them until they were just too destructive to ignore.

This modern delusion of liberation from nature points toward a second moral lesson, one that is even more disturbing in its implications. Our own bodies are porous to the ecosystems we inhabit. The physiological processes that keep us alive do so only by myriad exchanges—minute by minute, hour by hour, day by day—of compounds, nutrients, minerals, and other substances without which we could not survive. Our health depends on the permeability of our bodies to the very nature from which we imagine we might isolate ourselves. So when we fill the world around us with toxic substances, we fill our own bodies with those substances as well. More often than not, the unintended by-product of the resulting exposures is *pain*.

Here is the darkest insight of this dark book. Pain is nature's way of communicating in the most intimate possible way—through the nerves and fibers of our own flesh—the harm we do not just to nature but also to ourselves. It is the proof that our conscious selves remain tethered to our physical bodies and inextricably tied to the larger ecological universe even when we pretend otherwise in our dreams. The implications of this haunting insight reach far beyond the Japanese fields and factories of Brett Walker's *Toxic Archipelago* to touch the communities, homes, and bodies of everyone who reads this book.

PREFACE

For the past decade I have taught an environmental history of Japan seminar, first at Yale University and then at Montana State University. The seminar focuses on themes ranging from disease and the generation of scientific knowledge to perceptions of nonhuman animals and modern industrial pollution. Each year, I carefully attempt to sharpen my explanations regarding what drives environmental problems in Japan, even as my explanations, frustratingly, have become less specific as I increasingly reject reductionist explanations of our current environmental mess. That is to say, environmental problems in Japan, as in other industrialized societies, are not just caused by industrial greed or anchovy feeding habits or rural poverty or messy mining practices or religious beliefs or war and empire. Rather, they are caused by a combination of these forces, and many others, too. All these forces function as part of naturally occurring and anthropogenic levels in causal cascades or in linked ecological events that trigger, like carefully lined up dominoes, pollution episodes.

At certain moments in history, historical and natural drivers come together—serendipitously joining forces, one might say—to form what I label in this book as "hybrid causations." Hybrid causations, as we shall see, are the key to understanding environmental problems in Japan. You could stare under a microscope at a sample of the biocide parathion for weeks and never fully understand how it kills people or facilitates insect evolution. This requires historical context, or viewing how parathion operates in landscapes and bodies across human geographic space and historical time.

In my seminar, I encourage students to view environmental history—all history, really—in this broad manner, while still not ignoring history's focused explanatory power. My message on this score is a simple one: because historical inquiry can analyze, then narrate, diverse causal forces (and generally rejects forms of reductionism), it is an important means of understanding the multifaceted problems life on Earth faces. Embracing an analysis of complex causal webs offers a far more compelling explanation than an overly simplified history does. For example, to say that cadmium caused "its hurts, it hurts disease" in postwar Toyama belies the role that human politics, economics, technology, and culture played in environmental pollution and industrial disease. Was it really cadmium that killed? Or was it the refinery technologies that processed it? Or was it the overseas war and empire building that demanded it? Or was it the eating habits of Japanese farmers? Or was it related to Japanese women's notions of beauty and skin complexion? Or was it all these factors acting in concert? Because human activity is so prevalent on Earth, environmental pollution and industrial disease cannot be understood without an exploration of the specific human activities—the human stories and histories—that drive these changes. This, too, is an important lesson that I try to relay to students in my seminar. In many respects, this book attempts to demonstrate how the hybrid causation model elucidates problems related to environmental pollution and industrial disease in Japan. The hybrid causation model does not shirk focused analyses and careful explanations in favor of descriptions of the big picture, rather it simply acknowledges that environmental history is moved by many forces, and so understanding our past demands that we acknowledge these forces as well.

Writing history is not a hybrid exercise, but it is certainly a collaborative one. I would like to acknowledge those friends and colleagues with whom I brainstormed, or who proofread and even edited substantial portions of this book. Without their kind collaboration, whether offered casually at the poker table or formally in academic settings, this project would not have been possible. Julia Adeney Thomas carefully read the entire manuscript and offered substantial comments and encouragement. To say that she greatly improved it would be an understatement. Her eyes see historical nuances far better than mine do, so if any interesting ones have been elucidated in the pages ahead, she is probably responsible for them. Michael Reidy also read the entire manuscript. In his usual no-nonsense manner, he pushed me to use the book to establish new terminologies and vocabularies for how both historians and ecologists speak of such phenomena as "trophic cascades" and other so-called natural events. If, Michael queried me, history and culture are just as powerful a force in ecological systems as energy distribution or food webs—what we traditionally view as natural forces—then establish a new way of talking about pollution events that reflects this hybrid reality. I have not been altogether successful in this, but the astute reader will discern the attempts to do so with such terminology as "hybrid causations." Timothy LeCain and Dale Martin also read either all or substantial portions of the manuscript. They steered me clear of some silly mistakes regarding mining techniques and technologies. Dale also hand-drafted the one beautiful map in the book. Timothy George and another careful reader for the University of Washington Press improved the manuscript in many ways. At the press, William Cronon, Julidta Tarver, and Marianne Keddington-Lang were, as usual, absolute pleasures to work with, as was the copy editor, Pamela Bruton.

I am also grateful to James Bartholomew, Alex Bay, Rob Campbell, Susan Cohen, Kristen Intemann, Arne Keeling, Bridget Kevane, Nancy Langston, Paula Lutz, Michelle Maskiell, Ian Miller, Gregg Mitman, Mary Murphy, Kevin O'Neill, Sarah Pritchard, Ed Russell, Bob Rydell, Billy Smith, Conrad Totman, Robert Wilson, and Donald Worster. While presenting chapters at institutions around the United States, I received too much thoughtful advice to list here. Those institutions are the Massachusetts Institute of Technology (2005), University of British Columbia (2005), University of California, Berkeley (2006), Ohio State University (2006), University of Kansas (2006), Brandeis University (2007), Montana State University (2007), Columbia University (2007), and Yale University (2008). I also received helpful feedback during panels at the Columbia History of Science Group Annual Meeting (2004), the Association for Asian Studies (2005), and the American Society for Environmental History (2007, 2008). I took copious notes during these lectures and panels, and surely the insights of many are reflected in the pages ahead. Early versions of parts of chapters 1 and 2 first appeared as "Sanemori's Revenge: Insects, Eco-System Accidents, and Policy Decisions in Japan's Environmental History," in "New

Perspectives on Public Health Policy," edited by James Mohr, special issue, *Journal of Policy History* 19, no. 1 (2007): 113–44. I completed this book while serving as department chairperson, which is testimony more to the patience and extreme competency of my two administrative assistants— Diane Cattrell and Deidre Manry—than to any administrative skills that I may possess. These two are wonderful people to work with.

I received generous funding from several institutions and agencies. I serve as principal investigator for a National Science Foundation–funded project titled Technological Symmetry and Hybrid Environments at the Ashio and Anaconda Copper Mines. Timothy LeCain is the co-PI on this project. Obviously, much of the research for and insights gained from the NSF project bled into chapter 3 of this book, which investigates the Ashio copper mine. At the NSF, I appreciate all the careful advice I received from Fred Kronz, who directs the program for social, behavioral, and economic sciences. I also received funding from a generous Vice President for Scholarship, Creativity, and Technology Transfer Research Grant (Montana State University), a Research Enhancement Award (College of Letters and Science, Montana State University), and the College of Letters and Science (Montana State University). I also benefited from an extremely fruitful trip to the Harvard-Yenching Library, sponsored in part by a Harvard-Yenching Travel Grant.

At the Montana State University's Renne Library, the interlibrary loan staff proved unsurpassable in their ability to produce rare Japanese-language sources on everything from insecticide use to mercury poisoning. Miwa Munehiro at Kyushu University made rare documents related to the Hōjō colliery explosion available. I also benefited from visits to the Minamata Disease Municipal Museum, the Tagawa Coal Museum, Kamioka's Mining Museum, and other small museums, libraries, and archives scattered around Japan.

Yet, despite the efforts of so many people dispersed across so many places, mistakes surely remain, and as is customary, I take full credit for every last one of them.

PROLOGUE

On 7 February 2005, in the Nemuro Straits, off the Shiretoko Peninsula of eastern Hokkaido, near the small town of Rausu, a pod of twelve orcas became hemmed in between a fast-moving, wind-blown ice floe and the jagged coast. In the morning, Rausu residents could hear the orcas crying out from the ice as they tried to escape, the sound piercing the howling North Pacific winds. This part of Japan is ice-cold country in the winter. By afternoon, however, the whales had visibly tired and their cries had grown discernibly weaker. Rausu residents, armed with ropes, tried to dislodge the whales and did manage to free one adult female the next day. She was last seen swimming slowly in open water; the ice floe crushed to death the rest of her pod. The water around the remaining whales turned a pinkish color as the rocky shore sliced and ripped their smooth cetacean bodies.

The dead consisted of one adult male, five adult females, and five calves. Veterinary experts performed necropsies on nine of these whales. The results were even more disturbing than the image of an entire pod being crushed to death along the rocky coast of Hokkaido. In the blubber of the whales, PCB (polychlorinated biphenyl) and mercury concentrations were estimated to be eleven times higher than normal for whales in Japanese coastal waters.[1] As wolves of the sea, orcas sit squarely at the top of most marine food chains, and the toxins had bioaccumulated in their bodies. Milk was discovered in the stomachs of the calves, and this was one toxic pathway, from mother to child. Deeply disturbing were reports by an underwater cameraman (who had helped retrieve the carcasses) that the largest adult female had died while hovering above one of the younger whales, apparently protecting her calf. Her huge flippers remained wrapped around the body of the younger whale. Early reports indicated that two of the calves had parasitic illnesses, but it is more likely that they suffered birth deformities caused by the elevated mercury and PCB concentrations. One calf had a sore on its jaw, while the other had problems with its adrenal glands and kidneys.

We will never know for sure why these normally sea-savvy creatures were trapped between ice and shore. An early speculation that the ice, driven by high winds, had caught the cetaceans by surprise while they hunted seals seems facile: orcas can swim fast (at about fifty kilometers per hour in bursts). I think it is more likely that the calves suffered from birth defects caused by industrial toxins and that they slowed the pod down. The pod's decision to stay with their deformed calves even as the ice moved quickly toward shore cost them their lives.

I must confess that, partway through writing this book, when I heard the story of this destroyed orca pod, a darker tone began to permeate parts of my analysis and narrative. The image of a mother orca trying in vain to protect her deformed calf was hard to shake, particularly because I assume some blame, as a member of *Homo sapiens industrialis*, for their destruction. These whales and the other souls like them that suffer from elevated industrial toxins in their bodies represent the legacy of industrialized Earth. Just as the mother orca bequeathed poisons to her calf, we bequeath the legacy of our toxic bodies to our offspring. I tried to exorcise the darker side of this book during later editing and rewriting, but I was unable or, quite possibly, unwilling to do so. No doubt, when they read the pages ahead, some of my colleagues will cry out, "He narrates environmental declension!" And rightly so, I should add.[2] But I remain unapologetic: I am a historian and I am calling it as I see it, and I see environmental decline and deterioration everywhere. In the end, this book, though analytically so much more, became the story of one nation's contribution to the profound environmental mess in which we find ourselves. It is the story of the birth of Japan's toxic archipelago.[3]

TOXIC ARCHIPELAGO

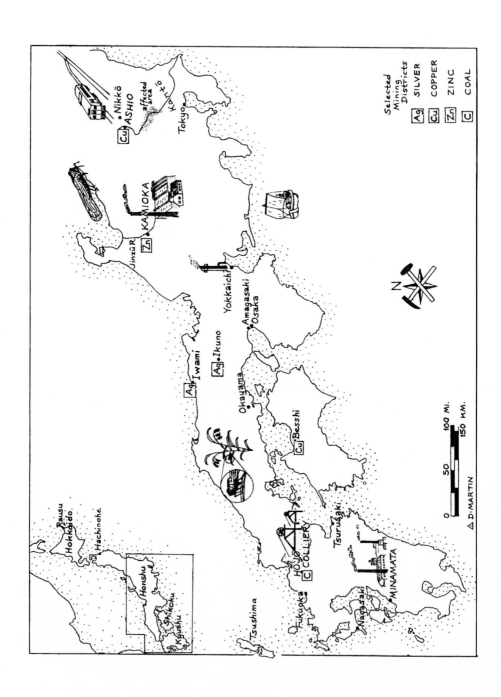

Selected
Mining
Districts

Ag	SILVER
Cu	COPPER
Zn	ZINC
C	COAL

N

0   50   100 MI.
0   150 KM.

△ D·MARTIN

Hokkaido.
Usu
Hachinohe
Honshu
Shikoku
Kyushu
Tsushima
Tsuruzaki
Fukuoka
HOJO COLLIERY C
Nagasaki
MINAMATA
Okayama
Besshi Cu
Amagasaki
Osaka
Ikuno Ag
Yokkaichi
Iwami Ag
Jinzū R.
KAMIOKA Zn
Tokyo
Kantō
affected area
Nikkō
ASHIO Cu

INTRODUCTION: KNOWING NATURE

One of the most celebrated stories in Japanese history is that of the Akō Incident. Like most samurai stories, it portrays pride, revenge, and, quite noticeably, a lot of agonizing pain. It also portrays sacrifice. In the story, pain, in the form of *seppuku*, or ritual disembowelment, serves as a gory expression of personal loyalty. In turn, personal loyalty serves as the glue holding together Japan's early modern order, based as it was on Confucian filial piety and vassalage. One of the most visceral manifestations of the importance of loyalty to Japan's early modern order was glorified pain through disembowelment. Before you discontinue reading in disbelief that I would start this book with a samurai story, remember that some cultures ascribe nobility to this kind of death: it is hard to question a man's sincerity for a cause when he is, on the most dramatic of occasions, tearing out his entrails with his bare hands to demonstrate it.[1]

In 1701, the lord of Akō Domain, a country samurai named Asano Naganori (1667–1701), got into a dangerous squabble with the shogun's court etiquette master, Kira Yoshinaka (1641–1702). Though the precise reasons for Asano's "grudge" remain a mystery, the standard explanation, relayed by the Confucian scholar Muro Kyūsō (1658–1734), is that the "Asano house had failed to give an adequate bribe to Kira in return for his guidance in matters of etiquette," and Kira consequently snubbed the Asano House.[2]

Apparently, Asano sought to settle the matter by attacking Kira inside the Edo Castle precincts. "Do you remember my grudge from these past days?" he shouted, according to one witness. In striking Kira with his blade, Asano broke the law, and after considerable deliberation, councilors granted him the privilege of taking his own life by disembowelment. When he did so, he left behind a handful of vassals who eventually avenged their lord's death by killing Kira on a snowy winter evening in 1702. They presented Kira's severed head to their master's grave at the Sengakuji Temple. Flummoxed by the clash between private filial ethics and brazen public disobedience, the Tokugawa shogun's chief Confucian councilors granted them, too, the honor of cutting open their bellies. Supposedly, they took their own lives to preserve Japan's precarious burgeoning nation: they sacrificed themselves to maintain the uneasy balance between warrior ethics and the development of early modern law. As Eiko Ikegami writes, the judgment of the Tokugawa shogunate "placed the values of law and order above those that had governed the medieval lives of the samurai."[3]

Now, fast-forward two and a half centuries to a different kind of national sacrifice in 1966, this one for Japan's industrial order. Imagine a poor, elderly man appearing and disappearing as he walks slowly between the towering shadows cast by the Daikyō Petroleum Refinery in Yokkaichi, on the Pacific coast of Japan's main island. He enters his home never to be seen alive again. When Lord Asano sliced open his belly at the dawn of the eighteenth century, Yokkaichi was home to modest fishing villages and was a prominent post station along the Tōkaidō, or Eastern Sea Circuit. By 1966, Yokkaichi had transformed utterly: it boasted large petroleum refineries that fed Japan's new industrial hunger pangs. Colossal facilities, these refineries were part of a *konbinato*, or Soviet-style industrial center, and stood as powerful symbols of Japan's postwar economic recovery. Like Japan's early modern order, however, they also demanded forms of sacrifice. The refineries destroyed the small village of Isozu, located along the Suzuka River: the Tsukiji fish market in Tokyo declined its stinking catches and the lungs of its inhabitants burned from sulfur dioxide. Isozu's fishermen protested, even trying to plug an industrial drainpipe on one occasion; petrochemical corporations and the local government brushed them aside. Once again, Japan faced an ethical impasse, not between warrior ethics and early modern law, but between unbridled industrial growth and public health: sacrifices were required.[4]

One of those desperate souls sacrificed was Kihira Usaburō, the lone, wandering seventy-five-year-old man described earlier, whose home was in the shadows of one of the largest refineries. Mired in poverty and lungs burning with pain, he hanged himself in July 1966. His would not be the last sacrifice. In December 1966, Okabara Hanji, a refinery employee, died of acute bronchitis at the age of twenty-nine. In June 1967, Sugimoto Shōichirō died when his acute bronchitis worsened to a condition known as pneumothorax (a dangerous concentration of gas or air in the pleural cavity). On 23 June 1966, Ōtani Kazuhiko, who had carried Kihira's picture during the funeral procession, complained in his diary of relentless coughing. One year later, his body quaked even more severely with violent, sulfur-dioxide-induced coughs. On the morning of 13 June 1967, Ōtani committed suicide at his workplace, a sweet-red-bean confection shop, in the shadows of the monuments of Japan's industrial order. He left behind these words: "Today again the air looks bad." Then, in October 1967, a third-year middle school girl, the all-too-young Minami Kimie, died of respiratory complications.[5] There would be others as well.

These two sacrificial episodes, though different in so many obvious ways and separated by over two and a half centuries, share a handful of less-obvious similarities, ones that expose dangerously subversive themes that, as we shall see, thread their way through Japan's history. They become visible, however, only when we focus our analytical attention on Japan's relationship to the physical environment. To begin with, both episodes exemplified ultimate sacrifices to the state, one an early modern order and the other a capitalist industrial one. Both episodes took place at symbolically poignant sites, one an ancestral-grave temple, evidencing a Confucian civilization, the other a petroleum refinery, which evidenced a fossil-fuel one. Both episodes chafed at nerves exposed during certain tumultuous historical moments: the former case symbolized allegiance to a changing vassalage system; the latter, allegiance to an entrenched industrial one. Both episodes were also painful. As their blades sliced their bellies, the pain experienced by the Akō samurai was a visceral connection to their early modern regime, which had ordered their deaths. Similarly, the pain experienced by the victims of Yokkaichi asthma, as they dangled by their slender necks or coughed their way into crematoriums, linked them to the current industrial regime.

These two tragic episodes capture many of the themes explored in the pages ahead. My themes are the relationship between pain and the nation; the ultimate causes of the colossal toxic pollution that saturates our modern landscapes; and the manner in which pain caused by pollution insults our always-porous bodies. It is the historical nature of the Japanese relationship to their toxic archipelago that is my principal concern. Toxins sicken bodies because industrialization, with the aid of the modern state, simplifies and rationalizes in a manner that eases production, and this simplification requires engineering the environment, whether around mines, factory sites, or rice paddies. Once environments have been simplified, toxins move through them more easily and, in effect, directly to human bodies. Toxins cause pain in bodies, and certain kinds of pain serve as internal "biological indicators" of a poisoned landscape. By contrast, toxins move less easily in less simplified environments, such as naturally occurring ones. For our purposes, the critical moment in Japan's environmental history is the nineteenth century, when the manner in which Japanese interacted with themselves, nonhuman organisms, and the environment was transformed. With the nineteenth century came the advent of *Homo sapiens industrialis* on the Japanese Islands, a new breed of human utterly penetrated, engulfed, and transformed, often at the molecular level, by the engineering, industrializing, and poisoning of the environment in and around it.

PAIN AND NATURE

All of us, like Kihira Usaburō, understand our inseparable connection with nature best through our bodies, most especially through our bodies when we suffer physical pain. Pleasure, while rooted in the body, often eludes our consciousness of its bodily origins and finds a comfortable spot in ordinary social practices such as eating and talking. Ecstasy, which may have no place in the social order, can find expression beyond the body in language, in art, and in flights of imagination. But excruciating pain allows no escape. It is embedded in the body and remains relentless and beyond representation—unless, of course, the pain is not your own. The more distant the pain—that of the Japanese enemy melting during the atomic bombings of Hiroshima and Nagasaki or, even more distant still, that of a genetically engineered, hemophiliac beagle strapped to a stainless steel table and undergoing a vivisection—the more we tend to deny it.[6] Those souls most distant or different from us suffer pain the least in our undeniably self-centered perception of the world.

Nonetheless, pain serves as one of the basic drivers for the pursuit of modernity and civilization. Julia Adeney Thomas has written that Japanese political theorists, such as Maruyama Masao (1914–96), believed that "true modernity provides individuals with autonomy by liberating them completely from nature." Therefore, we might extrapolate that pain caused by environmental pollution, a result of the body's embeddedness in nature, reminded those Japanese who suffered pain, or even who merely heard about those who suffered pain, that they had stalled "at the threshold of this great historical adventure from nature to freedom."⁷ If Thomas is correct on this point, as I believe she is, the victims of industrial disease and environmental pollution became subversive symbols of Japan's (and, at a certain level, everybody else's) everlasting enslavement to nature. Because the victims of industrial disease and environmental pollution lived and died in the shadows cast by such modern edifices as petrochemical refineries, they became even more subversive: antimodern ghosts shrieking from the modern industrial landscape. Their cries tell us that true modernity, for all its lofty promise, is a cruel fantasy.

People, and I include most scholars, too, tend to view themselves as outside or beyond nature, even while eating and digesting other living things. When eating, every human on Earth connects to nature through chewing and digesting plant and animal flesh. Michael Pollan observes that the act of eating "represents our most profound engagement with the natural world." Nevertheless, because organisms, when placed in agricultural, industrial, or laboratory contexts, resemble technologies more than they do natural objects, eating is perceived as a technological exercise as opposed to an ecological one, the product of human ingenuity as opposed to a celebration of the natural bountifulness of Earth. In recent decades, industrialized nations have so processed their food that, as Pollan explains, it "appears as pure products of culture rather than nature." Presenting food as culture rather than as nature is done through obscuring the histories of different foods, which includes their exposure to deadly toxins or heavy metals or dangerous pesticides.⁸ But our inseparable, and quite natural, relationship to the "biological" in these biotechnologies, such as engineered farm animals and grains, becomes apparent when we experience pain.

As William Cronon famously argued, we tend to think that "the place where we are is the place where nature is not."⁹ This perspective weakens significantly, however, if the "place" is between the jagged teeth or in the intestinal tract of a large carnivore. David Quammen, who has studied such carnivores, explains that "alpha predators have kept us acutely aware of our membership within the natural world. They've done it by reminding us that to them we're just another flavor of meat."[10] But in our modern world, most big carnivores are gone as a result of our attempted vanquishing of nature and its toothy pain-givers. "Civilized man will not tolerate wild beasts that eat his children," remarked one famous zoologist.[11]

Often, however, the pain and suffering that remind us of our relationship to nature is caused by the modern technologies and engineered environments that are meant to shelter us from certain kinds of pain, meaning that, paradoxically, the more technologically driven modern life becomes, and the more alienated from nature it thus appears, the more we are reminded in painful ways of our timeless connection to nature. Linda Nash has written about the material connections between bodies and environments in the Central Valley of California. "Ironically," she observes of industrial agricultural lands, "it has been in the most industrialized landscapes—those landscapes that are typically taken as symbolic of the human alienation from nature—that these connections become most clear. As humans have industrialized the land, the land has, in turn, industrialized them."[12] Our bodies are porous and easily insulted—easily industrialized—inescapably tied to the environments we inhabit: not only the food we eat but the air we breathe and the water we drink can prove dangerous. In this respect, modernity and its technologies and engineered landscapes have not distanced us from nature, as Maruyama and other theorists imagined they would. Rather, they have exaggerated connections, particularly at the interfaces of the organic and inorganic. Industrial toxins that travel to bodies through interfacing layers of engineered and naturally occurring food webs allow us to see our connections to the natural world as never before.[13] Despite the considerable ink spilled trying to tell us otherwise, we can never be liberated from nature.

This is particularly true of Japan, a country where, since the mid-nineteenth-century Meiji Restoration (1868), such slogans as *bunmei kaika* (civilization and enlightenment) and *fukoku kyōhei* (rich country and strong military) drove forms of social, biological, and environmental engineering and technological advancement. Nonetheless, intense, physical pain has been a constant companion to this civilizing mission, and the pain of the Japanese people should remind us all of our connection to the natural world. Chemical toxins dispensed in hybrid, engineered industrial and agrarian environments have served as haunting harbingers of our inability to truly distance ourselves from nature—despite the fact that nineteenth-century Japanese oracles, such as Fukuzawa Yukichi (1835–1901), insisted that distancing humanity from nature was the key indicator of nineteenth-century civilized life.[14] In the late nineteenth and early twentieth centuries, polluted environments became dangerously common in Japan as a result of such attitudes, as did industrially diseased bodies.

However, as we saw at the outset of this introduction, pain is an important part of participation in national communities, including the Japanese one. I argue that pain ranks even higher than national myths and a shared language in creating Japan's national community, because it is so undeniably visceral. Japanese do not have to learn in school to feel pain, as they learn shared myths and language, but they do have to learn how to interpret its meaning as a form of dignified (and preferably quiet) sacrifice on behalf of their nation, just as Kihira Usaburō demonstrated when he silently hanged himself. At this juncture, let me sound a note of caution: I am not trying to resurrect some late-nineteenth-century myth that Oriental societies are inherently more primitive, naturally embedded, violent, and, hence, painful than Occidental ones.[15] Rather, my point is that all modern nations, including the Japanese one, require pain and acceptance of that pain from their subjects and citizenry, particularly at key historical moments. The act of interpreting and contextualizing such pain as dignified national sacrifice is critical to state legitimacy; but pain caused by industrial pollution is less easily interpreted and contextualized as dignified and so can prove, as I have suggested, dangerously subversive to the nation and those who tell its stories. Chiefly, pain caused by Japanese toxins tortures marginal groups, such as poor fishers and farmers, which has also made it easier to ignore by those who write the nation's history.

It occurs to me that pain has long been part of Japan's national experience, though a careful distinction must be made between premodern and modern politics and notions of sacrifice. Take some prominent examples. Individual samurai from the twelfth through the nineteenth centuries sliced open their bellies in ritualized disembowelment to display their bloody loyalty to overlords and family honor, because loyalty both to lords and to extended families held together Japan's premodern state structure.[16] Here loyalty to the medieval and early modern states was measured by the endurance of individual pain, such as the pain suffered by the Akō samurai. In the Meiji years, mass sacrifice, rather than individual sacrifice, was made explicit as imperial command in the Imperial Rescript on Education (1890), when the imperial household ordered its subjects to offer themselves "courageously to the State."[17] Considering that, in 1890, Japan teetered on the eve of over five decades of brutal empire building and conflict, mass sacrifices to the state would be measured in collective pain: the pain suffered by men dying in droves on battlefields throughout the Asia-Pacific region, by mothers hearing the tragic news months later in their home villages (or not being vouchsafed the news at all), and by women and children incinerated in their wooden homes by bombs carefully designed to do so.

Pain has shaped Japan's national experience in other ways as well. In the wake of the destructive Nōbi earthquake of 1891, which violently shook rural communities in the agrarian heartland around Nagoya, Tokyo politicians and even the Meiji emperor traveled to the hardest-hit areas, in a symbolic gesture designed to ease the suffering of the people. When news of the devastation reached people throughout the country in newspapers, the pain of the people on the Nōbi Plain served to unite the sentiments of the nation, as did the magnanimous imperial relief effort. Before the birth of the nation, earthquakes caused local suffering; afterward, they became the grist for nationalizing "human emotions" and the act of sacrificing for the country. Portrayals of the Meiji emperor and Tokyo politicians shedding tears as they commiserated with people suffering physical pain only served to dramatize the collective suffering of the national body.[18] Pain in the bodies of Japanese subjects caused real, discernible pain in the body of the emperor: pain was a constant companion to Japan's hallmark nationalizing events in the nineteenth and twentieth centuries. Here is the crux of the matter, though: pain is an ultimate cause, not a proximate one. The interpretation of pain (i.e., that it can unite the emotional sentiments of the nation) occurs only after it has been inflicted, and so the imagined community, insofar as pain is concerned, is an attempt to make sense of the suffering that occurs in national contexts.

Decades later, when Japan lost the Pacific War, the emperor, only weeks before the Allied Occupation, told his subjects, in their burned-out cities, that the nation would "endure the unendurable."[19] But little did those filthy masses huddled around crude radios know that the suffering would continue after the Allied Occupation had packed up and left. Japan's postwar economic recovery was measured in another type of pain, one that seamlessly continued from nineteenth-century experiences with rapid industrialization. This was the pain inflicted by toxic pollution from critical industrial sectors. For the purposes of this book, the sources of this pain are the production and dissemination of chemical insecticides for scientific agricultural improvement; copper mining for the electrical infrastructure and trade; zinc and lead mining for military and civilian purposes; nitrogen fixation for fertilizers and plastics; and coal mining for energy needs. In every one of these critical sectors—critical to Japan's nation-building project in the Meiji period, the establishment of empire through war, and economic recovery in the wake of the Allied Occupation—the nation demanded sacrifice and, in doing so, inflicted pain on people.

There is an important lesson here. This pain, suffering, and sacrifice tell us something often forgotten in the context of participation in national communities, a topic of considerable debate among historians of Japan. Nations are not entirely culturally determined, invented entities, as is so often asserted: the effects of ecological transformation and pollution demonstrate that people really do physiologically experience nations' policies and priorities.[20] Just as bodies can become industrialized, so too can they become nationalized: cadmium concentrations in femoral bones and mercury damage in brains are physical inscriptions of the nation's policies on the body. Changes also occur in the land. Take a quick example from the eighteenth century, one that will be explored in the first chapter: the "wild boar famine" of 1749 in Japan's far northeast. Tracing the emergence of the "imagined community" in eighteenth-century Japan, Susan Burns writes that, through an exegesis of "native" Japanese texts in the context of the *kokugaku* (nativist or national learning) discourse, "'Japan' began to be constituted as the primary mode of community, one that transcended and subsumed other sources of identity, such as status, occupation, religion, region, village, and city."[21] She has indeed traced a powerful identity shift, one that probably did occur, but such a reconstitution of identity would have been largely confined to those who could read (certainly not a majority of the population). Even though an exegesis of certain texts surely built "Japan" as a discursive community, pain that occurred because of nationwide ecological shifts that caused the large-scale starvation (but localized in the northeast) witnessed during the wild boar famine provided a far more physical reminder to Japanese, especially illiterate ones, of their membership in a new form of national community. That is, sericulture in the Kantō, hundreds of miles away, directly touched Hachinohe farmers and transformed their relationship to the land: often, empty stomachs provide far more grist for self-reflection than full heads do. As we shall see, this is precisely how Andō Shōeki (1703–62), a local physician and philosopher, interpreted Hachinohe's painful plight during the wild boar famine, and so will we in chapter 1. Hachinohe and its hungry inhabitants became part of a protoindustrialized and early-nationalized natural environment.

That is to say, humans know nations through senses other than their discursive imaginations (though this does not discount the importance of ideas). Nations such as Japan, with their centrally planned economies, partially design industrial policy (the market, presumably, takes care of the rest); and pain, though culturally interpreted (by public health officials, for example), is only sometimes imagined. After the Nōbi shaker, the jagged red bricks that fell from the Nagoya post office sliced human skin in painful ways, cuts and bruises more heinous than traditional wooden architecture had caused, and they were the result of Meiji planning. The pain that nationally endorsed government and industrial enterprises inflict is real, as the food webs that are part of national ecosystems are real. There is, after all, nothing less imagined than one's own pain, and one of the most concrete impacts of the nation and its political economy, outside the extreme hardship of total war, is the pollution that poisons subjects and citizenry.

The bottom line is that many Japanese suffered from the emergence of a national ecosystem and, eventually, the poisons dispensed in it. Despite the hopes of such luminaries as Fukuzawa Yukichi and Maruyama Masao, we remain as deeply embedded in nature as ever before.

JAPANESE BODIES SUFFERING

When I really want to hammer home to students the horrors of industrial toxins, I show them short clips from a video titled *Igaku to shite Minamatabyō: Shiryō to shōgen* (Minamata Disease: Sources and Testimonies). Some years ago, a Japanese professor visiting from Kumamoto University left the tape with me before departing, and it has, over the years, become a standard in my classroom repertoire. A grainy documentary, the video depicts victims of Minamata disease at the Kumamoto University Hospital as they are being observed by doctors, one of whom is the internist Tokuomi Haruhiko. The doctors all wear thin black neckties, sixties-style horn-rimmed glasses, and carefully starched lab coats. Everything about the doctors, but in particular the dispassionate manner with which they observe the suffering of the victims, suggests that these are men of science. The only part of their conduct that suggests anything other than a dispassionate, scientific gaze is the fact that they often know the victims by name, particularly the children, whom they refer to with the affectionate Japanese suffix *kun*.

The most disturbing scenes in the documentary show these lab-coated men watching hospital footage on a movie screen of a parade of victims trying to perform simple tasks such as walking, smoking cigarettes, and drinking water; they also watch as the victims writhe, shudder, and shake. Often, the sufferers' hospital gowns fling open during their delirious episodes, revealing adult diapers or an exposed breast. One woman's eyes turn so far back inside her head that they reveal only eerie white orbs as she jumps on her bed. Meanwhile, the men in white lab coats observe the footage while Tokuomi comments on the fact that none of the victims, because of the severity of their disease, proved able to perform the ordinary tasks that the doctors asked of them. Without the Japanese informational subtitles, it would have been hard to determine, given the agonizing content of the footage—both the ghastly images and the weirdly dry commentary—whether the lab-coated men were medical caregivers, university researchers, or even torturers.

The documentary also depicts frame after frame of diseased, or what were called "dancing," cats. Some, with quivering hind legs, careen backward and fall to the floor from tables; others turn in circles or run full-speed into concrete walls. The documentary depicts a torture chamber of feline medical horrors. It shows researchers digging for shellfish in the grotesque mercuric sludge of Minamata Bay and feeding portions to cats in a laboratory. Once sick, researchers place the cats in strange situations: they force one cat to confront a large red rooster, while another, partially paralyzed and blind, has a white, beady-eyed lab rat dragged across its body by the rat's long, pink tail. The documentary shows the cats crying out; but their voices are silenced in favor of the dry scientific commentary of the researchers. When the cats move near lab assistants to be held or to rub against them as cats famously do, the assistants resituate the cats so that the filming of their "dancing" can continue apace. Even if the human or nonhuman victims had uttered anything during the filming, the editors silenced their voices in favor of the voices of the researchers. Researchers, not the victims, explained the pain.

Nonetheless, the victims' facial expressions remain absolutely haunting. All the victims, but in particular the children, such as Kamimura Tomoko, possess painfully stretched, imbecilic smiles. "This is called the laughter of obsessional neurosis," one researcher offhandedly remarks. To me, it appears to be the grimace caused by day after day of relentless, searing, dizzying pain and delirium. It requires a great deal of pain, for example, to force you to claw your way through a concrete hospital wall, which is precisely what one victim attempted to do. When I observe the footage, rather than search for dispassionate objectivity, as historians are supposed to do, I search for ways to express my rage.

It is just as well that the documentary spares the viewer the wailing voices of these human and nonhuman victims in favor of the explanation of scientists, given the complex nature of the articulation of lasting pain: pain's "inexpressibility." Elaine Scarry has written that the nature of intense pain is so hard to articulate for the sufferer that it represents the complete "destruction of language," because the sufferer, in order to express him- or herself, often reverts to "the cries and screams of human hurt." To hear such utterances, in turn, represents the "shattering of language" for the listener. Scarry writes: "Physical pain does not simply resist language but actively destroys it, bringing about an immediate reversion to a state anterior to language, to the sounds and cries a human being makes before language is learned." And physical pain differs from other sensations in that it does not have a "referential content," because it is not *of* or *for* anything. Unlike being afraid of something or hungry for something or desiring someone, pain has no referential content, and so its expression occasions "the process that eventually brings forth the dense sea of artifacts and symbols that we make and move about in."[22] In other words, pain creates the cultural milieu we inhabit.

Scarry argues that, because of its inexpressibility, moreover, pain is often objectified by weapons, the tools designed to open bodies and that "can lift pain and its attributes out of the body and make them visible." Humans tend to "recognize" pain in the weapon itself rather than in or on the victim's body.[23] This raises an interesting question: what if the pain is caused, not by a projectile or knife, but by a poison that dissolves in saltwater and enters the body of women and unborn children clandestinely, through normal behaviors such as eating, drinking, and even breathing? What if one's own national community, the members of *Homo sapiens industrialis,* was partially responsible for the toxins that caused pain? In this case, the weapon becomes modern life itself. When artifacts of modernity cause the pain, the factory or mine, and the nation that supports and depends on it, convert from artifacts of modernity to weapons, a conversion most people are unwilling to accept because it represents a challenge to the world as they know it. This is particularly true of Japan, where, since the late nineteenth century, factories have served as icons of national and cultural splendor.

In the early twentieth century, for example, Osaka was not disdained as the Capital of Industry or the Capital of Smoke but rather celebrated, despite the dangerous ambient concentrations of sulfuric acid, ammonia, and chloride. Indeed, in Osaka, between roughly 1912 and 1925, the combined amounts of combustibles and ash exceeded amounts in London and rivaled those in Pittsburgh.[24] To destroy factories or nations or even to recognize them as weapons, as opposed to icons of modern progress, is to defy Japan's entire modern experience. For this reason, openly talking of modern pain in Japan's history is subversive: it presents Fukuzawa Yukichi, oracle of modern civilization, as an idiot, and Osaka as a borderline Superfund site. In Japan and elsewhere, therefore, the price of this recognition is simply too high, and so the pain of the victims of industrial disease is transformed into a form of less-than-dignified, and certainly not always empathetically shared, sacrifice for the nation. Pain is safer expressed this way, rather than as a civilization-destroying natural impulse. In one sense, those suffering from industrial disease, having the potential to destroy our world, become ghosts. They haunt us because we do not sequester their tired souls in shrines, like those of the Japanese soldiers (some of whom are war criminals) at Yasukuni Shrine in Tokyo, for example; rather, we unleash them, unceremoniously, to wander endlessly in our national subconscious, their suffering never adequately contextualized. This is when the imagined community becomes malignant.

In the documentary *Minamata Disease: Sources and Testimonies,* even though the writhing patients and the doctors are in the same room, their experiences are truly worlds apart. So intense are the flickering images that, when I show them in class, both students and I unwittingly suspend belief and deny that such levels of pain can exist, even though the pain, as represented by the contorted faces and clawlike hands of the sufferers, appears so obvious. I assure the students that the filmic images are people, not celluloid phantoms, but even I remain unsure at the end of the hour. I safely file the video on my office shelf to await another year's viewing.

There is no single explanation for why really big, painful environmental problems occur. They are, in effect, the product of complex hybrid causations and obey no single reductionist trajectory of reasoning or disciplinary methodology. They are, like so much in history, the aggregate, macro-effect of many independent causal drivers.[25] Therefore, it should come as no surprise that the idea of hybrid contexts and causations, both topical and analytical ones, permeates this book. Whether read individually or together, the six chapters make one simple overriding assertion: physical pain caused by industrial pollution is the product of toxins that navigate naturally occurring ecosystems and technological systems that are seamlessly intertwined and indicative of highly engineered environments. My principal argument is that, at a certain level, Earth has become a gargantuan hybrid environment in which we are deeply embedded, one interlaced with complex, historically constructed ecological pathways that, in inauspicious instances, eventually lead from industrial facilities to human consumers. Industrial toxins that flow through engineered Earth and its technological systems render useless academic ruminations on the differences between wilderness areas and cities, organic and inorganic, nonhuman and human, biology and technology, or even nature and artifice. Industrial toxins, when finding their way to human bodies, reject such boundaries—even placental boundaries—so it makes sense that we should, too, when tracing them. Everything on Earth, living or otherwise, is integrated into one interconnected, bufferless web that is neither artifice nor nature. Parsing the differences between natural and artificial agency in the creation of environmental pollution is a fool's errand, because the circumstances that produce, transform, transport, and concentrate deadly toxins are usually the result of a complex mixture of agencies. Some agencies are naturally occurring, and others are anthropogenic: both remain relevant to understanding how industrial toxins function, sicken bodies, and cause pain.[26]

When I visited Minamata City during one rainy week in the spring of 2006, I hiked around the entire Chisso chemical factory complex in an attempt to take a single picture. What I remember most was being drenched and cold, because of the relentless rain. To this day, the Chisso Corporation is an economic pillar of Minamata, but it wins precious few accolades for operational transparency, as the formidable walls, moats, rusting barbed-wire fences, hedges, trees, and guards around the entire industrial campus demonstrated. At one point, though, I watched for nearly an hour with absolute wonderment as a small crab crept out of the filthy moat that surrounds Chisso and, after avoiding an oily flotilla of discarded plastic Coke bottles and 7-Eleven convenience store grocery bags, carefully maneuvered out onto the sidewalk. Fifty years ago, this would have been the beginning of one biotechnological leak, I thought: the beginning of a tiny, creeping organic pathway that could have easily brought trace amounts of pollutants from the engineered drainage ditch of the factory, once used to discard mercuric effluence, to human consumers, because crabs are within the complex marine food web that sustains the region. But much, much bigger leaks existed, because the Chisso factory depended on nearby waterways, such as the Minamata River, to flush massive quantities of mercury-laden waste into the bay and out of its industrial system. There can be no separation between the artificial and the natural within an industrial system such as the Chisso complex because all such industrial systems are embedded in the natural systems around them. This is the nature of the industrial metabolism, of which we are a part.

Take insecticides, the topic of the second chapter: when sprayed, insecticides become part of insect bodies and alter their evolution by inducing resistances. But, even more germane, these toxins become part of the paddy ecosystem that insects inhabit, leading to systemic "normal accidents," as Charles Perrow calls them, which result from the complex, tightly coupled nature of modern agriculture. That modern environmental pollution needs to be seen as an "ecosystem accident" is another important dimension of this book. Perrow says that ecosystem accidents result from the "interaction of systems that were thought to be independent but are not because of the larger ecology." Chemical companies such as Chisso operated as if pregnant women and their fetuses were buffered from the mercuric catalytic operations of their factory, but the story of Minamata disease proves that they were not. Another of the unforeseen and unanticipated consequences of dumping tons of mercuric effluent is the biomagnification of mercury in the living tissue of organisms.[27] Perrow writes: "Eco-system accidents illustrate the tight coupling between human-made systems and natural systems. There are few or no deliberate buffers inserted between the two systems because the designers never expected them to be connected."[28] This is especially true of less engineered ecosystems, where there are no "designers." The point about there being "no deliberate buffers" in hybrid systems is an essential one as we navigate the pages ahead.

I plan to make my argument with six chapters. The first two chapters trace the history of health problems caused by insecticide application in Japan. Here the hybrid causation in question takes the form of biotechnologies, such as certain insects, as well as the engineered paddies that other, more pesky bugs inhabit. Insects such as silkworms better fit the taxonomies and categories of technology than biology, as do the carefully terraced paddies where cultivators grow Japan's rice. But toxins flowed through both the bodies of buzzing biotechnologies and the trophic tiers of engineered paddies to human and nonhuman consumers. In the Shimotsuke Plain, for example, sulfuric acid from the Ashio copper mine smelters first killed silkworms by contaminating mulberry leaves. In this sense, silkworms, the bodies of which represented ages of agrarian engineering through selective-breeding practices, served as biological sentinels that signaled toxic troubles in Japan's rural lands.[29] Later, in the immediate postwar years, companies such as Sumitomo Chemical produced biocides that, much like the sulfuric acid from the Ashio smelters, navigated engineered paddy lands and food webs until they interfaced with people. My case study is parathion, a poisonous organophosphate, which became the insecticide of choice in the 1950s and 1960s. Parathion poisoned people in ways that should have been easily anticipated: it killed things that came into direct contact with it. But it killed in less anticipated ways as well, such as when it naturally morphed in certain circumstances, such as in intense sunlight, or when reasonably well-intentioned government warnings alerted suicidal people to the chemical's killer qualities.

The third and fourth chapters focus on the Ashio and Kamioka mining complexes, the former an important copper mine, the latter a system of lead and zinc mines. With these two mining complexes, the hybrid causation in question is that which seamlessly interfaced smelters and the ore flotation technologies deployed at both sites with surrounding riparian ecosystems and paddies in the Watarase River and Jinzū River basins. Cultivators downstream from these two mines had centuries earlier utilized these rivers to support their highly productive paddies. But, with the advent of Japan's industrially driven mining industry in the late nineteenth century, these two rivers came to serve other purposes: they flushed away heavy metals such as cadmium. Bettering the ore flotation technologies deployed at these two mines to improve yields was measured in ever-finer degrees of pulverization in order to extract higher percentages of desired metals. But finely pulverized metals naturally oxidized easier when flushed away as tailings. Oxidized metals such as cadmium traveled through naturally occurring river currents and engineered irrigation channels to rice paddies, where they entered plant stocks and, eventually, the bodies of rural people. But the ecological process by which toxins entered people intertwined with cultural idiosyncrasies to socially construct industrial disease. That women in the Jinzū River basin, like most Japanese women throughout the ages, sheltered themselves from the sun and hence deprived themselves of an important source of vitamin D (which metabolizes calcium and helps bones) meant that they suffered the effects of cadmium more than men. But this is only one in a series of cultural factors that shaped the nature of intense pain—or "it hurts, it hurts disease"—downstream from the Kamioka mines.

The fifth chapter investigates Minamata disease, or methylmercury poisoning. Here the hybrid causation takes the form of intertwined biological and industrial metabolisms, a system comprising cascading layers of ecological relationships in the marine food web. By taking a careful look at the environment around Minamata, this chapter highlights the bioaccumulation that occurred throughout trophic tiers, but in particular in certain prominent shellfish and anchovies that served as the heart of local fisheries. The biological metabolism of shellfish and anchovies, specifically the means by which they filter oxygen and nutrients from saltwater, made them deadly efficient vectors for methylmercury dumped by the Chisso plant, where engineers used mercury as a catalyst. But human fetuses filter nutrients from placentas in the same way shellfish and anchovies do from their marine habitats, and when mercury disrupted stem-cell migrations during the development of unborn children, the results took the form of the horrific birth defects portrayed in *Minamata Disease: Sources and Testimonies.*

The final chapter investigates a deadly coal-dust and methane-gas explosion at a Japanese coal mine in north-central Kyushu in December 1914. Killing 687 people in an instant, it still stands as the worst mining disaster on Japanese soil and one of the worst anywhere. The Hōjō colliery, owned by Mitsubishi, was situated in the rich coalfields around Tagawa City and, in the first two decades of the twentieth century, deployed some of the best mining technologies available in the global marketplace. The hybrid causation in this chapter is the Hōjō colliery itself. Although collieries are essentially engineered spaces, particularly their subterranean areas, they are subject to only partially foreseeable natural factors, such as hydrology, coal-dust accumulation, methane-gas concentration, cave-ins, and a dependency on both human and nonhuman labor. At the Hōjō colliery, it took coal dust, methane gas, one improperly assembled "safety lamp," and, by some estimations, an imbalanced ventilation system to spark the explosion. In May 2006, thumbing through the nearly seven hundred death certificates held at Kyushu University reminded me of the pain caused by this tragic event, which was not totally the fault of Mitsubishi but stemmed from the sheer technological complexity of the hybrid space of the Hōjō colliery. Like insecticide use, copper, zinc, and lead mining, and plastics and fertilizer production, coal needed to be mined to satisfy the energy needs of the modern nation. It is part of an essential industrial system, like all the systems discussed in this book. Like the zinc that galvanized warships or the lead that served as bullets or the chemicals that improved agricultural production or the plastics that democratized consumption, high-calorie coal from Hōjō fueled modernity.

The reader should be cautioned in advance that the chapters often touch on themes that are not immediately recognizable as essential to the core assertions made in this book. In essence, to better historicize the topic, the chapters take a page out of the Hmong storyteller's repertoire: they "speak of all kinds of things" related to the six episodes under consideration. The Hmong storyteller, writes Anne Fadiman, believes that the "world is full of things that may not seem to be connected but actually are; that no event occurs in isolation; that you can miss a lot by sticking to the point; and that the storyteller is likely to be rather long-winded."[30] The world looks this way to the history teacher, too, I have discovered. The history teacher, who can also be irritatingly long-winded, spends the better part of his or her career lecturing on the unanticipated and unforeseen relationships that connect events in the past, often insisting that nothing exists in isolation. Any seasoned teacher knows that "you can miss a lot by sticking to the point," and so I have remedied this by letting my narrative wander a little in the pages ahead. I ask the reader to bear with me. Just as there are ecological webs that interconnect organisms, so too are there cultural and material webs that interconnect historical experiences.

When making my argument about hybrid spaces, industrial pollution, and human health, I embed each case study within Japan's history. The first chapter explores Buddhist attitudes toward insects, for example, because the notion of the transmigration of the soul informed how Japanese viewed insect emergences in paddies. Historically, Buddhist cosmologies constructed the notion of agrarian entomology as much as the biological sciences or applied chemistry did. The third and fourth chapters situate copper, zinc, and lead mining within the broader context of Japanese overseas commerce and imperial conflict because, to a large degree, trade and war fueled mining in Japan. Zinc, when mixed with copper, created brass for equipment on naval vessels and for shrapnel cases, while lead dug from the ground was carefully reconstituted into bullets that, when propelled from rifles into Chinese bodies, violently forged an empire. Chapter 4 also connects industrial disease to traditional Japanese values regarding beautiful skin complexion and idealized female behavior. In the fifth chapter, the fetal mutilations caused by methylmercury poisoning in Minamata take on new meanings when placed in the context of traditional Japanese attitudes toward pregnancy, medical culture, Confucian and Buddhist notions of fetal development, and ancient stories of strange birth defects and what they portended. In the final chapter, although the 1914 explosion at the Hōjō colliery serves as the centerpiece of the investigation, the chapter begins with an exploration of medieval Buddhist renditions of hell that bear a striking resemblance to life, and death, inside a coal mine. Traditionally, many Japanese imagined the subterranean as a Buddhist hell.

This is only a small, but representative, sampling of some of the broader cultural and material connections established in the chapters ahead. These cultural and material connections embed in nature and history Japan's struggle with environmental pollution and industrial disease.

1 THE AGENCY OF INSECTS

This chapter, though not without a handful of human actors, stars four insects: a tachinid fly and the Japanese beetle it eats, silkworms, and mosquitoes. Their actions, or the actions on them by humans, demonstrate how cultural values become ecological reality in engineered landscapes. Insect behavior also exposes how Japan's nineteenth-century entrance into the international arena had immediate environmental consequences, as Japanese beetles (and other six-legged brethren) transcended the ecological boundaries of their island home to become serious agricultural pests in the United States and elsewhere. Beetles established empire far earlier than their human counterparts.

Beetle populations blossomed in the United States after they escaped their biogeographical context. U.S. entomologists learned after traveling to Japan that re-creating elements of the beetle's native habitat, namely artificially reintroducing it to natural predators and disease, could serve as a biotechnology of insect control. But knowledge of beetle predators needed to be discovered, and it was done, as we shall see, by tapping into the ancient Japanese hobby of gathering and raising insects. As for silkworms, we shall discover how cultural values specific to Japanese aesthetics and Confucian cohabitation practices drove their evolution. Eventually, the silk industry transformed Japan's caterpillars and landscapes, a process in which silkworm cultivators need to be seen as biological engineers whose activities helped morph organisms and craft a national landscape in the eighteenth century. Finally, we shall turn to the metaphysics of Buddhist cosmologies and arbovirus (arthropod-borne virus) dissemination to trace how religion and entomology intersected at different moments in Japanese history to raise havoc with human health and cause pain. Our case study is Japanese B encephalitis.

Problems with insects principally occur within hybrid spaces, where human practices and knowledge creation merged with engineered ecological conditions. Had they not merged where they did, the episodes discussed in this chapter would not have occurred. Not only is history scribed onto documents, but it is also inscribed onto the bodies of humans and insects, as well as sliced, shoveled, and excavated into landscapes around the world. One breathing canvas on which we paint our histories is insects and their habitat. As Gregg Mitman argues, the "actions of nonhuman actors such as rats, lice, or fleas are connected to, not independent of, histories of knowledge production through which such objects gain new meaning and power in the world."[1] The lesson is that historical research is central to understanding evolution and insect-borne pestilence. Given that Earth is a gargantuan, engineered space, as suggested in the introduction, today's ecology is history, because that value-laden engineering took place over historical time.

JAPANESE INVADERS

The Japanese beetle (*Popillia japonica*) invaded the United States in the summer of 1916 when the hungry chafers established a beachhead at a nursery in Riverton, New Jersey. When compared to the "helmeted beetles" (*Allomyrina dichotoma*) that children in Japan collect and raise in small, plastic terrariums and whose shells resemble the ornate armor of medieval samurai warriors, the Japanese beetle is ordinary in everything except for its reflective golden color and voracious appetite for the same crops that humans tend to cultivate and eat. Evolution has made it an economic competitor, not an insect that contributes to human economies such as silkworms or bees. The United States deployed insecticides in earnest to kill Japanese beetles in mass numbers, chemicals that became popular in Japan in the 1950s and that will be discussed in the next chapter.

According to entomologists, in the first year of its invasion the beetle inhabited a modest area of about one acre; by 1941, the year Japanese Zeros strafed Pearl Harbor, beetles had made far more impressive gains than Japan's skilled pilots and inhabited some 20,000 square miles of soil in the American homeland. East Asian farmers rarely considered the Japanese beetle a serious pest; but once the beetle arrived in New Jersey—its grubs tucked clandestinely in the bundled roots and soil of a shipment of azaleas—the lack of native predators and diseases meant that it quickly went to work on crops across the country, destroying everything from soybean and clover to apple and peach trees. In the early 1920s, other "Oriental" invader species followed the gains made by the Japanese beetle, including the camphor scale (*Pseudaonidia duplex*) and the Asiatic garden beetle (*Autoserica castanea*).[2] The six-legged Yellow Peril invasion from the East was on. These insects, but mostly the Japanese beetle, represented a scourge on the civilized face of the planet, much as the American propaganda machine famously depicted the Japanese people to be once the Pacific War got under way. Sadly, the rhetoric deployed to justify destroying Japanese beetles and Japanese people was basically interchangeable during this period. This is because, at their most basic level, American racism and agricultural entomology were based on supposedly fixed biological principles.[3]

By 1945, even though the United States had subdued, though not eradicated, "Louseous Japanicas" with incendiary bombs and atomic weapons, the Japanese beetle continued to molest crops unimpeded throughout rural America. Rachel Carson, in *Silent Spring* (1962), featured Japanese beetle eradication campaigns in the Midwest as among the most egregious examples of the dangers of chlorinated hydrocarbons when sprayed indiscriminately over America's pastoral landscapes. As is so often the case, chlorinated hydrocarbons poisoned the very constituencies they were meant to protect (and continue to do so). In 1959, for example, specially equipped airplanes doused about 27,000 acres in southeastern Michigan with aldrin, a highly toxic and relatively inexpensive insecticide, reportedly to manage the beetle infestation in that area.[4] Despite the fact that some local entomologists questioned the necessity of the program, the aldrin dusting continued apace, and although the beetles survived the bombing, such birds as the American robin did not. People's lawns were strewn with dead songbirds. Similarly, between 1954 and 1961, Illinois dusted some 131,000 acres with dieldrin, which, in laboratory tests, proved some fifty times more toxic than the infamous DDT (dichloro-diphenyl-trichloroethane).

Here songbirds and household pets began dying throughout the sprayed areas as well.

What made such campaigns of "annihilation" and "extermination" so tragic is that the Japanese beetle, after about 1954, had, in most instances, ceased to be a serious agricultural pest, as populations had started to stabilize after the initial invasion, largely because of the importation of biotechnologies: predatory insects and bacterial "milky" disease from the beetle's native habitat. When those first Japanese beetles made landfall in New Jersey in the earthy roots of azaleas, they arrived in an environment free of at least ten of their mortal insect enemies. In Japan, a kind of tachinid fly (*Centeter cinerea*), through its own reproductive activities, tirelessly kept "golden coin insect" numbers in check through an ecological equilibrium between the two species that is centuries old and actually quite gruesome. Indeed, the fly's unwieldy Japanese name is *mamekoganeyadoribae*, or "the fly that lives in the Japanese beetle." The name says it all. In their native habitat, a variety of knotweed (*Polygonum reynoutria*) is one of the favorite haunts of Japanese beetles. In this bushy, lush world, tachinid flies hunt for unsuspecting (and usually love-struck) beetles on the leaf tops. So terrified of tachinid flies are Japanese beetles that, if they catch a glimpse of one, they quickly drop from their leafy cover to the ground rather than risk confrontation with this ruthless predator. Sometimes the two engage in a gripping life-or-death struggle. For this reason, tachinid flies have compensated by normally preying on mating beetles, which usually prove too preoccupied to notice a stalking fly.

Japanese beetles have good reason to fear these small flies. Tachinid flies do not immediately kill and eat beetles. (Remember, this is the fly that lives *in* the Japanese beetle.) Instead, after observing the mating beetles for some time, a female tachinid identifies the female beetle and, in a lightning-fast diagonal run, quickly maneuvers herself to lay several eggs on the thorax of the female beetle. In the early 1920s, U.S. researchers from the Bureau of Entomology who were visiting Japan noticed that in certain parts of northern Japan nearly all of the Japanese beetles inspected had such eggs around their thoraxes. Having attached her eggs to the beetle's thorax—or "provisioned her eggs," as entomologists say—the female fly's work is basically done; but now the beetle has been served with a nine-day death sentence. The larvae within the eggs develop in about two days, and rather than hatch externally, the larvae employ rasplike teeth to bore through the shell of the egg and directly into the thorax of the beetle. Eggs mistakenly deposited on more armored and, therefore, better-protected parts of the beetle's exoskeleton often prove unable to penetrate the body cavity and quickly perish. Once in the thoracic cavity, the larvae molt and then move into the main body cavity, attaching themselves with a perforated hook to air sacks in order to breathe. The beetle, being eaten alive from the inside, usually buries itself in the ground. In the body cavity of the beetle and underground, the larvae then move back into the thorax, mercifully killing the beetle-host in the process; later, still living inside the beetle, the larvae eat the entire content of the body cavity. Four days after the beetle has died and nine days after the female fly originally attached her eggs, the larvae morph into pupae and survive in the buried cavity until they emerge in the early morning hours some ten months later. Once mature, the female flies then search for other love-struck female beetles on which to lay their eggs and procreate.

The engineers at chemical giant American Cyanamid (responsible for the development of the pesticide parathion in the United States, featured in the next chapter) could never have even dreamed of such an effective insect-killing machine, particularly one with so little collateral damage. Because of the tachinid fly and other predatory insects, Japanese beetles never posed much of a threat to Japanese farmers, unless, of course, these farmers unwittingly used chemicals that killed tachinids, which they often did. The increase in Japanese beetle populations as a result of the killing of tachinid flies with pesticides is an example of a trophic cascade in the agrarian food web perpetrated by humans.

Starting in 1921, the team from the Bureau of Entomology paid over two hundred Japanese children to collect parasitized specimens of the Japanese beetle to be released at ground zero in Riverton, New Jersey. The Japanese children must have enjoyed making money while engaged in their age-old hobby of netting insects. As far back as the early eleventh century, Japanese courtiers wrote nostalgically of the ringing songs of the bell cricket (*Homoeogryllus japonicus*), which they described poetically and, in typical Japanese fashion, onomatopoeically. Courtiers sometimes collected these emotionally evocative insects and then set them free in their gardens. In the thirteenth century, Tachibana Narisue, in his *Kokon chomonjū* (Notable Tales Old and New; 1254), described an excursion in 1095 to the fields of Saga near Kyoto to catch insects. Everybody from the head priest downward gathered horses from official pavilions and departed the capital carrying stylized bamboo cages with dangling decorative cords. The party dismounted at Toyomachi and proceeded on foot. They caught insects until evening and then returned to the capital, where they fed the crickets and other creeping creatures leaves from bush clover and other perennial plants (*Patrinia scabiosaefolia*). Once back in the palace, the courtiers raised their saké cups and composed poetry to celebrate the occasion.[5] The fictional Prince Genji had autumn insects (perhaps caught on an expedition similar to the one described by Tachibana) released into his garden in order to create a lonely mood that evoked, as Heian courtiers often wanted to do, a Buddhist sense of impermanence and transcendence.[6]

Later, in the eighteenth and early nineteenth centuries, the admirers of insect songs learned how to cultivate crickets from how-to books. Raising the eggs of the pine cricket (*Xenogryllus marmorata*) proved relatively simple and something that any enthusiast could do.[7] The ability to cultivate insects led to the business of insect vendors (*mushi uri*) in some towns and cities. In the nineteenth century, Kitagawa Morisada (b. 1810) described the practice of selling insects as one of the "modern customs" of Tokugawa Japan. On city streets, decorative bamboo cages dangling from colorful insect-vendor kiosks contained singing bell crickets (*Homoeogryllus japonicus*), giant katydids (*Mecopoda elongata*), pine crickets (*Xenogryllus marmorata*), buprestid beetles (*Chrysochroa fulgidissima*), and others.[8] These insects served early modern Japanese as pets.

Culturally speaking, Japanese children and their parents knew about collecting, keeping, and appreciating the habits of bugs because it was part of Japan's history, and U.S. entomologists tapped into this history to collect and deploy Japanese biotechnologies for scientific reasons. By 1924, after releasing beetles with eggs around their thoraxes, entomologists spotted parasitized Japanese beetles within a twelve-mile radius of Riverton.[9] The fate of the Japanese beetle in the United States was sealed, but chemical companies and their political allies, as we shall learn, still pushed hard for the use of chemical insecticides, both in the United States and abroad in the 1950s and afterward.

When U.S. entomologists released Japanese beetles parasitized with tachinid fly larvae in Riverton, they deployed insects as a kind of biotechnology: they tweaked, if ever so subtly, the insect predator-prey landscape in North America. Indeed, the cultural knowledge of agricultural entomology, insect behavior, and insect gathering gained over centuries in Japan was utilized by U.S. entomologists and exported across the Pacific in this ecologically driven reengineering scheme, where it was used to control

Japanese beetles in orchards and other crops. For entomologists, using tachinid flies as a biotechnology required learning about local Japanese ecologies (and trying to reproduce them elsewhere), tapping into ancient Japanese cultural practices, recruiting eager children to net parasitized insects, and strategically transcending global biogeographies, just as the Japanese beetle had originally done on its own. As the story of the Japanese beetle also demonstrates, what necessitated this reengineering project in the first place was Japan's nineteenth-century entrance into the international arena, after centuries of relative seclusion.[10] "Opening Japan" to the United States had immediate ecological consequences. But Japanese did not just observe, catch, raise, and adore evocative bugs; they manipulated their evolution through selective breeding to serve their aesthetic and market needs. Here is where our story of the silkworm begins.

SILKWORMS

One point of topical congruency between this chapter and chapter 3 is the environmental impact of the Ashio copper mine, specifically the deleterious effect it had on silkworm nurseries downstream and downwind in the Shimotsuke Plain. In this instance, silkworms served as unwitting biological sentinels, or highly sensitive alarms in hybrid spaces. Think of their untimely deaths as flashing red lights on an environmental dashboard. In the carefully tended working lands of Shimotsuke, spring's unnatural silence portended environmental havoc as early as the 1880s. What makes the relationship between the mine refineries and silkworm nurseries of interest is that silkworms died because of an "ecosystem accident," wherein the complex, tightly coupled relationships among extracting ore, smelting, photochemical processes in the atmosphere, acid rain (or acidic deposition), the location of mulberry plantations, and the monophagous habits of silkworms killed the insects and thereby caused economic hardships among farmers downstream from the mine. This is an example of the hybrid causation discussed in the introduction. But, in the case of Japanese villages, traditional economic and social systems that had evolved over centuries and that interfaced with the ecosystem also shaped the nature of environmental crisis in the Shimotsuke Plain. To be sure, all these systemic couplings, from rural lending practices and kinship patterns to mining interests and local ecologies, were mostly unanticipated by mine operators, farmers, and, of course, the unsuspecting silkworms themselves while they munched on mulberry leaves. Silkworms are the key to our story.

Silkworms (*Bombyx mori*) not only serve as biological sentinels downstream and downwind from mines but survive as organisms that humans have, over centuries, transformed into purely industrial technologies: they are utterly dependent on human beings. That is, as historian Edmund Russell, a major proponent of "evolutionary history," has argued, organisms such as silkworms have "changed in historical time" due to intentional and unintentional human meddling with three keystone Darwinian factors: variation, inheritance, and selection. Russell contends that investigating the manner in which human histories have shaped the evolution of other organisms allows us to "historicize organisms themselves," which, refreshingly, carves out a new place for historians in generating knowledge about the current state of evolution and the natural world.[11]

Today, tucked away in "stock centers" at a handful of major East Asian universities are hundreds of Mendelian mutations of the silkworm, most of them spontaneous and discovered by cultivators and then preserved; other mutations have been induced by scientists through irradiation techniques and chemical mutagenesis. Many of these mutations represent "improved strains," or silkworms that exhibit economically desirable characteristics such as rapid growth rate, large cocoon size, good silk filament quality, and disease resistance. Silkworms from southwestern China, for example, have proved desirable because of their hereditary resistance to toxic fluoride levels in mulberry leaves, an environmental condition caused by the vibrant brick industry in that region. This is historical evolution in action: the brick industry produced environmental toxins that over historical time induced selection among silkworms, leading to evolutionary mutations among the organisms; in turn, scientists isolated and preserved this beneficial gene for future breeding purposes. In the case of Japan, stylistic idiosyncrasies that have evolved since Heian period (794–1185) female courtiers wore some eighty pounds of silk clothing carefully chosen to match the season influenced the evolution of silkworms as well, because only certain bugs produced the desirable high-quality filament.[12] Today, functional genomics has allowed institutions to engineer silkworms that produce specialized silks, as well as recombinant proteins that are made in the silk glands and possess beneficial pharmacological qualities. Indeed, within certain institutions, Japanese scientists have accumulated entire silkworm DNA sequences and distribute clones internationally for commercial and scientific use.[13] Because no wild silkworms exist (their closest relative is *Bombyx mandarina*), they represent one of the oldest examples of historical evolution and organisms being used as industrial technologies. Certainly in Japan, silkworms have depended on their human providers for millennia (and in China for much longer).

In the 1880s, Japanese farmers in the Shimotsuke Plain noticed that wild insects no longer chirped and buzzed in their rice paddies, and those involved with sericulture became dismayed when painstakingly tended colonies died in household nurseries after eating mulberry leaves tainted with sulfuric acid originating from upwind smelters. A sulfuric acid film covered these leaves, one created through unanticipated photochemical mechanisms in the atmosphere and disseminated through the air and brought to Earth's surface by normally beneficial precipitation. In the dawn of Japan's industrial age, who could have anticipated that mines could kill silkworms many miles away or that normally beneficial rain could spread corrosive acid? Who would have thought that advanced industrial technologies and the sericulture industry were tightly connected in this manner? Most farmers involved in sericulture shared their homes with silkworms, raising them from eggs that agents from the silk industry delivered every spring and early autumn. Since ancient times, silkworms have held an important place in rural Japanese economies; they have lived together with cultivators and have coevolved to provide for their economic needs.

Silkworms have long been in Japan, as evidenced by ancient creation mythologies. During one divine encounter narrated in the *Kojiki* (Record of Ancient Matters; 712), the intrepid, but also quite hungry, deity Susano'o kills the food deity, Ōgetsuhime, because he thought she sought to pollute him by pulling various foodstuffs out of her nose, mouth, and anus. From Ōgetsuhime's divine corpse grew various vital grains—the foodstuffs on which Japanese have endured for centuries—but also silkworms, evidencing the importance of silkworms in Japan's ancient economy.[14] "In the corpse of the slain deity there grew [various] things: in her head there grew silkworms; in her two eyes there grew rice seeds; in her two ears there grew millet; in her nose there grew red beans; in her genitals there grew wheat; and in her rectum there grew soy beans."[15] Japanese wove silkworm cultivation into the deepest fibers of their cultural fabric; the caterpillar's domestication paralleled the domestication of Japan's earliest food crops.

Preindustrial rural households tended their silkworm nurseries with the same care that they bestowed on their rice, millet, bean, wheat, and soybean fields, and acidic deposition in the Shimotsuke Plain, when it tainted mulberry leaves and poisoned silkworm nurseries, proved economically devastating. No doubt, losing silkworms proved emotionally troubling as well, because sericulture constituted a form of animal husbandry in a country that boasted few large herds or flocks of hoofed organisms. For about the past two centuries, when rural households purchased silkworm eggs, often they exchanged no money and the agent simply deducted his proceeds when the worms had spun their precious silk cocoons. Often as many as twenty thousand of these eggs were spread out on wooden trays; once hatched, farmers carefully brushed the squirming larvae on to rearing trays using a soft feather so as to not crush their tiny bodies. Farmers covered the rearing trays in wet rice husks to provide the necessary humidity and then spread out a layer of chopped white mulberry (*Morus alba*) leaves for the silkworms to munch on. Often families sacrificed their sleeping space to provide comfortable accommodations for these bugs. They did so because the enterprise could be profitable.

Generally, for about three days, the larvae devoured the carefully cut mulberry leaves; on the fourth day they hibernated. But then they shed and were reborn, with gauzy skin and bright stripes down their bodies. Such metamorphic qualities—their ability to change into completely different creatures—became potent symbols of Buddhist notions of transmigration: when the soul, in the cycle of birth and rebirth, travels to the next life after this one. Eighth-century mythmakers marveled in the *Kojiki* at the metamorphic quality of silkworms as well. "Among the insects raised by Nurinomi [a fourth-century immigrant to Japan], there is a strange variety of insect that changes three ways; first it becomes a crawling worm, then again it becomes a cocoon, then once again it becomes a flying bird."[16] As with the East Asian writing system (called *kanji* in Japanese) and other technologies and institutions, sericulture had no doubt been perfected elsewhere and brought to Japan by migrants, mainly from the Korean Peninsula, between the fourth and eighth centuries.

In the nurseries, by the fifth or sixth day, the worms grew to the point where cultivators needed to carefully spread them out on even more trays, with an ever-ready supply of fresh mulberry leaves. Silkworms grow at a tremendous rate, and by the time they spin their silk, they weigh about ten thousand times their weight as larvae. The silkworms eat and molt and eat and molt four times in all, until, after their final metamorphosis, they prepare to spin their cocoons by eating steadily for six days straight. By this time, the silkworms measure about one to two inches in length and walk reasonably dexterously for having eight sets of legs: three sets of jointed legs, with a single claw at the tip, and five sets of fleshy leglike protrusions with hooks for climbing and clinging. They also sport a lavishly decorative short "anal horn" on their backs. In the larval stage, silkworms prefer the delicate shoots from the tops of the mulberry; when adults, they eat everything even remotely mulberry: the twenty thousand larvae cultivated by one rural household would have consumed a total of thirteen hundred pounds of leaves. In their final six days, silkworms become vulnerable to weather shifts, humidity levels, naturally occurring infections, and anthropogenic toxins, and families pampered the insects by monitoring temperature and humidity levels using charcoal braziers and damp rice husks.

Farmers set aside hundreds of acres for growing mulberry to feed hungry caterpillars, often where there was barely enough land to grow grain and vegetables to feed people. Indeed, the industry expanded exponentially throughout the Tokugawa period, particularly after the shogun restricted imports of raw silk from Qing China in 1685. Narita Jūhyōe, a sericulture expert, estimated that silk production had doubled during the seventeenth and early eighteenth centuries and then quadrupled by the early nineteenth century.[17] In eighteenth-century Shindatsu (Fukushima Prefecture), farmers reengineered mulberry trees by crossing strains (the Yamaguwa and Shiraguwa varieties) so that the new, hardier trees could be grown in more places.[18] Because of the economic potential of sericulture, in the early eighteenth century Hirosaki Domain provided farmers with loans to establish mulberry plantations. Yonezawa Domain encouraged the development of the sericulture industry by establishing twelve nurseries designed to propagate mulberry seedlings.[19] In the most dramatic example, between the late nineteenth and early twentieth centuries, farmers in the Shimoina region (Nagano Prefecture) replaced subsistence farming with sericulture farming as their principal occupation. As Kären Wigen notes, the displacement was so thorough that, as the local population grew, the "county as a whole increasingly depended on imported grains and pulses" because farmers devoted so much arable land to mulberry. In 1884, Shimoina farmers committed 7 percent of arable land to mulberry production. In 1921, they devoted 50 percent.[20] This transformed the temporal and spatial rhythms of agrarian life: more time (particularly women's time) and space were now devoted to these little, hungry caterpillars.[21]

With more land devoted to sericulture and less to grain crops, the demand for food to feed hungry urban populations (part of the ecological footprint of Edo, present-day Tokyo, to be discussed in chapter 5) forced distant areas such as Hachinohe Domain, in the far northeast, to redesign local agriculture toward export monoculture (to supply Edo), setting the region up for devastating famine when soybean crops failed because of weather and, in one bizarre instance, exploding populations of hungry wild boars.[22] This is the essence of coevolution: in this case, humans changed their behavior to feed hungry bugs on which they had come to depend.[23] Japanese farmers reprioritized time and arable land to make room for more mulberry plantations, refashioned lending patterns, risked awful debt, kept children at home, and sacrificed their living space just to nurture silkworms.

When silkworms began spinning, families designed frames for them to hang from. Timing was critical at this stage, because if the special frames were not ready when the worms began to spin their cocoons, they simply destroyed the cocoons of others and ruined the quality of the silk. Over the next several days, the family watched as the worms went to work on their beautiful translucent cocoons made from thread excreted from special glands: a piece of evolutionary hardware that has allowed these creatures to be treated with such complete care. Once they completed the cocoon, they began to molt one final time, and eager farmers raced the cocoons to the silk agent to collect their money. Farmers boiled poor-quality cocoons to make silk thread for their own clothing; some ate the plump, protein-rich insects or fed them to fish in communally tended ponds. Little was wasted in preindustrial Japan. Later, in the period just before the Pacific War, silk agents paid high prices for cocoons. (One cocoon could produce over 1,500 feet of valuable silk thread.) Obviously, when entire colonies of silkworms perished as a result of toxins, it financially wiped out these already deeply impoverished rural households, who famously produced no less than 70 percent of Meiji tax revenues through crushing land taxes.[24] Rural families shouldered the financial burdens of Japan's industrialization; they suffered the environmental ones, too.

Even more than tachinid flies, silkworms provide an excellent example of an industrialized organism whose life has been shaped by economic systems, social networks, ecosystems, and evolutionary history in general. They also offer an example of a biotechnology that, if indirectly, began to shape Japan's national landscape in the eighteenth century. Consider this perspective: Japanese desired certain silk fabric from certain kinds of caterpillars because of traditional cultural sensibilities, ancient ones that defined what silk was beautiful and what silk was not. Japanese bought silkworms in the manner they did, by borrowing eggs, because of the development of rural financial institutions. Japanese women, rather than men, raised silkworms because of labor patterns, Confucian kinship expectations, and their dexterity.[25] One entrepreneur from western Japan wrote: "Lots of silkworms can be found in every province. . . . This is a woman's enterprise and does not require input from men so it can be performed with the labor not needed for cultivation."[26] Similarly, Kanō Tanboku, in *Yōsan hiroku* (Confidential Record of Silkworm Rearing; 1803), emphasized: "Sericulture is the work of women, and it does not sacrifice the labor of men." The caterpillars, he wrote, are "frail creatures that demand the most minute ministrations."[27] And, in some instances, silkworms died of industrial poison as biological sentinels because of Meiji economic priorities, including a prioritization of industrial work over cottage industry, and unanticipated ecosystem mechanisms.[28] It is the sheer weight of history that determined evolution in the case of silkworms: this is why historians remain so central to discussions regarding the evolution of biotechnologies and ecological health on Earth.

INSECTS, BUDDHISM, AND JAPANESE B ENCEPHALITIS

Biologically, silkworms underwent three distinct transformations on their way to their final destination of becoming moths. For this evolutionary talent Japanese associated metamorphic insects such as silkworms, butterflies, cicadas, and mosquitoes with the cyclical nature of human existence according to Buddhist cosmologies. Insects such as silkworms and cicadas started out as eggs, they hatched and became hungry larvae, they matured to even hungrier pupae, and, in their final transcendence, they sprouted wings and spent the remainder of their often-short lives fluttering from flower to flower as a butterfly or moth or, when chance might have it, were quickly devoured by a hungry crow or crazed until death by the glare of a bright oil lamp or electric light. Once, while camping with a friend named Tsuchiya Tatsuhide at Lake Shikotsu (on Hokkaido), we watched for an hour or so as cicadas emerged from the ground and shot skyward, attempting to seek shelter in the mixed conifer and evergreen forest that surrounded the lake. But crows waited patiently in the trees and, as far as I could determine, intercepted and ate every last bug that shot from the soil. It was quite sad. Japanese felt this melancholy emotion, too. Indeed, Japanese literary classics are littered with insect references, usually alluding to the sadness or the impermanence of this transient world.[29]

In the nineteenth century, Lafcadio Hearn (1850–1904), an American living in Japan, wrote lengthy meditations on insects and Buddhist notions of impermanence. Hearn lived in Japan in the metamorphic Meiji years, when Japan itself shed its skin, and he lamented the cruel destruction of an older Japan in favor of the new industrial order. As David Lurie explains, much like the silkworms and cicadas that he observed, Hearn too underwent a metamorphosis while living in Japan, where he adopted the Japanese name Koizumi Yakumo and, in his own mind, sprouted wings of national liberation and became in many respects "Japanese."[30] When writing about butterflies, Hearn retrieved ancient Japanese and Chinese myths about people wandering this world in the form of butterflies, sometimes eavesdropping on former lovers. According to other stories, butterflies also descended on the ancient capital of Kyoto by the thousands in the tenth century and, in doing so, portended the countless men to be killed and resurrected as insects during the rebellion of Taira no Masakado (d. 940).

Hearn also tied the fate of mosquitoes to the fate of the older Japan he cherished. Some of the mosquitoes that infested his Tokyo neighborhood originated in a deeply spiritual place, in a nearby cemetery, where, at the foot of ancient, moss-covered Buddhist tombs, worshipers placed water in *mizutame* (cisterns) so that the souls of the dead, when reborn and preparing for their journey to the next realm, could satisfy their insatiable thirst. The standing water in thousands of cisterns and flower receptacles provided excellent breeding habitat for mosquitoes and, according to Meiji Japan's hygienic standards, posed a health risk. The mosquitoes that so pestered Hearn and other Tokyoites rose "by the millions from the water of the dead," he wrote. He speculated that "some of them may be reincarnations of those very dead, condemned by the error of former lives" to wander Earth as bloodsuckers. He marveled that "some wicked human soul had been compressed into that wailing speck of a body."[31]

Here, Buddhist orthodoxies seamlessly intersected with, and thereby influenced, ecological conditions; the cisterns and vessels left at the cemetery provided water for transmigrating souls as well as prime breeding habitat for mosquitoes. Religious institutions and cultural sensibilities interfaced with ecological conditions to cause an urban health crisis.

Consider this intricate web of causation: had it not been for the religious demand for cisterns, the cascading and unforeseen "ecosystem accidents" that were caused by these cemeteries would not have occurred. Indeed, these swarms of Japanese insects represented a serious threat in the eyes of a Meiji state increasingly concerned with national discipline through the health and hygiene of Japan's citizenry. Some of the mosquitoes (*Culex tritaeniorhynchus*) born in these Buddhist cisterns carried the arbovirus (arthropod-borne virus) that causes Japanese B encephalitis. Normally, these mosquitoes live and breed in the marshy paddy lands of rural Japan, but standing water in cities, such as in drainage ditches, attracts them as well. One reason the mosquito-borne disease thrived in rural areas, and later came to the outskirts of cities, was because this peculiar virus spends part of its life cycle in the bodies of pigs, which serve as an "amplifying host." With the advent of modern agriculture, vast numbers of pigs came to live near human populations.[32] Between 1926 and 1938, about the same time that several high-profile Japanese B encephalitis outbreaks occurred, Japan witnessed nearly a 100 percent increase in its pig population, from 504,758 to 997,980. Although small rural cultivators raised most of these pigs, some large-scale producers, according to later Allied Occupation documents, were "located on the outskirts of the large cities," where the animals had easy access to garbage for feed.[33] Obviously, the decision to place large concentrations of pigs near cities (with their mosquito-ridden cemeteries and other favorable environments, as well as large human populations) set Japan up for ecosystem accidents in the form of Japanese B encephalitis epidemics.

Mosquitoes sucked the blood of these pigs and transported the blood-borne, amplified virus to other pigs and eventually to human hosts. Normally, most people do not develop severe symptoms when infected with the Japanese B encephalitis virus, but when they do, the disease can be devastating, causing death or brain damage and paralysis. In 1924, some 6,000 reported cases of encephalitis left 3,800 people dead in Tokyo alone; that same year, the disease also occurred in Kagawa District of Kyushu, where 60 percent of those who contracted the affliction—some 3,500 souls—died of fever and brain swelling. Japanese B encephalitis was also one of a host of afflictions that plagued Japan immediately after the surrender to the Allies in 1945 (table 1).[34]

Of interest to our story of social institutions and unanticipated consequences is that Ishii Shirō (1892–1959), an eccentric young Japanese biologist, invented the filtration device that proved instrumental in isolating and identifying the Japanese B encephalitis virus. But his career later proved a sinister one, as he applied his scientific expertise in water impurities, filtration, arboviruses, and insects to develop Japan's biological weapons program in China.[35] Although outside the scope of this book, the biological weapons program that Ishii oversaw in China during the Pacific War, among other activities, raised bubonic plague–carrying fleas in nurseries (much in the manner that villagers had raised silkworms), packed them in bombs in swabs of cotton, and then released them over Chinese cities such as Ningbo (27 October 1940) and Changde (11 April 1942).[36] Japanese killed

TABLE 1 Postwar Japanese B Encephalitis Statistics

Year	No. of victims	No. of deaths
1946	201	99
1947	263	228
1948	4,757	2,620
1949	1,284	1,177
1950	5,196	2,430
1951	2,188	956
1952	3,545	1,437
1953	1,729	720
1954	1,758	732
1955	3,699	1,373
1956	4,538	1,600
1957	1,793	744
1958	3,900	1,349
1959	1,979	723
1960	1,607	650
1961	2,053	825
1962	1,363	568
1963	1,205	566
1964	2,546	524
Total	45,604	19,321

Source: Suzuki Takeshi and Ogata Kazuki, *Nihon no eisei gaichū: Sono seitai to kujo* (Japan's Hygiene and Insect Pests) (Tokyo: Shinshichōsha, 1958), 37–38.

thousands of Chinese civilians with this biotechnology. This personal and institutional linkage between killing anthropoids and arthropods should not surprise us, however. The same European and American companies that developed chemicals and aerial dispersal technologies to kill bugs transferred them easily to human battlefields during times of war.[37]

NATIONAL ECOLOGIES

Earlier in this chapter, I conjured an image of silkworms, tucked in well-humidified, thatch-roofed rural households, being fed tender, carefully cut mulberry leaves. The caterpillars thrived when rural cultivators transformed rice paddies and vegetable fields into mulberry plantations to feed them. Famously, cultivators in Shindatsu (Fukushima Prefecture) doted over their silkworms with "the most minute ministrations," as Kanō Tanboku observed. Those who served as middlemen in the sericulture industry eventually transformed into a new category of farmer, called *gōnō,* or "wealthy peasant."[38] The wealth of these middlemen did not go unnoticed. In 1866, Shindatsu experienced uprisings because of a reviled silk tax (mainly on raw silk and silkworm-egg cards) that was said to be the brainchild of wealthy peasants—a "wicked plot" by "rascals"—not Tokugawa ministers. The violent uprising in Shindatsu constituted one of the unanticipated socioeconomic consequences of the coevolutionary partnership between people and their bugs.[39] Those who did not have the economic wherewithal to prosper from serving as middlemen in the sericulture industry, though they often husbanded the bugs, saw this biotechnology as a serious threat to the traditional social stability of their communities. That is, silkworms facilitated a redistribution of wealth in rural Japanese villages.

But there were other consequences of silkworm cultivation near Edo even more unanticipated than uprisings. When agricultural lands were replanted with mulberry, the burden for raising food crops, such as soybeans, weighed on more distant areas. By the eighteenth century, Edo, with its more than one million mouths and stomachs, had started to devour resources from distant domains and provinces, such as Hachinohe Domain, in the far northeast, which had begun to raise soybeans to feed the hungry urban populations to the south. Later, in the nineteenth and early twentieth centuries, this was precisely how the Third World was created on a global scale: the jolting process whereby "peripheral," usually colonial, holdings were forced into monocrop regimens in order to supply food and other resources for distant, better-organized metropolitan populations.[40] As Mike Davis has shown, colossal famine was often the result of this brutal integration into Western-controlled global food markets. Davis writes of these late Victorian famines: "Millions died, not outside the 'modern world system,' but in the very process of being forcibly incorporated into its economic and political structures."[41] As a result of economic growth in the Tokugawa years, Japan began economically colonizing itself, creating a regional Third World in peripheral domains and, on occasion, famine.[42] In turn, central Japan and the silkworms that lived there with their human providers became the First World, at least within Japan. This proved to be the national ecological footprint, at least in part, of silkworm cultivation and other forms of cash-crop farming.

In 1744, at the same moment those cultivators began to devote more time and arable land to mulberry, a little-known scholar named Andō Shōeki (1703–62) arrived in Hachinohe Domain to serve as a *machi isha*, or "town doctor." Unlike salaried physicians, town doctors needed to be skilled and entrepreneurial to survive in the competitive medical marketplace that was eighteenth-century Japan.[43] Andō proved up to the task and quickly made a reputation for himself as a doctor and lecturer. His skill as a doctor was exceeded only by his deep knowledge of Buddhism and Confucianism, and in time, he attracted the attention of town elders, domain administrators, and the local intelligentsia. One listener remarked that Andō, when giving lectures on the True Way, proved "superior even to the sages of antiquity." Unfortunately, only fragments of his life in Hachinohe can be pieced together, but Andō appears to have garnered quite a reputation while in the northeast, and he wrote several treatises with a strong, orthodox Neo-Confucian flair. Hachinohe, however, was a tough place in which to live in the eighteenth century, and as the conditions around him deteriorated, his taste for Neo-Confucian thought (or any sort of philosophical orthodoxy for that matter) soured, and he set out on the path of a more unorthodox vision of the human place in the natural world. In effect, he called for agrarian sustainability and a more equitable form of social justice.

Similar to other northeastern domains, Hachinohe suffered four major famines in the eighteenth century (1702, 1749, 1755, and 1783), caused by a combination of climatologic conditions and early modern economic integration. Cold, eastwardly winds called *yamase* occurred within the context of a global Neo-Boreal (Little Ice Age, 1450–1850) and damaged crops in northeastern Japan. In the Tenmei famine (1783), about half of the population of Hachinohe died of starvation or malnutrition. Grisly paintings of cannibalism remain among the most enduring legacies of these harsh decades in Japanese history. Of these eighteenth-century Hachinohe famines, the *inoshishi kegachi*, "wild boar famine," of 1749 was surely among the most bizarre: the famine was the result of a trophic cascade that was embedded in the web of factors presented in this chapter and stemmed from the relationship that people in central Japan had with their silkworms. More silkworms (and, hence, the demand for more mulberry plantations near cities to feed them) meant, on at least one occasion, more wild boars (*Sus scrofa*), because boars thrived in the slash-and-burn landscapes created when peripheral areas, such as Hachinohe, began raising soybeans to feed urban populations. Ultimately, boars competed with Hachinohe's poor seasonal workers for sources of nutrition. Along with environmental circumstances, political circumstances also contributed to the increase in boar populations: Tokugawa Tsunayoshi (1646–1709), the "Dog Shogun," had restricted hunting throughout Japan in 1687 with his *shōruiaware*, or "clemency for living creatures" order, which meant that, even sixty years later, there were just more boars around. The number of the boars' traditional predators, namely the Japanese wolf (*Canis lupus hodophilax* Temminck, 1839), appears to have been in decline in the northeast as well, possibly as a result of the eighteenth-century rabies epizootics.[44] The convergence of factors meant the perfect ecological storm: in 1749, the wild boars won their deadly competition with farmers in an undisputed knockout.

To feed Edo's population, Hachinohe farmers seized the moment and planted soybeans. The trade routes were already in place: the legumes traveled along well-navigated shipping routes that, since the early eighteenth century, had hauled furs, dried fish, and other products from Ezo (present-day Hokkaido), where Japanese had acquired them in trade with Ainu.[45] Hachinohe farmers created *yakibatake*, or "slash-and-burn fields," for soybeans, and when they exhausted the soil's nutrients, weedier plants such as arrowroot (*kuzu*), wild yams (*yamaimo*), and other starchy tubers thrived in the fallow fields left behind. Normally, the boars that inhabited Hachinohe ate acorns and chestnuts; but the denuding of hillsides in the wake of slash-and-burn farming left boars to uproot tubers in fallow soybean fields, which they easily did with their sharp tusks. Once the wild boars had eaten all the wild tubers, they then turned to what remained of agricultural crops; they even invaded the Hachinohe castle town on at least one occasion. In the end, some 3,000 people (about 10 percent of the domain's population) and countless boars died in the conflict. (In the third month of 1751, for example, hunters killed 2,923 boars throughout Hachinohe.) This interspecific war meant that it was a disturbing time to be a town doctor in Hachinohe: infanticide, heaps of dead bodies, unpredictable weather, malnutrition, and butchered boars, deer, and macaques everywhere.[46] Intellectually, Andō rejected the Neo-Confucian orthodoxy he once championed: he never again would be accused of being "the Confucian Master Andō."[47] Undeniably, his intellectual transformation was an unintended consequence of the rise of sericulture in central Japan, Edo's booming population, and the cascading effect it had in Japan's far northeast.

For Andō, the torturous wild boar famine of 1749 birthed a powerful critique of Tokugawa rule and the burgeoning national economy. In his critique, he yoked social justice to the nature of agrarian production to criticize the fabricated hierarchies of early modern governance. Cruel famines, such as the one witnessed in Hachinohe, occurred because people no longer pursued chokkō, or "Right Cultivation." In his mind, people in eighteenth-century Japan were out of balance with Earth's natural rhythms; they no longer heard the soft voice of nature, only the louder demands of profit and desire. People mined metals in the mountains for coinage, which fostered desire. They turned grain cultivation into cash-crop farming, which also fostered desire. Andō focused on the need for Japanese to conform to (rather than engineer, resist, or even fight) the rhythms of nature. For example, Andō famously critiqued the Jōkyō calendar (implemented in 1684), which Shogun Tsunayoshi had ordered astronomer Shibukawa Shunkai (1639–1715) to craft in order to establish a single, unified calendar for the entire realm. According to Andō, writing around 1754, the Jōkyō calendar, though certainly an effective "self-serving law" (shihō) devised to establish "national policy," was inappropriate for farmers living in the far northeast and elsewhere because it disrupted the sustainability of Right Cultivation. Crafting calendars should be about synchronizing people with natural rhythms, not "self-serving" political ones.[48] This may seem trite today, but in East Asia designing calendars remained one of the fundamental prerogatives of rulers: calendars set the temporal rhythms of dynasty.

Andō insisted that people needed to synchronize their behavior with Earth's natural rhythms because those rhythms are embedded in a larger cosmic order. In the magisterial *Shizen shineidō* he wrote: "Human beings are the perfect manifestation of Heaven-and-Earth [*tenchi*]. Since this is so, he who is ignorant of the essential nature of the production and birth of Heaven-and-Earth is ignorant of the birth and death of his own body and mind."[49] Not only are humans embedded in the environment, but they are the environment. To be ignorant of nature, in other words, is to be ignorant of one's own body and mind. (Note the difference between Andō's insistence on knowing oneself through knowing nature and Maruyama Masao's insistence, as discussed in the introduction, on knowing the modern self through liberation from nature.) Because people are embedded in nature, Andō repeatedly asserted that all natural disasters are in fact man-made ones. Human desire manifested itself as a pollutant that swooshed up into the heavens, soiled "Heaven-and-Earth," and disrupted natural cycles and caused disasters: more evidence that people are embedded in nature, not separate from it. In *Tōdō shinden* he wrote: "Natural disasters are created by humankind and return to humankind."[50] His unwavering belief in the "unity of opposites" meant that there existed, as he wrote in *Shizen shineidō*, "no triumph of one element over another." Therefore, feudal hierarchies, such as those codified in Japan's Neo-Confucian order, were unnatural (despite the claims of their architects to the contrary) and, hence, unjust. "After the distinction between the great ruler and his small followers was established," Andō wrote, "the great devoured what the smaller produced, and then the next greatest ate what the next smallest produced, on down the line, until the entire world followed this practice. This is the practice of the world of beasts."[51]

In his writings, Andō crafted a historical dualism. There was *hōsei*, or "the world of laws," which represented Andō's corrupt day, the world of elaborate governments or, in his words, "the world of exploitation and chaos brought about by the self-serving law." The age prior to "the world of laws" was what he called *shizen kasshin*, or the world of the "self-acting living truth," an age of marvelous spontaneity. (The word *shizen* is also commonly translated as "nature," rendering his utopia a "natural living truth.") This represented the "age before the appearance of the sages and the Buddha, the age when humanity lived according to the upward energy of the Truth and all followed the Heavenly Way of Right Cultivation."[52] To consume what one does not produce was outrageous. Even the historical Buddha, though compassionate, by "greedily consuming food that he did not cultivate," showed himself to be nothing more than a "great thief."

To Andō, rulers and the wealthy were nothing more than thieves because they failed to participate in Right Cultivation and fattened on the labor of others.

As an environmental philosopher, Andō would have agreed with Richard White's assessment: "Humans have known nature by digging in the earth, planting seeds, and harvesting plants. They have known nature by feeling heat and cold, sweating as they went up hills, sinking into mud. They have known nature by shaping wood and stone, by living with animals, nurturing them, and killing them." Indeed, Andō equated work, not with environmental destruction, as many U.S. environmentalists have, but rather with Right Cultivation and a rejection of the corrupt world of laws. Hypothetically, if Andō was asked by an unemployed logger in Forks, Washington, "Are you an environmentalist, or do you work for a living?" I am confident that Andō would have replied: "I'm an environmentalist *because* I work for a living."[53] He rejected rulers and governments, not farmers and laborers, as sowing the seeds of violent revolt and social discontent. If societies must have rulers, he suggested pointedly, people should "determine the proper amount of land for the ruler and require him to cultivate it."[54] It is little wonder that Andō became the darling of some early left-leaning historians of Japan.[55]

Moreover, Andō's deep compassion for the nonhuman world of "beasts" remains moving. He lamented the trapping and selling of birds, for example. In one dialog from his *Hōsei monogatari* (Tales of the World of Law), a black-faced bunting remarks: "What can they be thinking that they fail to understand how it would feel if they were put in a cage, if their wife and children were put in cages, and taken to be sold! No, they do not deserve to be regarded as human beings." A horse laments the birth of the equestrian arts: "Men put steel bits in our mouths and stuck hot peppers into our anuses, they cut and trimmed our hooves and branded our hides, they rode us to exhaustion and refused to allow us to eat as we liked. These were sufferings hard to bear." Andō was outraged by animal husbandry, what little of it was practiced on the Japanese archipelago. "Though beasts eat each other," he wrote, "beasts do not capture other beasts alive, pen them up, and keep them. The sages and wise men of the World of Law, though, do just this, and then kill these beasts, declaring that it is for their own nourishment, or as a sacrifice to Heaven." Andō asked: "Can there be any god in Heaven who would rejoice at having the very beasts that he gave life to killed and offered up to him?"[56]

Born from the environmental upheaval of the wild boar famine of 1749, Andō's critiques of political power, social hierarchies, nationalization of the economy, and cash-crop farming are retrospectively powerful ones, because his writings were not published in his lifetime. He recognized that political power, social inequality, and the unequal distribution of wealth—no matter what form they took; no matter how justified by laws; no matter how natural they seemed—were tied to Earth and access to its resources. This is what made animals superior to the people of Andō's day. "In the world of beasts there is no need to worry about bad harvests or famine, or being able to scrape together the annual tax and tribute, or of repaying loans," he lamented.[57] Concerns over famine and poverty Andō reserved for human society and its world of law, the proximate forces that caused boars to run wild in the streets of Hachinohe and cause so much death, destruction, and pain in emaciated bodies.

But Andō, for all his genius, could not have anticipated the new kind of pain and suffering that modern agriculture would bring to the Japanese archipelago. The rise of sericulture, the dislocation of seasonal farmers (caused by the emergence of cash-crop farming), soybean monocrop regimens in the far northeast, Neo-Boreal weather patterns, and terrible famine proved painful. Emaciation is quite painful: it hurts when the lining of the stomach slowly decomposes, when the abdomen protrudes because of the gasses created by the decomposition process, and when protein deprivation reddens hair and weakens bodies. The wild boar famine of 1749 was a local event that was indicative of a national trend and that demonstrated the interconnection between Japanese in the far northeast and silkworm (and other cash-crop) cultivators near Edo. This is precisely what Andō had wanted people to see. To sum up, changing environmental conditions in central Japan had unanticipated consequences in the environment of Hachinohe: early modern Japan had witnessed the birth of a fledgling national ecosystem.

Nonetheless, it was the introduction of chemical insecticides, discussed in the next chapter, that provided the chemical means to trace elaborate threads in Japan's national ecosystem and food web. Chemical insecticides moved clandestinely through food webs, killing human consumers in both anticipated and unanticipated ways. They, more than the rise of sericulture before them, highlighted that Japanese were embedded in a national ecosystem, and the key physical indicator of participation in this new national experience was, of course, pain.

2 THE AGENCY OF CHEMICALS

I f Buddhist beliefs regarding the transmigration of the soul shaped outbreaks of Japanese B encephalitis, they also determined how Japanese countered the threat posed by insect-borne crop damage and famine. Insects not only harbor deadly disease but also eat many of the same crops that people do. But because insect bodies harbored the souls of historical figures, the explanation for what motivated insect damage to crops was not entomological but rather historical and theological. That is, the prominent personalities of Japan's past—as understood through legends, histories, and hagiographies—determined the behavior of insects, not eons of evolution or their microscopic, though sophisticated, brains. Disgruntled generals who had been slain on the battlefield could return to the sites of their deaths to wantonly punish, for example. Consequently, how farmers and agronomists tackled the threat of insects was also determined by history and Buddhist attitudes—until, that is, the advent of scientific entomology, which ascribed insect behavior to different causes and thus radically reconfigured insect eradication campaigns. Starting in the Meiji years, Japanese began experimenting with chemical insecticides. In the second half of this chapter, we shall turn to the deployment of parathion in Japan to highlight how organophosphate chemicals operated within hybrid spaces to cause human pain on a national scale. My analysis will be as much ecological as historical or theological, because we need to trace parathion as it meandered through eddies and pathways of modern food webs in industrial agricultural settings to finally reach industrialized human bodies.

EARLY MODERN JAPANESE FAMINES AND INSECTICIDES

The Kyōhō famine of 1732, one of Japan's three great famines of the Tokugawa period (1600–1868), was partially caused by insects.[1] The famine ravaged central and western Japan, including the islands of Kyushu and Shikoku. *Unka*, or plant hoppers, were the principal troublemakers. In the beginning of the sixth month of the lunar calendar, farmers reported massive emergences of one species of rice plant hoppers (*Sogatella furcifera*), and about two weeks later, a different species (*Nilaparvata lugens*) also emerged. To this day, these delphacid insects represent a serious threat to rice crops throughout much of Asia. They travel on seasonal winds from southeastern China, their arrival corresponding serendipitously to the transplanting of lush, green rice crops in spring and early summer. In temperate climates, such as those of Korea and Japan, the hoppers do not survive the winter.[2] Hoppers are not that much different from other invader species such as Japanese beetles, though their agency, specifically their locomotion, differs. Japanese beetles resemble the fire ants of the American South: they relied on people, disruption, broken soil, nurseries, and the global economy to travel to the United States.[3] Plant hoppers, by contrast, took matters into their own hands by taking wing on seasonal winds. We call this natural agency, though both forms of relocation, as we shall learn, were the product of hybrid causations, as were the environmental results of the hopper's arrival in Japan.

In 1732, hoppers, hitching their tiny wagons to atmospheric locomotion, coordinated their arrival perfectly, and farmers reported widespread crop damage as a result of these two waves of insect invaders. In Komatsu Domain, in Iyo Province on Shikoku Island, farmers reported insect damage in the form of *mushigui,* a reference to hoppers infesting rice stalks and sucking these plants dry of their life-giving juices until they withered, turned brown, and died. So many hoppers swam on the surface of the paddies that the water turned "the color of soy sauce." During the day, the hoppers stayed on the rice stalks, contently sucking the juices; at night, however, when farmers inspected the crops with pine torches, they saw that the insects had moved to the heads of the plants, where they ate the precious grain itself. Despite prayers offered at temples and shrines to disperse the insects, crops died; farmers watched helplessly as insects less than an inch long consumed bushel upon bushel of the gold standard of Japan's eighteenth-century economy.

Not only cultivators in Komatsu but those in Hiroshima Domain experienced hopper infestations in 1732. They peaked around the sixteenth or seventeenth day of the seventh month of the lunar calendar. Farmers described the hoppers as having risen up from the "earth's vapors" to resemble giant plumes of noxious smoke hovering over the crops. Farmers also noticed, however, that during the first ten days of the eighth month, when temperatures dropped, the hoppers died off: they coped poorly with Japan's temperate climate. Farmers in the five home provinces around the ancient capital of Kyoto, the Kinai region, reported infestations of large hoppers (probably of the leaf hopper *Cicadula sexnotata*) that resembled the "golden coin beetle," the pesky insect known as the "Japanese beetle" that we encountered in chapter 1. Farmers described these flying insects as sporting an exoskeleton that resembled protective armor; in one night a swarm of them could eat the equivalent of tens of thousands of bushels of rice. In the Kinai, farmers compared the hoppers to the "golden coin beetle," but in the western provinces they referred to the pest as Sanemori: just as Lafcadio Hearn had ruminated on the transmigratory lives of mosquitoes in a nearby cemetery, farmers in Japan's western provinces believed that the insects were actually the spirit of the vengeful general Saitō Bettō Sanemori (1111–83), who, in the twelfth century, had died in the fields of Shinohara, Kaga Province, at the hands of his rival Tetsuka Mitsumori.[4] Farmers believed that Sanemori continued to hold a grudge against the farmers of western Japan and that he came back in the bodies of plant hoppers to ruin their rice crops: this was their Buddhist-inspired, historical explanation of insect behavior. Historical personalities and circumstances (such as the bitterness of a shamed, defeated warrior), not insect behavior or migratory patterns (such as the cognitive or instinctual capacities of their brains), determined the nature of Japan's early agricultural entomology. It also shaped how early modern Japanese entomologists sought to eliminate the threat caused by these pests.

In order to drive off these dangerous pests, a farmer needed to know something about Sanemori. After all, his disgruntled soul sought revenge in the tiny, buzzing bodies of these insects. In response, farmers from the western provinces fashioned frightening scarecrows, which they placed along coastal shorelines and on the borders of their villages and rice paddies. When Sanemori (perhaps better armored than in the twelfth century) ignored these straw men, farmers employed what they referred to as the "oil extermination" technique: they poured rapeseed or whale oil on the water of their paddies to suffocate hoppers that fell. This oil extermination method represents one of the first uses of insecticides in Japan. Rural lore explained that resourceful farmers invented the technique in Chikuzen Province, on Kyushu Island, in 1670 but later improved on it. A treatise on "insect control" by Ōkura Nagatsune (1766–1860) contains illustrations that depict farmers burning hoppers with pine torches and brushing them into oily water. Apparently, the method was discovered when a man named Yahiro, while lighting temple lamps, noticed that hoppers flew into the lit oil and died, and so desperate farmers replicated the technique on a larger scale by erecting giant pine torches in their paddies (fig. 2.1).

In Fukuoka Domain, in Chikuzen Province, farmers called the hopper infestations a "vision of Michizane's Dazaifu spirit," a reference to legendary classical scholar and statesman Sugawara no Michizane (845–903). On being exiled by political rivals to Dazaifu, capital of the western provinces (in present-day Fukuoka Prefecture), Michizane died in disgrace, but shortly after his death, his rivals in Kyoto began dying, too, and so north of Kyoto a shrine was erected in honor of "Tenman Tenjin," his posthumous, deified name. His spirit remains associated with rigorous scholarship and continues to grace smart young Japanese entrance-examination takers to this day. Farmers in Fukuoka, close to Michizane's grave, no doubt assumed that he had taken the form of hoppers, much as farmers believed that Sanemori had in Kaga Province.[5] For these Japanese farmers, entomology was a condition of history.

Ōkura Nagatsune's insect control treatise, titled *Jokōroku* (1826), presents fascinating examples of the methods used by rural cultivators to protect their crops and exterminate plant hoppers and locusts. He began the treatise by observing that, in times of unseasonable weather, hoppers and other rice-eating insects (*unka*) appear on rice crops and severely damage them, which often results in famine. Famine, he insisted, was the "number one affliction of the realm." Given that hundreds of thousands often died, he was right. He continued: "Farmers must learn the methods of preventing [damage caused by] plant hoppers" if the realm-wide scourge of famine was to be eliminated. Ōkura's principal example of the dangers of insects and

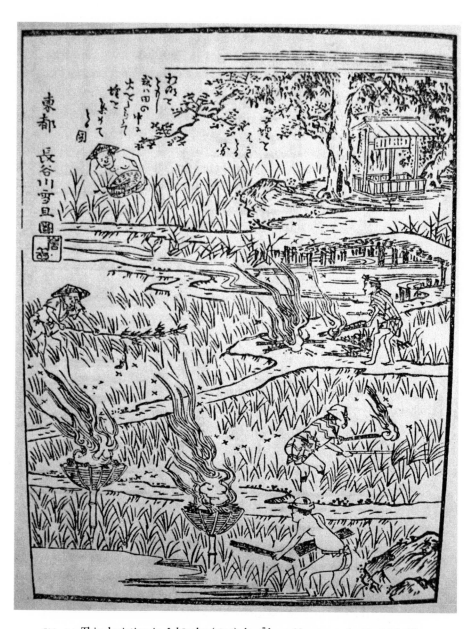

FIG. 2.1 This depiction in *Jokōroku* (1826), by Ōkura Nagatsune (1766–1860), illustrates farmers burning hoppers with oil and pine torches. *Source:* Ōkura Nagatsune, *Jokōroku* (Record of Insect Control), in *Nihon nōsho zenshū* (Complete Works of Japanese Agricultural Writings), vol. 15, ed. Shadan Hōjin Nōsangyoson Bunka Kyōkai (Tokyo: Nōsangyoson Bunka Kyōkai, 1977), 51.

famine was the Kyōhō episode; but he recalled the intense hardships of the Tenmei famine as well, specifically the unseasonable weather of 1783 and 1787, when he was a young child growing up in Hitashi, in Bungo Province, present-day Ōita Prefecture (historians estimate that over one million died in the Tenmei famine). He knew from personal experiences the tragedy of famine and sought to prevent it through the use of insecticides. Ōkura was no armchair entomologist. He sought firsthand knowledge about the effectiveness of different insect-killing techniques. When plant hoppers infested crops in Kyoto and eastward along the Tōkaidō travel circuit in 1825, Ōkura traveled to the region around present-day Shizuoka Prefecture. Farmers there were unable to procure whale oil to spread on their paddies, so they used rapeseed oil instead, which proved less effective. One farmer from Kami Shinden Village had gone so far as to experiment with different amounts of rapeseed oil by dividing his paddies into sections—turning his paddies into an experiment station of sorts—but, basically, the results proved the same: rapeseed oil just did not work all that well.

Protecting rice crops from hoppers proved "extremely difficult," and there were few substitutes for whale oil.[6] But even when whale oil was available, if farmers failed to apply it at the first signs of hopper infestation, it was ineffective against the tenacious pests. Ōkura also discussed rural lore regarding the weather and seasonal habits of hoppers. One older farmer relayed to him that insects usually ravaged crops during inclement weather in the spring and early summer, particularly in times of drought, a pattern that resembles devastating locust swarms in the American West.[7] Many illustrations of different methods of protecting rice paddies from hoppers grace Ōkura's text (fig. 2.2). For example, farmers dispensed whale oil in paddies and use brooms to sweep hoppers off the rice stalks and onto the water's oily surface, where the bugs suffocated. Farmers also lit pine torches to attract and burn insects. Both methods were labor intensive, and farmers had to be careful not to damage the plants with their brooms.[8]

During the Kyōhō famine, farmers tried these and other methods of insect control. Fukuoka farmers applied nearly one gallon of fish oil per acre to rid their paddies of the angry Michizane, an example of how Japanese refashioned fish and whales into technologies of insect eradication. In a sense, they were entomological Ghost Busters, vanquishing the spirits of Michizane, Sanemori, and others. The technique developed in Fukuoka quickly spread throughout the provinces of western Japan, such as Matsuyama Domain, in Iyo Province, where farmers reportedly tried the tech-

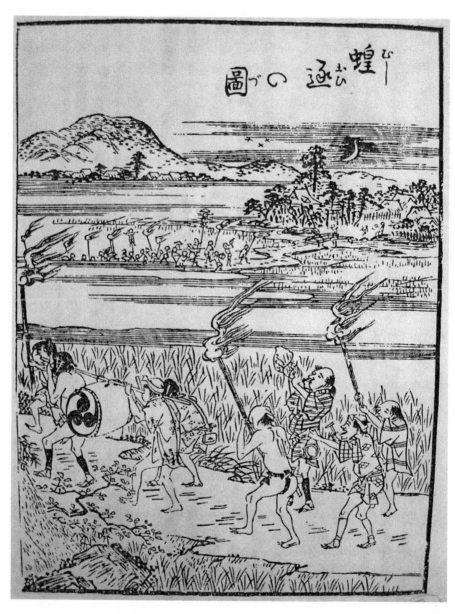

FIG. 2.2 Ceremoniously "driving away insects," or *mushioi no zu*, as depicted in *Jokōroku* (1826), by Ōkura Nagatsune (1766–1860). *Source:* Ōkura Nagatsune, *Jokōroku* (Record of Insect Control), in *Nihon nōsho zenshū* (Complete Works of Japanese Agricultural Writings), vol. 15, ed. Shadan Hōjin Nōsangyoson Bunka Kyōkai (Tokyo: Nōsangyoson Bunka Kyōkai, 1977), 23.

nique in their paddies as well. But fish and whale oil proved expensive and beyond the economic means of most farmers; and the fact that domain lords, and even the Tokugawa shogun, ordered prayers at various temples, though magnanimous indeed, probably did little to stem the hopper tide. The shogun had also associated insects with disgruntled ghosts and, in an official governmental response, ordered prayers at Japan's most sacred sites, including the Ise Shrine, the Grand Shrine at Izumo, Buzen Usa, Hitachi Kashima, Katori, Iwashi Mizuhachiman-gū, the Nikkō mausoleum, the Enryakuji Temple at Mount Hiei, and Gojiin. When domain lords formally reported the damage done to crops, the shogun generously reduced their *mononari*, or yearly rice tribute, and even offered loans to the most devastated areas.[9]

However, the cool temperatures in the eighth month that stemmed the tide of the hungry hoppers also destroyed what remained of western Japan's rice crops. The combined damage from insects and weather hit Matsuyama Domain particularly hard. In 1732 the lord reported that 3,489 people had died of starvation, along with 1,694 oxen and 1,403 horses. (Officials recorded a total mortality of 12,072, while 2,646,020 people suffered from hunger and malnourishment.)[10] What makes the Kyōhō famine important for our purposes is that, in the midst of the deadly crisis, Japan's earliest entomologists experimented with oils and other techniques to rid crops of hungry hoppers. Two principles underlay their eradication techniques: theology and history prompted farmers and officials to offer prayers, while a more empirical understanding of crops and insects prompted the use of oils (see table 2).

The approach taken by Japanese farmers and the Tokugawa shoguns in tackling the deadly Kyōhō famine is striking: they set up scarecrows on the coastline, conjured spells, worshiped at temples and shrines, anthropomorphized insects with the transmigrating spirits of past generals and statesmen, and relied on whale and rapeseed oil as an insecticide. These techniques expose how Buddhist sentiments, historical personalities, agrarian systems, and Tokugawa governance drove famine relief, the geography of disease, and causes of premature mortality in Japan. Here cultural systems intersected seamlessly with natural ones: an example of the manner in which historical legacies, religious orthodoxies, government institutions, and technologies manifest themselves in the physical environment. In the previous chapter, we saw how silkworms evolved in historical time as a result of anthropogenic forces such as manipulated breeding; they also

TABLE 2 Pre-Meiji Methods for Insect Control

874.8	The imperial court dispatched a special envoy to Ise Province after reports of insect damage. Envoys presented Shinto offerings and prayers to avoid calamity.
1641	In Izumo Province the effects of a secret family insecticide recipe designed to exterminate leaf hoppers were demonstrated.
1670.7	Yoshiemon, from Onga County in Chikuzen Province, exterminated leaf hoppers by sprinkling whale oil on the surface of rice paddies.
1720.7.7	Ōmaru Genshirō rediscovered the "oil extermination method," or the use of whale oil to exterminate leaf hoppers.
1732	Yahiro, from Mikasa County in Chikuzen Province, rediscovered the oil extermination method while filling sacred shrine lamps with oil.
1733	The Tokugawa shogunate notified western provinces of a "curse on rice-eating insects."
1769	Domain purchased whale oil to experiment with the extermination of rice-eating insects.
1778.10	The Tokugawa shogunate notified magistrates (*daikan*) regarding methods to exterminate the aquatic invasive weed *hirumushiro* (*Potamogeton distinctus*) from rice paddies.
1781.6.12	Takeda Chōhei established the drug company Yakushushō (today's Takeda Yakuhin Kōgyō).
1787	The Tokugawa shogunate notified various domains to use whale oil when insect damage occurs in rice paddies.
1796	The Tokugawa shogunate again notified various domains to use whale oil when insect damage occurs in rice paddies.
1855	In Gifu Prefecture, cultivators Murase Heizaemon and Nagai Magohei invented a method to disinfect wheat seeds.

Source: Matsubara Hiromichi, *Nihon nōyakugakushi nenpyō* (A Historical Chronology of the Development of Agricultural Chemicals) (Tokyo: Gakkai Shuppan Sentā, 1984), 23.

Note: The dates in the first column are calculated according to the lunar calendar; e.g., 1720.7.7 = 7th day of the 7th month of the year 1720.

evolved because of social networks, household organization, religious attitudes, and agrarian practices. This should remind us of one of the more famous tenets of "chaos theory," which states that any single action, no matter how minute or seemingly inconsequential, when amplified through a system, can have unintended consequences somewhere else in that system because it is all interconnected at some level.[11]

History works in this fashion, too. When Saitō Bettō Sanemori made his fatal misjudgment and was slain in the battlefields of Shinohara, that event set in motion unintended consequences that resonated through the natural and supernatural worlds. They transcended time and space to alter the physical environment centuries later. Sanemori's defeat led to the crafting of historical memories that, when coupled with Buddhist theories of the transmigration of the soul and with insect migration habits, underpinned speculation about the motives of insects and, thereby, determined the response to insect emergences and insect-caused famine. Why did insects emerge to ravage laboriously tended crops? Because they—or rather the souls inhabiting their bodies—were furious about a military defeat they suffered centuries ago. They had a score to settle. In other words, insects as biological agents are only part of the story, because they buzzed and hopped through the hybrid spaces of the Japanese imagination, which is a rich landscape indeed.

MEIJI INSECTICIDES

Plant hoppers, locusts, scale insects, and other insect pests proved no less dangerous during the Meiji regime (1868–1912) than they had under the Tokugawa shoguns. But Meiji modernizers felt more pressure than ever to increase agricultural yields on croplands because, with industrialization, more people transferred from rural areas to newly constructed urban factories to work as laborers. Increased yields also boosted badly needed tax revenue. So, in essence, Japan's working lands needed to feed and thereby fuel a growing industrial population with fewer people actually cultivating them. For this reason, fertilizers and insecticides proved invaluable to Japan's modernization designs: in effect, farmers boosted yields with chemical fertilizers and, through increased use of insecticides, hoped to share fewer of their painstakingly produced calories with always-hungry six-legged competitors. Early modern farmers processed whale blubber and rapeseeds and turned them into agents of insect control; Meiji Japanese sought other remedies to eradicate pests, ones more chemical in nature. Sadly, caught in the friendly fire of Japan's turn to chemicals to eradicate bugs was the spiritual life of nature: an exorcising from the national mind-set of the belief that Michizane and Sanemori could inhabit insect bodies, or any other part of nature for that matter, in favor of a new scientific view of nature's agency. In this sense, Meiji's simplified, rational, and scientific approach realized what Carolyn Merchant has referred to as the "death of nature" in other contexts.[12] Insects were no longer fleshy bodies and crunchy shells possessed by historical spirits; they were reduced to fleshy, crunchy, soulless automatons that acted on instinctive impulses.

Unlike whale or rapeseed oil, chemical insecticides operate more deeply in social networks and ecosystems and, therefore, have the potential for more deep-seated alterations of the environment and human bodies. Systems, organizations, institutions, and networks became even more elaborate and widespread after the Meiji Restoration, because modern states rely on more rational forms of governance and social control than premodern states do. Meiji Japanese deployed chemicals because the way they viewed these bugs and agriculture had changed: in the modern scientific order, casting spells, offering official prayers at shrines and temples, and setting up scarecrows smacked of a superstitious past. Chemicals, by contrast, represented the promise of Euro-American science, a new form of magic, much as Buddhism had been centuries earlier. Modern science was rooted in economic entomology and advanced chemistry, not theories regarding the transmigration of Sanemori's bitter soul.

The Meiji approach favored Euro-American science over rural folk remedies and resulted in experimentation with simple chemical means of killing insects in the context of a more industrialized agricultural regimen.[13] Nowhere in nineteenth-century Japan was modern, industrialized agriculture more coveted than on the newly acquired island of Hokkaido, where the Hokkaido Development Agency (Kaitakushi; 1869–82) hired foreign experts from the United States and elsewhere to assist in the creation of modern agriculture on that island.[14] The United States, with its network of land-grant colleges, extension agencies, experiment stations, and state and federal development officers, provided the model institutions for nineteenth-century agricultural modernization in Japan.

In the United States, as early as the 1840s, economic entomologists began pushing for a greater role in the agricultural sciences. That is, they no longer wanted to be seen as quirky men with thick glasses whose homes were cluttered with case upon case of pin-impaled insect specimens. They wanted to contribute to practical science and did so by conjuring a war against insects in America's agricultural lands. Their call to arms was not without foundation: increasing urbanization had demanded more mono-crop agriculture to feed people, which made crops more susceptible to insect and weather damage. This is one of the lessons of the Hachinohe wild boar famine of 1749, discussed in the previous chapter: monocrop agriculture dangerously puts all caloric eggs in one basket, particularly for subsistence farmers. In 1854, the U.S. federal government hired a lone entomologist to travel the country cataloging and collecting information on noxious insects. By 1868, the same year as the Meiji Restoration, some states followed suit and hired entomologists as well. That same year, the journal *American Entomologist* was begun, which for its short life span peddled the economic entomologists' agenda. In the nineteenth century, among the insecticides sprayed on crops throughout the United States were "Buhach" (the American proprietary name for pyrethrum powder), "Paris green" (a copper acetoarsenate), "London purple" (basically, calcium arsenate), "lead arsenate," and "Bordeaux mixture" (discussed below). Signs of trouble related to the use of such insecticides appeared early. In 1891, for example, a public health scare related to poisoned grapes and Bordeaux mixture rocked New York City; later, public health officials debated the degree to which arsenic, which cultivators sprayed liberally on fruit crops, caused chronic health problems among consumers. This is an important point: the use of arsenic as an insecticide forced the medical community to grapple with the long-term chronic health consequences of insecticide poisoning.[15] Arsenic, as a "civilization-destroying" weapon (to use Elaine Scarry's language), killed slowly, clandestinely.[16]

Drawing on the U.S. experience, Hokkaido's working lands became nothing less than laboratories where the Hokkaido Development Agency tested newly imported agriculture technologies, including chemical insecticides. One of these technologies was an inorganic carbon-sulfur compound used to combat scale insects in orchards and "rust" on wheat crops in 1874. The compound "lime sulfur," as farmers commonly called it, proved effective against wheat crop and apple orchard diseases, such as fungal head blight (*Gibberella zeae*), wheat leaf rust (*Puccinia triticina*), and powdery mildew (*Podosphaera leucotricha*), as well as insects such as red mites (*Metatetranychus citri*) and arrowhead scales (*Unaspis yanonensis*). In 1881, moreover, Meiji modernizers began importing pyrethrum powder from England (made from chrysanthemums); four years later, they imported seeds for insect-repelling chrysanthemums from the United States and began cultivating the plants throughout the country. The plants proved so successful that by 1898, Japan, with the support of the Meiji government, became an exporter of dried chrysanthemum flowers to the United States. Simultaneously, Japanese scientists experimented with a variety of chrysanthemum-based chemical insecticides, including mosquito incense. In 1901, Japanese agronomists developed a "chrysanthemum-petroleum emulsion" that farmers used as an insecticide throughout the country. More importantly, Japanese scientists participated in the development of "pyrethroid," a synthetic version of the naturally occurring pyrethrum. This chemical became one of the four big insecticides of its day.[17]

In 1897, Japanese institutions devoted to erasing crop diseases—such as the Japanese Association for the Prevention of Plant Disease (Nihon Shokubutsu Bōeki Kyōkai) and the Japanese Association for Research into Regulatory Chemicals (Nihon Shokubutsu Chōsetsuzai Kenkyū Kyōkai)— also experimented with Bordeaux mixture at experimental grape vineyards in Japan. Bordeaux mixture, developed by Pierre-Marie-Alexis Millardet (1838–1902) in the 1860s, is a fungicide and bactericide made from copper sulfate and hydrated lime. Other simple-chemical-compound insecticides and bactericides experimented with were hydrocyanic gas fumigants, Horumarin soil disinfectants, and arsenic acid; naturally occurring insecticides included sulfuric acid, nicotine, and rotenone.

At experiment stations and elsewhere, Meiji Japanese tested a variety of new chemical insecticides, a project closely tied to modernization and industrialization. Simply put, workers and soldiers needed calories for Japan's new modern endeavor. In Meiji Japan there was also an intimate relationship between war and economic expansion, as will be tracked in subsequent chapters. Its interest in insecticides set the Meiji government apart from its early modern predecessor. Through such institutional appendages as the Hokkaido Development Agency and agricultural experiment stations situated throughout the country, not to mention a variety of agricultural research associations, the Meiji government directly supported elaborate national modernization projects and, in the realm of agriculture, established a precedent followed for decades for state-supported insecticide production and saturation—a further nationalization of the landscape. In the twentieth century, an institutional triad shaped the nature of insecticide production and application: the government, large chemical corporations, and cultivators. Unlike the Tokugawa shoguns, who displayed their support for insect eradication through prayers at sacred sites, the Meiji government offered resources to a wholly new belief system—Euro-American science—lending economic support and bringing to Japan the technologies and human resources required for the development of a domestic chemical industry.

The case of chrysanthemum-based chemicals is important. In just under two decades, Japan transformed from an importer of chrysanthemum powder from England to an exporter of dried chrysanthemum flowers to the United States. As we shall see, the same scenario holds true for the production of parathion in the 1950s. At first, the chemical giant Sumitomo Chemical imported the highly toxic insecticide from the United States and Germany, but after some prodding by a Japanese government concerned with skyrocketing trade deficits after the Allied Occupation (1945–52), the company began domestic production in earnest by mid-decade. Let us now turn to the case of parathion.

THE AGE OF CHEMICAL INSECTICIDES

Chlorinated hydrocarbons and organophosphates caught on in Japan after the Pacific War. Whale oil was an insecticidal technology obtained by boiling the blubber of whales; deploying tachinid flies to fight the Japanese beetle, by contrast, was an issue of overcoming island biogeographies. In the Meiji period, nicotine or chrysanthemums sufficed. But postwar insecticides proved altogether different from earlier eradication technologies in the way they interacted with insect bodies, the environment, and always-porous human bodies. Japanese farmers possess little fertile land and, therefore, need to make it as productive as possible, and so they spray their crops with liberal helpings of preharvest insecticides. For example, in the 1980s, American farmers dusted each acre with, on average, 0.65 pounds of insecticides, while their Japanese counterparts used a daunting 12.5 pounds per acre. In the 1980s, Japanese farmers used just over half the tonnage of insecticides sprayed by their American counterparts, even though they cultivate only one-seventy-fifth the land. Americans use more pesticides in the postharvest phase, when food is stored and shipped long distances across a vast country. Fears of postharvest chemicals are among the main obstacles that American-grown rice faces with Japanese consumers.[18]

The lethal organophosphorus ester insecticide parathion ranked among the most deadly poisons in the world and among the favorites of Japan's postwar farmers, pesticide companies, and people who sought to commit suicide or homicide.[19] It was a biocide of international renown. As Linda Nash has shown, it was a favorite among the fruit growers of California, for example. As early as 1949, California farmers applied parathion to their fields and orchards; that same year, in Marysville, California, twenty-five migrant workers became seriously ill after entering an orchard that had been sprayed with parathion. Nash has stressed nature's unanticipated agency when it comes to the toxicity and human health threat represented by such chemicals. She writes, "A study of parathion decay conducted in the 1970s revealed that pesticide residues in the same fields could vary as much as 90-fold, depending upon the time of year the chemical was applied." In other words, "Once introduced into the environment, OP [organophosphate] chemicals were subject to the uncontrolled agency of nature."[20] Of course, this is precisely the type of unanticipated, unforeseen ecosystem accidents described by Charles Perrow at the outset of this book.

In Japan, parathion injured people and environments in a similar fashion; but it also did so by means of unanticipated, social system (as opposed to ecosystem) accidents. That a government warning of the dangers of parathion's extreme toxicity served to alert those who wanted to commit suicide of its effectiveness is an excellent—if grim—example of the unanticipated manner in which policies and information crosscut different social networks to say different things to and have different consequences for different people. The numerous suicides resulting from consuming parathion and its relative paraquat are systematically related to government and corporate efforts to stem accidental exposure to the insecticide through the dissemination of information regarding its toxic qualities. This is the essence of chaos theory: a single action (no matter how benign) performed in a complex, interrelated system, particularly a social system, can have unintended consequences.

The German chemist Gerhard Schrader (1903–90) developed the first organophosphate chemicals at the Farbenfabriken Bayer facilities in 1937, and the Nazis continued their development as a chemical weapon. Though several generations removed, parathion is related to Sarin gas, which the Japanese cult Aum Shinrikyō, led by its spiritual leader Asahara Shōkō (b. 1955), used to murder twelve and injure thousands of Tokyo subway riders in March 1995. Chemists developed parathion in 1944, and it began replacing DDT (dichloro-diphenyl-trichloroethane) in the 1950s, mainly because of its suitability as an insecticide: it persisted well in the environment and did not break down in sunlight or water.[21] As Nash pointed out, it morphed, too, intensifying under certain circumstances. Obviously, these same resilient qualities made it a dangerous environmental polluter—it haunts environments for ages, not to mention alchemizing into even deadlier forms under nature's auspices.

Japanese imported parathion from Bayer and American Cyanamid in 1951. When Japanese farmers began spraying parathion on their rice crops, they noticed quick results as yields soared. Originally, farmers used parathion to kill rice-eating bugs, such as Asiatic rice borers (*Chilo suppressalis*), stinkbugs (Pentatomidae), and plant hoppers; but later they also targeted fruit and vegetable eaters, such as aphids and leaf folders. Quickly, the Ministry of Agriculture and Forestry (Nōrinshō) hailed the effectiveness of the chemical against the Asiatic rice borer and appropriated ¥40 million for experiments in mass extermination.

One doctor overoptimistically declared that, as a result of parathion, Japan's perennial postwar food shortage had been "solved." Two high-profile incidents alerted people to its dangers: a little girl from Shizuoka Prefecture and an agricultural reform advocate from Hyōgo Prefecture died from parathion poisoning.[22] In response, lawmakers passed laws to alert people to parathion's toxicity. Better yields came at a high cost: in a period of six years, between 1953 and 1958, physicians reported nearly ten thousand instances of parathion poisoning, and three thousand of those proved fatal.[23] Parathion, it turns out, also caused pain on a national scale. As with all organophosphate esters, parathion is a cholinesterase inhibitor (it blocks the activity of cholinesterase enzymes in the brain, inhibiting nerve impulses). In large doses, it can kill, and in smaller doses, it can injure reproduction; the symptoms include muscle twitching (fasciculation), breathing difficulties, profuse sweating, and urinary and bowel problems.[24] It should not be surprising, then, that early on, some Japanese researchers suspected parathion as being responsible for fetal deaths and other health problems. In the 1950s, the Japanese government distributed some fifty thousand grams of a substance used in the moderately successful "oxime" therapy to treat potential cases of parathion poisoning. With one treatment requiring between one and two grams per patient, the Japanese government, we can assume, anticipated tens of thousands of cases of accidental parathion poisoning.[25]

Even before the importation of parathion, however, the government had passed the Agricultural Chemical Control Law (Nōyaku torishimari no hōsei; 1948), but it had more to do with increasing production of chemicals and improving their quality than with prohibiting the circulation of highly toxic chemicals. As Gerald Markowitz and David Rosner document, in the United States, big chemical companies had the undivided attention of politicians.[26] The same was essentially true in Japan. But the Japanese government voiced its good intentions, and its statement is worth quoting, if for no other reason than to emphasize the degree to which none of the promises regarding safety would be kept. It reads: "This law establishes a registry system for agricultural chemicals, and beyond acting to control their sale and use, it normalizes the quality of agricultural chemicals and ensures proper use of them to promote safety. It also stabilizes the production of agricultural chemicals and contributes to the protection of the health of the citizenry, together with contributing to the preservation of the living environment of the citizenry."[27] Ultimately, the law would be revised on three occasions (1951, 1962, and 1963). It was not until October 1972 that it was given any real teeth. Five years after the original law was passed, the Ministry of Health and Welfare and Ministry of Agriculture and Forestry started enacting tougher "control laws" to educate people about the dangers of agricultural products, particularly parathion and methyl parathion. In August 1955 the government listed parathion as a "special toxin" (*tokutei dokubutsu*), one year after Sumitomo Chemical began its domestic manufacture.[28]

Sumitomo's corporate histories published as late as the 1980s gush that the development of parathion provided a "valuable service" to "our country." According to these histories, Sumitomo discovered the economic promise of parathion in July 1950 after the company president visited the headquarters of American Cyanamid. In September of the next year, American Cyanamid sought to establish international economic ties to Japan and tapped Sumitomo to peddle the chemical in East Asia more broadly. Initially, the strategy was that American Cyanamid would offer Sumitomo parathion to sell in Asia and, over time, nurture a robust market for the insecticide. Then, once market share had been created, Sumitomo would be taught how to manufacture the chemical itself. In June 1951, at about the same time that American Cyanamid tried to expand the parathion market to East Asia, Bayer began marketing Folidol (their proprietary name for parathion) in Japan as well. Subsequent tests in agricultural experiment stations proved that the chemical killed Asiatic rice borers in rice paddies, dryland crops, and fruit orchards: not surprisingly, the government approved Folidol for use in Japan. Its toxic effectiveness was a far cry from that of the whale-oil insecticides used during the Kyōhō famine, and so was the effectiveness of the institutional systems by which it was disseminated from chemical corporations to agricultural lands to human bodies. Tokugawa ministers maintained ties to temples and shrines; modern ministers maintained ties to corporate chemical giants and big agriculture.

Meanwhile, Sumitomo's relationship with American Cyanamid continued to expand. In March 1952, Sumitomo became American Cyanamid's "Japan delegate" for the marketing and manufacture of parathion. Later, in September of that same year, the two companies jointly decided that Sumitomo would construct parathion factories in Japan to manufacture parathion but that, until that time, Sumitomo would import and sell the American product. By November 1953, Sumitomo was importing and selling American Cyanamid's parathion. Importantly, there was a slight difference between the parathion produced by American Cyanamid and Bayer: the former manufactured ethyl parathion; the latter, methyl parathion. Ethyl parathion is more toxic, though both, if handled improperly (or even properly), can prove deadly. To Sumitomo, the Bayer product appeared more appropriate to Japan's small farms, and so the company sought a licensing agreement with Bayer. Postwar economic conditions in Japan prompted the government to try to limit the number of imports and begin more domestic production, and this policy extended to the chemical industry. With the government urging Sumitomo to begin the immediate domestic production of parathion, the Japanese company acquired licenses to manufacture American Cyanamid's product in May 1953 and Bayer's product a bit later, in October.

Production began at Sumitomo's Tsurusaki Plant. The site proved optimal for two reasons: the company already stored the raw material paranitrochloro benzene (PNCB) at the site, and facilities at the site that had once produced monochloro benzene (but had been idle since 1951) could be put back into use. By March 1954, Sumitomo was producing some thirty tons of ethyl parathion each month at the Tsurusaki Plant. To boost production, Sumitomo's Okayama Plant, which produced monochloro benzene, an ingredient in ethyl parathion, was fully automated for remote operation. By March 1955, Sumitomo had begun the production of Bayer's methyl parathion at the Tsurusaki site as well. That year, Sumitomo manufactured some fifty tons of ethyl and methyl parathion at the Tsurusaki Plant.

In April 1955, Sumitomo, realizing the government's ambitions for more domestic production, manufactured enough parathion to halt importation of the chemical from the United States, and eventually it supplied all Japanese domestic consumption of the pesticide. Manufacture of the insecticide expanded at a staggering pace: in 1955, the Tsurusaki Plant boasted a monthly production of 630 tons; by 1960 that number had increased to 1,000 tons. Starting in September 1957, Sumitomo marketed parathion throughout Japan under the Bayer name Folidol. Sumitomo established the Parathion Research Group (Parachion Kenkyūkai) in 1954 and, presumably in response to the highly toxic nature of the insecticide, the Parathion Poisoning Remedy Research Group (Parachion Chūdoku Chiryōhō Kenkyūkai) in 1955.[29] Parathion became a ubiquitous part of Japan's chemical industry and agrarian landscapes, from dryland crops and orchards to terraced paddies. But few advocates of the chemical anticipated the ecosystem accidents and social system accidents that began to occur.

In some aquaculture paddies, for example, parathion and methyl parathion killed fish. Compared to other Asian countries, Japanese raise few fish in their irrigated paddy lands. Japanese farmers who did raise fish in their paddies principally cultivated common carp (Cyprinus carpio); before modern, high-intensity rice monoculture in Japan, raising fish made sense because the fish provided cheap protein and their excreta fertilized the rice plants. Also, carp consumed many pesky insects such as hoppers, and the higher levels of water needed to raise fish cut down on rat infestations in the paddies. Carp also contributed to the historical evolution of silkworms by consuming undesirable caterpillars (and thereby weeding out certain traits undesirable to human providers) discarded into the ponds. On average, farmers practicing such aquaculture released between one thousand and two thousand fingerlings per 2.5 acres; the average fish yield in Japan is between 129 pounds per acre without artificial feeding and 204 pounds with it. But chlorinated hydrocarbon insecticides applied directly to the water killed or contaminated most of the fingerlings, which proved quite susceptible to the poison.[30] Sadly, though, it was not just carp that died by parathion poisoning. As Table 3 reveals, hundreds of people also suffered.

But in a ghoulish twist to our story, in Japan accidental poisoning by

TABLE 3 Parathion Production, Poisoning, and Death Rates, 1952–66

Years	Production amount (tons)	People poisoned	People killed	People killed by suicide or murder
1952	436	106	—	5
1953[a]	7,825	1,564	70	121
1954[b]	16,874	1,887	70	237
1955[c]	17,585	899	48	462
1956	20,208	706	86	900
1957	18,158	570	29	519
1958	19,256	816	35	522
1959	22,029	484	26	470
1960	23,838	537	27	468
1961	25,475	564	32	470
1962	19,562	320	25	434
1963	16,539	183	20	374
1964	13,064	142	14	315
1965	9,059	67	15	293
1966	7,711	72	12	253

Source: Uemura Shinsaku et al., Nōyaku dokusei no jiten (Dictionary of Toxic Agricultural Chemicals) (Tokyo: Sanseidō, 2002), 146–47.

[a] Beginning of the Organic Chemical Injury Prevention Campaign (Yūkirin seizai kigai bōshi undō); passage of the Toxic and Harmful Substance Control Law (Dokubutsu oyobi gekibutsu torishimaru hō).

[b] Sumitomo Chemical begins domestic production of parathion.

[c] Parathion designated as "special toxin" (tokutei dokubutsu).

parathion proved to be only part of the public health threat posed by the insecticide. In 1957, two years after the government designated parathion as a "special toxin," accidental death rates plummeted from eighty-six people in 1956 to twenty-nine people. In 1956, however, the use of parathion to commit suicide or murder nearly doubled. Obviously, the designation "special toxin" spoke to two different social networks: for some it was a warning, but for others it served as an advertisement. Table 4 lists the kinds of incidents that occurred in Japan as a result of the use of parathion.

The use of parathion and related agricultural chemicals for suicide is most striking. Japan remains a country that stresses social conformity, which has, according to some specialists, contributed to its dubious distinction of having one of the highest suicide rates on industrialized Earth. Social conformity places a lot of pressure on young people. In the 1950s, the ingestion of large doses of parathion was one method of choice for those hoping to end their lives. By the 1980s, however, the herbicide known as paraquat had become the poison of choice. Chemists developed paraquat in 1882, but its propensity to kill pests was not discovered until 1959. This bipyridyl herbicide ranks among the most deadly pulmonary poisons

TABLE 4 Types of Accidents Involving Parathion Insecticide from 1956

Type of accident	Poisoning	Death	Total
Group application	1,566	25	1,591
Individual application	128	23	151
Repairing application machine	3	0	3
Transport	4	0	4
Entering application area	37	0	37
Entering vicinity of application area	94	1	95
Drifted from application area	24	4	28
Mishandling	16	7	23
Poor storage	3	5	8
Other	11	5	16
Suicide	0	237	237
Total	1,886	307	2,193

Source: Matsunaka Shōichi, Nihon ni okeru nōyaku no rekishi (Japan's Agricultural Chemical History) (Tokyo: Gakkai Shuppan Sentā, 2002), 66.

known and so has attracted an enormous amount of scientific attention.[31] Basically, paraquat releases oxygen-free radicals that painfully destroy lung and kidney tissue. In Japan, the number of suicidal, homicidal, and accidental deaths from paraquat increased steadily in the mid-1980s: from 594 in 1984 to 1,021 in 1985. Of the 1,021 deaths reported in 1985, over 96 percent were suicides. A series of indiscriminate, and highly sensational- ized, soft drink poisonings that left seventeen dead in 1985 made young people contemplating suicide aware of its lethal properties; also, in the 1980s, paraquat was readily available in Japanese garden shops and was listed as a "special toxin" by the Japanese government. Today, the Japanese government has severely restricted use of the chemical to only those people with proper documentation and has laced the herbicide with vivid colors and rancid odors to make it less palatable to those who might drink it.[32]

RESTRICTING PARATHION

In both May 1965 and May 1966, the Ministry of Agriculture and Forestry directed that nonmercuric pesticides replace mercuric ones. In March 1966, Japan's Diet began taking steps against certain toxic insecticides, such as phenyl-mercury. By the summer of 1969, the government banned the sale of ethyl and methyl parathion; by December 1969, the government suspended the production of parathion and TEPP (tetraethyl diphos- phate). Sumitomo histories explain the suspension of parathion as caused by two factors: pesky insects such as the Asiatic rice borer had developed evolutionary resistances to the chemical, and it killed or poisoned too many people. But between 1954 and 1969, 6,648 tons of ethyl parathion and 3,960 tons of methyl parathion had been sprayed throughout Japan. The stuff saturated Japan's toxic archipelago. Sumitomo saw things differently, however: "Starting in 1955, our country's production of agricultural crops, particularly rice, increased: this was the contribution of these chemicals."[33]

In May 1971, the government prohibited the sale of DDT, while sales of BHC, endrin, dieldrin, and aldrin were restricted. One month later, the government prohibited the use of ethyl parathion, methyl parathion, and TEPP.[34] In 1972, the government passed a series of laws prohibiting or seriously restricting many highly toxic agricultural chemicals, as listed in Table 5.

TABLE 5 October 1972 Regulation of Agricultural Chemicals

Nature of regulation	Agricultural chemical name
Prohibited	Organic mercury (excluding use as seed and grain fumigants)
	DDT
	Parathion
	Methyl parathion
	TEPP
	BHC
Suspended	2,4,5 T
Designated as leaving residue on crops	V acid lead
	Endrin
Designated as leaving residue in the soil	Aldrin
	Dieldrin
Designated as water pollutant	Octachlorotetrahydro methanophthalan
	Endrin
	Benzoxepin
	PCP
	Rotenone

Source: Kankyō Hōrei Kenkyūkai, ed., *Kankyō kōgai nenkan* (Yearbook of Environmental Pollution) (Tokyo: Gakuyō Shobō, 1973), 141.

In the first chapter of this book, I described how Japanese beetles are parasitized and, eventually, eaten from the inside out by the ravenous young of tachinid flies. Let us suspend scale (but not necessarily belief) for a moment to put this in perspective: imagine a monstrous, heavily armored, flying creature of about one hundred pounds —about the size of a very large dog— catching you by surprise in the midst of sexual intercourse (after having stalked you for days) and then violently wrestling you to the ground. Before you can squirm free, the monstrous creature has positioned its abdomen near your head and, with a pumping and gyrating motion, laid its moist, sticky eggs on your throat and flown away with a loud buzz. You try but you cannot dislodge them. Sure, as a human you are clever: after this traumatic event, you can go about your business for a week in denial, maybe visit an ear, nose, and throat specialist, or even a grief counselor of some kind; but for all intents and purposes you are done. You will die a hideous death as the monster's young burrow inside you and eat your innards until only your flabby, lifeless skin remains. This sort of gruesome episode happens to smaller, less introspective and philosophical souls in your own backyard every day—to bugs of amazing varieties—though we miss it, because it is not of our scale: it happens (thankfully) on a different horizon.

In this chapter I raised the prospect of insects participating in alternative scales of time as well: that is, high-speed evolutionary time. The two species of plant hoppers mentioned in this chapter—*Sogatella furcifera* and *Nilaparvata lugens*—survive between ten and twenty days in the summer months and about twice that long in autumn. Under the proper conditions, they can lay several batches of eggs in one season. The Asiatic, or striped, rice borer (*Chilo suppressalis*), another insect pest we have met, can live between forty-five and fifty days, given the right environmental conditions. The point is that evolution occurs more rapidly in insect populations than it does in human ones, because their generational turnover is faster. Plus, there are millions more insects than us, which means that mutations—say, a serendipitous (for the insect) genetic resistance to a chemical insecticide or other anthropogenic force—are far more likely to occur in insects than in human or nonhuman animals. Insects are evolutionarily dynamic: this is why these small creatures are so subject to the ebbs and flows of our history. They are part of the landscape and, as such, are part of the biological canvas on which we paint our stories: they are flesh-and-blood historical sources.

Take *Chilo suppressalis* as an example. First, some basic entomological facts about this moth: one female Asiatic rice borer can lay several egg masses each season, with between 50 and 250 eggs per mass. In a controlled setting (i.e., without predators), scientists determined that between 60 and 90 percent of these eggs were fecund (though these numbers are surely higher than out in the paddies). From the moment the female lays these eggs to their metamorphosis into moths, about thirty-five days can elapse. Through this entire period—from egg to larva to pupa to moth—the borer eats, damages, and kills rice crops at an astonishing pace. The insect actually pupates within the rice stem, causing substantial damage in the process. In cooler climates, between one and two generations can live in one year; in warmer climates, six or more generations can live in one year. At the larval stage, the average dispersal distance is around one to two feet, meaning that the insects hatched from one egg mass stay within about a seven-foot radius of their natal plant.[35] Like the lives of any living organism, the life of *Chilo suppressalis* is hard to quantify into a neat formula. For the purposes of this investigation, however, the following numbers are important: a life span of fifty days and two generations in one year (which is average for most of the Japanese archipelago). The best methods for determining population densities are hotly disputed, but usually entomologists count larvae on stems and pupae in stems and capture adult moths in light traps (sometimes as many as 30,000 in a single night); borer population densities are determined by weather, previous population densities, and other factors. Parasites are important in culling borer populations: both *Trichogramma japonica* and *Phanurus beneficiens* eat borer eggs and larvae.[36]

When talking of hereditary resistances to chemical insecticides, the key components of which are mutation, selection, and evolution, the life span is less important than population density, the number of eggs laid in a single mass, and the number of generations in one year. We are using two generations per year, which means that some 149 hopper generations can live in the span of one Japanese life (the life expectancy for a Japanese person is 74.5 years). Thus, hoppers evolve nearly 150 times faster than their Japanese hominid counterpart. If we take into account population densities, this 150-times-faster number explodes upward exponentially: we are talking about hundreds of thousands of larvae, if not millions, in a single field. If a country such as Japan begins a nationwide program of spraying parathion for Asiatic rice borers, with so many bugs in so many fields producing so many generations per human life span, it will not take long for evolutionary resistances to occur in historical time. In any biological community, mutants are everywhere (but nowhere more so than in insect communities) and hence so too the potential for chemical-induced selection: evolution in the form of resistances to insecticides.

With such a short life span and so many generations, evolution can occur rapidly through both natural and unnatural selection in insect populations. Remember, one of the main reasons cited by Sumitomo Chemical for the suspension of production of parathion was insect resistances.[37] But take a small handful of other examples: flying scale insects, nematode worms, and some ticks have reportedly developed resistances to such powerful toxins as buquinolate, thiabendazole, and HCH/dieldrin in only a matter of a few generations. History can play various roles in evolution through selection. For example, federal officials, such as those in the Agricultural Research Service (a division of the U.S. Department of Agriculture), devised strategies to use insecticides based on certain economic and political considerations related to their ties to the chemical industry, and consequently, bugs developed hereditary resistances and evolved.[38] In Africa some mosquitoes have evolved in a manner that allows them to avoid DDT sprayed in village huts; other mosquitoes, such as the tenacious *Culex pipiens,* can withstand normally lethal doses of organophosphate insecticides because they actually digest the poison.[39]

The point is that everyday history drives evolution on Earth. There really are what we can safely call "Japanese insects," because their evolution has been, at least in part, driven by Japanese politics, society, and culture. That is, human ideas permeate the physical reality of the natural world. Japanese have inscribed their history on the bodies—on the very genetic predispositions—of these buzzing beings. Like firsthand observers of historical events, insects, too, are primary sources, though with natural agency of their own. Historians have considered how books and other documents take on independent lives in the public domain. Try interpreting a bug.

3 COPPER MINING AND ECOLOGICAL COLLAPSE

This chapter focuses on the Ashio copper mine, the site of Japan's first major pollution disaster. I begin by situating the mine within the broader assertions made in this book: that this technological complex, and the engineered environments it birthed, seamlessly connected to the naturally occurring Watarase River basin. The river fed downstream paddies that, in their own way, were engineered environments as well. As technology advanced, smelting and ore flotation devices that allowed miners and processors to extract ever-higher percentages of their desired metals and discard higher percentages of the undesirable ones caused pollution problems in nearby agricultural lands. But these pollution problems, particularly their consequences for human health, represent the product of hybrid causations, where naturally occurring photochemical processes in the atmosphere and oxidization processes in riparian ecosystems created the toxins that caused human pain. Poisonous silt from the mine rendered once-rich agricultural lands a moonscape, the result of devastating flooding. The disaster at Ashio is the first indication that Japan's unbridled push to be a rich country with a strong military in the Meiji years would not be without costs: in this case, intense human pain caused by environmental pollution, both water-borne toxins and relentless acidic deposition (forms of acid rain).

The Ashio copper mine sits near Nikkō, once the hub of an elaborate network of Tōshōgū shrines that deified the shogun Tokugawa Ieyasu (1542–1616) and thereby legitimized his family's authority to rule over the entire realm.[1] It also sits near the headwaters of the Watarase River, the beginning of an elaborate watershed that fed the Tone and Edo rivers and that provided fertile topsoil and irrigation water for the Kantō, still considered Japan's richest agricultural lands (though it is heavily urbanized). Today, Japanese know Nikkō more as a national park overrun by deer than as an elaborate political ruse designed to project feudal authority vertically and cast it as divine, but the site is also important for its nearby copper mine.[2] Copper extracted from Ashio has always been tied to state power, whether to that of the Tokugawa shoguns or the Meiji emperor. Copper extracted from Ashio adorned Edo Castle and the Nikkō mausoleum and, later, was used for currency (imprinted with "Ashi" for Ashio) and utilized for export purposes. In the nineteenth century, copper served as the conductor for transmission of electricity from one location to another; but it also brought badly needed foreign wealth to Japan. It and its alloys are also in the guts of most technological gadgetries, both military and civilian. Throughout the Meiji years (1868–1912) most copper mined was actually exported: silver and copper financed both Japan's early-seventeenth-century unification under the Tokugawa family and its nineteenth-century unification under the Meiji oligarchy. In the historical timelines such as the ones strung in this book, copper can be a connector and conductor.

If copper extracted from Ashio legitimized Tokugawa political authority vertically by projecting it toward the heavens and linking it to notions of divine rule, extracting copper required creating engineered subterranean environments that facilitated ore extraction and accommodated labor. These underground environments need to be seen as examples of hybrid realms. Within these realms and the surrounding terrestrial ones, raw ore, subsurface aquifers, machines, humans, donkeys, mulberries, silkworms, and other natural and unnatural actors constituted one holistic system. Mines—no matter how deep, carefully engineered, or painstakingly controlled—remain tied to their surface environments through an industrial metabolism fed by subsurface and surface technologies, usually ones with sublime vertical symmetry. That is, they are designed to bore deep into Earth's surface, transport ores upward to terrestrial processing facilities, and then discharge, through smokestacks, toxins into the atmosphere.[3] All this vertical symmetry, engineers thought, could limit horizontal surface pollution. But surface environments, somewhat predictably, proved more difficult to manage than their subsurface, vertical counterparts, even though mining engineers often applied the same simplified logic to their management. Engineers controlled the shafts well enough (unless, of course, miners rioted or rocks tumbled and crushed people), but once toxins left the Ashio site and, moving horizontally, washed downstream, events got out of control.

The Ashio complex interconnected humans and machines, much as the engineered, agrarian systems discussed in the previous chapter linked dangerous pesticides to bugs, their evolution, and, eventually, human consumers. Although technological innovations proved economically valuable, what made Japanese mines productive until the 1880s was not mechanical technologies but arduous labor. Mining is about energy extraction: miners expend it in the name of moving metals or minerals, in order to produce or transfer it. Over the course of global history, labor, as both work and giving birth, has been one means by which people encounter the natural world. Every time a miner's chisel or drill strikes an ore face, he encounters nature on gritty terms.

The labor at copper mines required caloric and, after industrialization, fossilized energy. Smooth-running turbines generated energy carried in wires crafted from the copper that labor extracted from the ground. In this sense, all machines, even those most removed from the labor and Earth that created them, are "organic machines," as their bodies (like the bodies of organisms) are fueled by recently living or long-dead life. If you want to find nature, explains Richard White, search no further than the steam engine's inner bowels or the transmission lines above your head or the computer's keyboard beneath your fingertips.[4] The organic always supports the mechanical and so, quite simply, Japan's age of "enlightened politics"— the Meiji age—required a more sustained encounter with nature through a better organization of labor and deployment of technologies (not a distancing from nature as Fukuzawa Yukichi and Maruyama Masao urged in the introduction). Partially naked miners who chiseled chunks of metal thousands of feet beneath the surface or who coughed black dust from their scarred, aching lungs knew nature well enough. Civilization does not separate people from nature; rather, it masks our interconnectedness behind layers of simplified geometric shapes, scientific engineering, and rational modes of production. In turn, people feel buffered from the natural world by these layers, only to be reminded of their connection to nature when industrial pollution easily navigates hybrid contexts, including food webs, to bodies to cause physical pain. We have already seen how this works with insecticides in carefully engineered rice paddies. Next we will examine how it worked in engineered landscapes in and around Japan's major mining sites.

COPPER AND UNIFICATION

We begin with a history of copper mining in Japan. Even earlier than the construction of the Tōshōgū shrines at Nikkō, the Ashio copper mine had been under direct Tokugawa jurisdiction. Two peasants discovered copper outcroppings at the site around 1610 and reported their discovery to the Nikkō Zazen'in, a Buddhist temple. The next year, the senior councilor of Shogun Tokugawa Hidetada (1579–1632), Sakai Tadayo (1572–1636), offered experimentally refined copper to officials in Edo, the shogun's capital. Satisfied with the quality of the refined copper, officials in Edo thereafter listed Ashio as an official copper mine of the Tokugawa family. To oversee the newly attained Tokugawa territories, Fujikawa Shōjirō became the magistrate of the Ashio mine, a position that went through several incarnations over the decades; but, all the while, the wealth generated at the site ensured that Ashio remained under tight Tokugawa control.[5] In this way, copper extracted from Ashio proved central to Japan's unification under Tokugawa rule. The two words that best describe the material buttress of Tokugawa power are "paddies" and "mines."

The Tokugawa shoguns quickly integrated Ashio in their overseas trading ambitions. They did so because influential Japanese warlords had long harnessed their military fortunes to the wealth generated at mines. In the middle of the sixteenth century, warlords, fueled by internal political and military rivalries, sought to expand trade with Southeast and East Asia. China supplied wealthy Japanese with valuable silk fabrics, but stepped-up production at Japanese silver and copper mines made buying expensive fabric possible. Competition between warlords sparked interest in new mines across the archipelago, because precious metals financed the military buildups and endemic wars during the Era of the Warring States (1467–1568). Powerful warlords developed mines in the middle of the sixteenth century: the Imagawa family, which entertained aspirations of unifying the country until a military fiasco in 1566, opened the Umegajima mine; the Uesugi family opened the Tsurushi mine on Sado Island; and the Ueda silver mine opened about this time as well. Takeda Shingen (1521–73), another powerful warlord, received gold from the Minamisaku and Suwa mines; and the Ōuchi family, with the help of copper merchants and mining engineers, developed the Ōmori mine, which eventually became one of the most productive sites in sixteenth-century Japan. Basically, the silver and copper trade with China financed Japan's civil wars during the Era of the Warring States, because the Chinese, though rich in silk fabrics, hungered for more silver, which Japanese warlords gladly supplied.

Just as Japanese silver and copper financed that country's Warring States civil wars, however, it also financed Japan's unification under the Tokugawa shoguns in 1600. The Tokugawa managed to mint a fairly unified currency system by the end of the seventeenth century that contributed to the country's political unification.[6] Of the three great unifiers of the sixteenth century, however, Tokugawa Ieyasu was not the only one to purchase political and military advantage with precious metals. During the legendary Kyushu campaign of 1587, Toyotomi Hideyoshi (1536–98), Ieyasu's flamboyant predecessor, departed for the southern island with 250,000 samurai to subdue powerful lords such as members of the proud Shimazu family of Satsuma Domain.[7] In order to finance the expedition, "twelve horses loaded with gold and silver" accompanied Hideyoshi and his colossal army. For warlords such as the Satake family of northeastern Japan, on the other hand, gold served as tribute and paid for required Kyoto lodging under Hideyoshi's early "hostage system," as well as for gifts for his closest confidants.[8] In other words, Japan's warlords harnessed the burden of Japan's domestic currency system, which financed political favor and the country's unification in the late sixteenth century, to gold, silver, and copper mines (and the laborers and environments that surrounded and sustained them).

Even though, as we learned in chapter 1, Japanese silkworms and humans busily worked together to supply the most important trade item—silk fabric, at least after 1685 and the Tokugawa restriction of imports of raw silk from Qing China, which boosted Japan's domestic production of raw silk, particularly in places such as Shinano Province[9]—it was actually fluctuating gold and silver values in East Asia that facilitated an increase in the volume of trade. After about 1400, China, after decades of failed monetary policy under the Yuan dynasty (1279–1368), used silver as a new monetary medium. As Kenneth Pomeranz writes, during this period of monetary reform, "Silver was becoming the store of value, the money of account (and often the actual medium) for large transactions, and the medium of state payments for this [China's] huge and highly commercialized economy." However, China had precious few silver mines, which made silver more valuable in China than gold or other trade items.[10] Thus, over the centuries, a robust silver trade occurred between Japan and China, despite the fact that the Ming emperor prohibited Chinese ships from trading at Japanese ports, even after a loosening of "maritime prohibitions" in 1560. But ample evidence from the 1540s and 1550s suggests that a thriving illicit trade proved vibrant enough to keep a steady stream of silver leaving Japanese mines. And Chinese pirates such as the infamous Wang Zhi allegedly made a fortune running silver between Japan and Malaysia until Ming officials executed the buccaneer in 1557. The shogun permitted the Sō family, on Tsushima Island, to trade silver with Korea, because of their assistance with Japanese pirate suppression; these stateless maritime bandits, known as *wakō* in Japanese, remained a perennial problem in the Japan Sea until the late sixteenth century. But Koreans already knew Japan possessed bountiful silver mines. Earlier, in 1542, the priest Anshin Tōdō, an envoy from the Ashikaga shoguns, reportedly boasted to his counterparts on the peninsula: "In the Hokuriku area of our country there is a mine, the name of which is Kaneyama [literally, "cash mountain"], producing much pure silver in recent years, one of the marvels of the world."[11]

The arrival of the Portuguese in 1543 on a Chinese ship changed the dynamic of Japan's heretofore-illegal silver trade with China. Once Portuguese carracks began arriving at Kyushu ports, these Great Ships unburdened their holds of the silks, saltpeter, porcelain, and mercury that had been loaded on the docks of Fujian and Guangdong and then returned to China with silver and other exports from Japan. Some Warring States lords on Kyushu, such as Ōmura Sumitada (1533–87), famously converted to Christianity in 1563 in order to accommodate the Portuguese and their financially and militarily advantageous China trade.[12] As early as 1570, moreover, Portuguese carracks began surveying the deepwater port at Nagasaki; by the following year the city became the principal port for the Portuguese trade between southern Japan and Macao (Aomen), which the Iberians had founded in 1557. The Great Ships served as the veins of the Portuguese trade with Macao; silver extracted from Japanese mines and transported to Nagasaki became the blood that pumped through them.[13]

In the 1580s, Japanese ships began calling on Southeast Asian ports as well, opening new silver markets in the Philippines, Vietnam, Cambodia, Siam (present-day Thailand), and elsewhere. Between 1586 and 1602, no fewer than thirty-nine ships traveled to Manila; between 1604 and 1635, some 356 Japanese vessels called on Chinese and Southeast Asian ports, their hulls loaded with silver from Japan's mines. With such a robust trade, it should not be surprising that Japanese settlements in Southeast Asian cities sprouted up. By the 1620s there were at least 3,000 Japanese living in Manila alone; cities such as Danang and Faifo in central Vietnam, Pinhalu and Phnom Penh in Cambodia, and Ayudhya, the capital of Siam, hosted other noteworthy Japanese settlements, which the silver trade, and hence Japanese mines and their environments, supported. Political conditions in some Southeast Asian countries made them particularly accommodating to Japanese settlements. In the late sixteenth century, for example, central Vietnam's Le dynasty had been restored, but the Trinh and Nguyen families actually divided rule of the country between the northern and southern sections, respectively. In order to finance their campaign against the Trinh in the north and Cham peoples in the rugged south, the Nguyen family looked to foreign trade, particularly with the Japanese, for weapons and badly needed finances. In 1601, the patriarch of the Nguyen even wrote Shogun Ieyasu directly, requesting that more Japanese ships call on his country's ports. The shogun obliged: more ships did make the journey, and they carried silver and copper, which blacksmiths used to make weapons or which purchased weapons from arms dealers elsewhere.[14]

Only after 1668, when Tokugawa shoguns prohibited the export of silver, did copper slowly emerge as Japan's leading base-metal export, finally doing so after about 1685 (see table 6).[15] When Japan pulled back exports of copper to China, it provided one motivation for the Qing emperor to colonize the Guizhou territory in order to provide safe roads to transport copper from mines in Yunnan Province in the 1720s.[16]

TOKUGAWA TECHNOLOGIES

With mining, the story is about labor and technologies: advancement in such areas as smelting made producing and exporting more metal possible and even more profitable. To supply silver to markets abroad and warlord

TABLE 6 Copper Export Sales to Chinese and Dutch, 1684–97

Year	Total copper exported (tons)	Chinese sales (tons)	Dutch sales (tons)
1684	3,389.43	1,765.566	1,623.864
1685	3,718.506	2,170.212	1,548.294
1686	4,339.236	2,940.762	1,398.474
1687	3,517.932	2,527.932	990
1688	3,049.596	2,224.596	825
1689	3,506.295	2,212.695	1,293.6
1690	3,443.136	2,445.282	957
1691	2,548.814	1,940.030	594
1692	2,686.365	1,440.245	1,188
1693	2,978.129	2,624.576	792
1694	3,319.206	2,170.014	1,102.2
1695	4,055.872	2,669.032	1,325.702
1696	5,839.352	4,572.299	1,209.755
1697	5,942.126	4,227.975	1,650
Total	55,333.995	35,931.216	16,497.887

Source: Kobata Atsushi, *Nihon dōkōgyōshi no kenkyū* (Research on Japan's Copper-Mining Industry) (Kyoto: Shibunkaku Shuppan, 1993), 155.

Note: Tons = U.S. (or short) tons.

coffers at home, silver and copper mines utilized new technologies, some developed at home but most imported from China. The first major breakthrough in Tokugawa mining practices came with the advent of *sunpō kiri,* or "survey mining." Survey mining required newly trained engineers to carefully survey veins or visible deposits while keeping in mind difficulties regarding extraction and drainage; they then determined the exact nature and dimensions of the shafts and tunnels needed to extract the minerals using mathematical equations.[17] Gradually, surveying done by newly trained engineers, individuals who specialized in discovering exposed and subterranean ore, replaced the earlier practice of excavating mostly exposed deposits (see fig. 3.1). Survey mining made much better use of available labor and produced infinitely more ore, because almost all ore lay buried beneath the surface. Even in Japan's preindustrial age, technological advancement in mining was principally about subsurface verticality: devising methods to reach ore tucked into subterranean veins.

When survey mining permitted miners to dig deeper into the subterranean environment, ventilation became an important consideration. Subsidiary shafts and tunnels for ventilation became necessary, as did side shafts so that miners could escape the smoke that inevitably accumulated in the mine from pine torches and other sources. By the seventeenth century, bellows in the form of "wind boxes" and "wind funnels" served to move fresh air into the mines as well. The development of "water shafts" and "water-collecting pools" aided drainage in the deeper mines, as did buckets hoisted by pulleys. Scroll paintings of the bowels of the Sado silver mine depict miners hand-cranking such hydrologic devices as Archimedean screws (*tatsudoi* in Japanese) that transported water upward into buckets that were then hoisted to the surface. This technology so resembles that deployed in ancient Mediterranean and European mines that some speculate that the technology was either introduced to China in ancient times, from whence it made its way to Japan, or was transmitted by Iberian merchants and missionaries who visited Japan in the sixteenth century.[18]

But the most important innovation in Tokugawa mining was in the arena of processing: the development of *haibuki,* or "cupellation smelting." In this process, dressed (i.e., processed) ore that contained traces of silver was melted together with lead, which bonded to silver. Once they had cleaned and cooled the molten alloy, miners reheated it and placed ash in the molten brew to absorb and remove the lead. (Lead's time had not yet come: it would be one of the metals of nineteenth-century empire building.) Once they had removed the lead-soaked ash, only silver remained; such smelting technologies meant that, by the mid-sixteenth century, the Iwami and Ikuno silver mines produced about one-third of the silver produced globally: just over forty metric tons. Once engineers added large "balanced bellows" to the smelting process, which, much like a giant seesaw in a playground, required one man on each end of a board balanced on a fulcrum, mine production and labor efficiency increased yet again. However, the fires that such bellows made possible required enormous amounts of timber for charcoal, and early on, localized environmental degradation occurred as a result of such technologies.[19] In typical Tokugawa fashion, at the Besshi smelters, which employed cupellation technologies, miners periodically dug up the floors to collect any copper or silver that might have dropped through the cracks, which served, in retrospect, as an environmental cleanup of sorts.[20]

Masuda Tsuna (d. 1821) was an employee of the Sumitomo family, which owned and operated the Besshi copper mine in Iyo Province (present-day Ehime Prefecture on Shikoku Island). Masuda's *Kodō zuroku* (Illustrated Record of Copper Smelting) serves as a guide to the technologies and human labor at the mine. The technical illustrations, by wood-block-print artist Niwa Motokuni Tōkei (1758–1820), of the individual processes involved make this a very valuable source. The technologies at the mine included lamps crafted from whelk shells and ventilation tubes for air circulation called *shakuhachi* (named after a five-holed bamboo flute). In the early stages, before the mine shaft entered solid rock, miners reinforced the shaft with wooden planks to avoid deadly cave-ins. Miners chipped at the ore face with hammers and chisels; they carried the ore out on their backs in straw baskets with shoulder straps. The *Kodō zuroku* suggests that, as a rule, good ore contained "one part of copper in ten" (or 10 percent), while poor-grade ore contained about half that amount. Once the ore had been hauled to the surface, women and elderly miners sorted the ore and discarded rock with low copper content. To remove sulfur and other impurities, miners roasted the ore in large kilns: they alternated layers of wood and ore and then capped off the kiln with a layer of damp straw. The kiln smoldered for about thirty days, the *Kodō zuroku* explains, before the roasting process was complete. Roasting ore releases a great deal of sulfur dioxide, and no doubt the process caused some regional environmental and human health problems.

A series of smelting processes separated the "black copper" crust from waste rock and other minerals. Later, miners smelted the black copper again and ran off the slag to obtain copper ready for refining. The *mabukidō*, or "refined copper,"·was obtained by smelting copper that contained no traces of silver. Miners then melted the refined copper in a crucible and cast it. The *Kodō zuroku* points out that copper cast in the shape of bars was principally used for trade with foreign countries. Copper for Japan's domestic market was cast in different molds. Before the Meiji Restoration, the refinement and monopolized sale of *wadō*, or "Japanese copper," was controlled by the shogunal Dōza, a kind of Bureau of Copper, located in Osaka and, later, in Edo and with a branch office in Nagasaki. After the Meiji Restoration, the Dōkaijo and Dōzankyoku assumed similar duties.

In a process that differed from the *haibuki* method, miners mixed lead with the copper that contained traces of silver to form *aibukidō*, or "alloyed copper." Miners placed alloyed copper in a furnace and heated it until the lead liquefied but the copper had not (which can be done because of the different melting temperatures: copper melts at 91°C while lead melts at 327°C). The copper that miners rendered was called *shiboridō*, or "wrung-out copper," and the silver was drawn out with the lead extract. This process, which the *Kodō zuroku* explains Sumitomo learned from an Iberian merchant, was called "Southern Barbarian smelting," a reference to the first Europeans arriving in southern Japan. Miners then separated the silver from the lead in a furnace lined with ash using a cupellation method.[21]

As we shall see in the final chapter, women proved a ubiquitous presence inside Japan's coal mines, but the technological configuration of the copper mines meant that women principally remained on the surface to dress ores, as the Sado scrolls and the *Kodō zuroku* illustrate. These early modern conditions persisted until both men and women were displaced by modern technologies, which caused changes in labor dynamics. At the Ashio mine, for example, technology and changing economic conditions had actually ousted women from the mine site altogether, relegating them to domestic chores in the lodges; but by the early twentieth century, technologies transformed labor conditions at the subterranean ore face, sparking a violent labor riot in 1907, in the final years of the Meiji emperor's life. The 1907 labor riot is worth investigating briefly, because its outbreak was, as we shall see, related to the modern industrial and technological changes occurring at the mine in the early twentieth century.

In the Meiji years, there was nothing new about violent labor strikes and riots at Japan's hard-rock and coal mines. In the late nineteenth century, the over 150,000 Japanese miners who worked in the industry often went on strike or even rioted: ten major strikes shook the horrific Takashima coal mine alone before 1887. "Mining brotherhoods," early labor unions of sorts, proved easily disrupted by the application of new mining technologies and painful cost-cutting and rationalization measures, such as feeding laborers poor-quality, imported rice. Having to eat this rice stung because it was associated with the dark-skinned, non-Japanese people who farmed it. Japanese rice was white and had long symbolized a distinct Japanese ethnic identity; some scholars had even likened eating rice to a religious experience. Nativist scholar Hirata Atsutane (1776–1843) valorized paddy cultivation as Japan's "ancient way" and believed that, as Harry Harootunian describes, "Japanese rice was superior to the rice of all countries, and those who consumed it took in a divine food that guaranteed their uniqueness and superiority over all others."[22] In other words, feeding workers imported rice proved a particularly egregious abuse of managerial power:

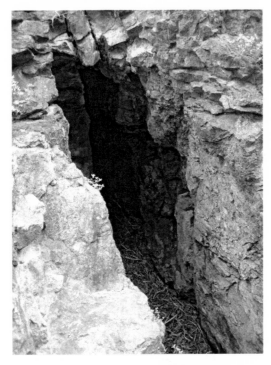

FIG. 3.1 Remnants of *tanuki-bori*, or "raccoon-dog holes." Often dug by husband and wife, these shallow, hand-hewn mines were common until the mechanization of the Ashio copper mine in the late nineteenth and early twentieth centuries. Photograph by author.

it violated long-standing cultural assumptions about food, spirituality, and ethnic identity.

Because of these conditions, Ashio miners rioted in a manner reminiscent of the "smash-and-break" outbursts of the Tokugawa age, when farmers ransacked the storehouses of wealthier peasants, an economic class created in Japan's protoindustrial age.[23] Unlike the Tokugawa disturbances, however, the Ashio riot erupted far underground. On 4 February 1907, miners commandeered the foreman's underground cabin and then proceeded to cut copper telephone cables, break electric lights, scatter and destroy papers and documents, and toss dynamite into the cabin and demolish it. Once on the surface, rioters clobbered Honzan shaft director Minami Teizō over the head, and from the floor of his lodge he saw them "smashing everything." He continued, "I heard a calmer voice among the rioters, who must have been one of the ringleaders, saying, 'Eat and drink your fill, but there must be no looting, because that would shame us. But let's make sure we smash everything thoroughly.'" Only after Prime Minister Hara Kei (also called Takashi; 1856–1921) dispatched three companies of soldiers did the violence subside.

Even though buildings lay in ruins, only one person, Takeuchi Takejirō, died during the riot, when he burned alive, apparently while drunk. There were many reasons for the outbreak of violence—poor working conditions, inadequate nourishment, imported rice, abusive "lodge bosses," long workdays, reduction in pay, and a litany of other complaints—but one was that the miners, much like the Chisso factory workers in Minamata discussed in chapter 5, worried that pollution control measures, such as those adopted in the 1897 Third Mine Pollution Prevention Order, threatened to close down the mine and deprive them of the means of making a living.[24] Indeed, the hard labor of Ashio engineers and miners produced toxic emissions and erosion that destroyed the product of the hard labor of farmers downstream who produced rice and, therefore, sacred calories that fueled the nation (except for the miners upstream, apparently). Rice and silkworm cultivators need to be seen as engineers, too, because they transformed either riparian systems or caterpillars into technologies of production, just as industrial engineers did with mining environments.[25] When these two engineered environments—agricultural and industrial—interfaced is when problems arose for human health in the region.

MODERNIZING THE ASHIO COPPER MINE

During a visit to the Ashio area in 2005, it immediately became clear to me that my approach to examining the mine and interpreting its history had been dangerously flawed, as have most other interpretations of the mine's past. Indeed, the Ashio mine is not an industrial abomination staining the natural landscape but rather a technological appendage, one seamlessly attached like a prosthetic to the natural environment surrounding Bizendate Mountain (1,272 meters, or 4,172 feet), the hub of the mine complex. Without exception, all Ashio shafts tunnel into the innermost depths of this single mountain. The mine and its processors are embedded in Bizendate: complicated networks of vertical shafts and horizontal tunnels anchor towering smokestacks to rich deposits of metallic ores like roots from an ancient tree. Even as it rusts, decays, and crumbles with age, the mine and its processors still represent sublime technological verticality.

If mine shafts and smokestacks anchored this technological prosthetic a century ago, today nature has thrust upward from Earth to secure Ashio's decaying infrastructure through rejuvenation and reclamation: long, slender evergreens provide a canopy to once-denuded hillsides (at least in the Kodaki area, where there was no significant smelting activity), and lower-growing vegetation pokes and protrudes through cracks in terraced stone lodging foundations (the lumber was carted away years ago) and crumbling community bathtubs (fig. 3.2). Wild grasses and shrub bamboo grow through broken beer and medicine bottles, as well as porcelain bowls, cups, and ornate toilets. The folks at Ashio worked in the mines, at the processors, or at schools and other facilities that supported the resident community. They lived in long, duplex wooden lodges—hundreds of them lined up on carefully terraced mountainsides (fig. 3.3). The women indulged themselves with cosmetics from small, hand-blown glass bottles with tin twist-on caps. The men, it seems, when not bathing at the community baths, ate, drank, took medicine, and urinated in porcelain toilets decorated with images of blue phoenixes. At least, this is what the archaeological evidence left behind suggests. The newly rejuvenated forest canopy hosted new primates: the only Japanese macaques (*Macaca fuscata*) I have ever witnessed in the wild climbed and foraged in these forests, above the cracked, moss-covered remains of this past industrial community. It occurred to me that they had triumphantly reclaimed this land: my hunch was confirmed by several people I talked to in the area who caustically challenged me to try and grow vegetables. I spent hours following and observing these monkeys: there are precious few macaques in Montana, where I live, so they enchanted me. They and the tree canopy they call home are also a part of Ashio's enduring hybrid history.

Like most places worth visiting in Japan, a "one-man car" diesel train takes you to Ashio. It departs the small town of Aioi and follows the meandering Watarase River through steep canyons to the Ashio complex. En route, some smaller paddies and vegetable plots terraced the canyon hillsides, as did occasional gravel pits. At the Ashio site, the complex comprises three main mines (Kodaki, Tsūdō, and Honzan), but there were other entrances into the side of Bizendate as well: Takanosu shaft, Honguchi shaft, Ariki (Honzan) shaft (1885), Tsūdō shaft (1885), and Kodaki shaft (1885) (fig. 3.4). The largest of the milling and smelting facilities was situated near the Ariki (Honzan) shaft; Kodaki once had processing facilities, not to mention schools and stores, but they are now only archaeological remnants. The inn where I stayed was located up the Koshingawa River, west of Tsūdō proper and near the Kodaki shaft site. Near the Kodaki shaft, the forests have recovered splendidly, accented by blooming mountain

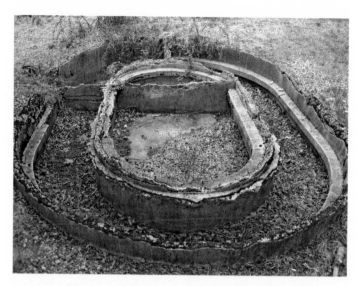

FIG. 3.2 An old cement bathtub is one of the few signs of past mining activities at the entrance of the Kodaki mineshaft at Ashio. Photograph by author.

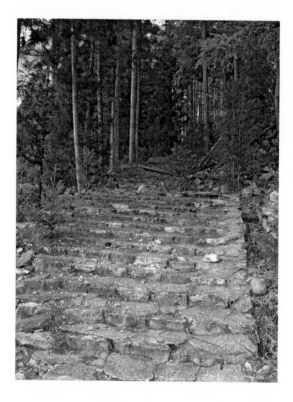

FIG. 3.3 It has taken about a century for trees, moss, and other undergrowth to reclaim this stairway, the drainage ditches, and the terraced foundations of the homes that provided lodging for tens of thousands of miners and their families working at the Kodaki mineshaft at Ashio. Photograph by author.

cherry blossoms and macaques. With its steep canyon walls and jagged rock formations poking through low-hanging clouds, the area resembles the exaggerated, toothy landscapes painted by such Chinese masters as Qu Ding (ca. 1023–56) and Wang Meng (ca. 1308–85). One day, I walked the circumference of Bizendate: it is not as far as it might seem, though it is destabilizing to fathom the history of a place whose circumference you can hike in a single day. By contrast, it would take years, if not decades, to navigate the environmental footprint of the mine. Walking the site made it easier for me to understand why the local environmental impact was so destructive. The region around the Ariki (Honzan) shaft resembles the upland desert landscapes of southern Idaho: the vegetation has yet to return and the mountains are still essentially barren (fig. 3.5). This stands to reason: this is where the main processing and smelting facilities were located since 1893. This is where the poisons accumulated.

Navigating the Ashio complex brings into focus the holistic, integrated nature of this site—its hybrid nature. The Ashio complex was an industrial system with four parts: labor that extracted ore from deep inside Bizendate; technologies that separated, processed, and smelted the ore; riparian ecosystems (the Degawa and Koshingawa rivers, which feed the Watarase River) that washed away the waste; and the engineered paddies downstream in the Shimotsuke Plain that received the waste.

This hybrid configuration was the result of a simplified modern mindset that swept Japan after 1868.[26] After the Meiji Restoration, Japanese modernizers had looked at Japan's many copper mines anew, from the vantage point of an age of "enlightened politics," both literally and figuratively. In the minds of such public intellectuals as Fukuzawa Yukichi, the individualism of "Occidental" philosophy had begun breaking the shackles of the stifling "Oriental" filial piety.[27] Engineers, like plastic surgeons stretching new sinews inside an old, worn-out body, had begun running elaborate networks of telegraph wires and, later, copper electrical wires to factories, cities, and even homes. Eventually, even telephone wires connected Japan's hinterland to Tokyo's metropolitan politicians.[28] In the twentieth century, these wires harnessed factories and households in Japan to the brave new era of twenty-four-hour lighting, industrial production, and bright, sparkling modernity. And if transmission lines harnessed factories and households to power plants, the electricity they transported harnessed workers, such as the "factory girls," who, with blistered fingers, carefully spun the

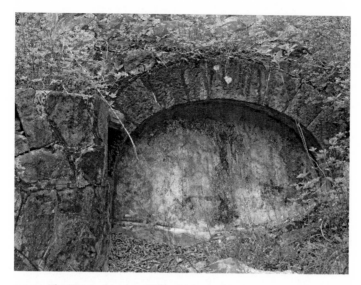

FIG. 3.4 The Honguchi mine shaft, which tunnels into Bizendate at Ashio. Today, the mineshaft is well hidden by thick brush, and the opening is cemented shut. Photograph by author.

FIG. 3.5 The hillsides around the main Ariki (Honzan) mine shaft and smelting facilities at Ashio are still denuded and scarred by erosion. Photograph by author.

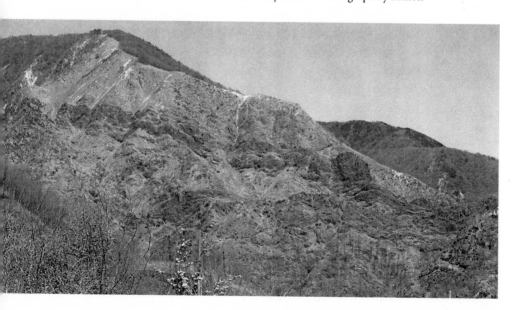

silk excreted by the caterpillars of chapter 1, to a new temporality of production: the twenty-four-hour workday.[29]

Itō Hirobumi (1841–1909), one of the architects of this sparkling modernity, reflected on the relationship between Japan's "enlightened politics" and technologies when he wrote that the purpose of the newly formed Ministry of Industry (Kōbushō; 1870–85) was to "make good Japan's deficiencies by swiftly seizing upon the strengths of the western industrial arts; to construct within Japan all kinds of mechanical equipment on the western model, including shipbuilding, railways, telegraph, mines and buildings; and thus with one great leap to introduce to Japan the concepts of enlightenment."[30] Under Itō's tutelage, the Ministry of Industry executed its vision of the importation of the mechanical arts to Japan; engineers completed the earliest stages of Japan's railroad (by linking Tokyo to Yokohama and Osaka to Kobe) and a nationwide network of telegraph wires by the 1880s. Eventually, the 32,000 factories built across Japan, employing no fewer than 800,000 laborers, 5,400 steam engines, and 2,700 electrically powered devices, thrust Japan into a new age of technology and mechanical production.[31] By 1895, 4,000 miles of copper transmission lines bound Japan tightly to its new modern endeavor. In 1910, in Kyoto, some private residences had electric lights installed. In her diary, Nakano Makiko, the wife of a Kyoto merchant, jotted down that on 12 January 1910, an electric light brightened her home. She wrote, "It was so bright that I felt as though I had walked into the wrong house."[32] By 1935, Japan led the world in electrification by providing 89 percent of its households with electric lighting, about the same as Germany (85 percent) and significantly more than Great Britain (44 percent) and the United States (68 percent).

However, Japan's use of residential electricity remained mostly confined to lighting, as in 1937 less than 1 percent of Japanese homes, nearly 13 million households, possessed electric refrigerators and washing machines.[33] Most Japanese acquired these "sacred treasures" of the domestic realm only after the Pacific War (1937–45), especially during the periods of high-speed economic growth in the 1960s.[34] But Tokyo politicians and social engineers required tons of copper and coal to transmit and fuel this transformation, much more than Tokugawa technologies and labor practices had ever extracted from Japan's mines. Such quantities could be acquired only through a moderate reorganization of human labor and, more importantly, a radical reorganization of technology. Verticality was again the key: this technology dug deeper into the bowels of Earth, extracting more copper than ever before from heretofore only imagined depths (such as that imagined in the medieval paintings of Buddhist hell that will be explored in chapter 6). In doing so, however, these technologies released hellish, hidden toxins that poisoned farmlands near the mines and caused human pain.

In 1877, the "Mining King of East Asia," Furukawa Ichibei (1832–1903), gained control of the struggling Ashio mine. At this juncture, laborers worked about 74 out of a total of 250 pits dug into ore outcroppings; the area reportedly resembled a "beehive" with its many "raccoon-dog" holes. Remnant Tokugawa technologies and poorly engineered mining areas failed to satisfy Japan's new copper needs. Soon after the financier Shibusawa Eiichi (1840–1931) offered his considerable financial backing, and after Furukawa struck a series of rich veins in the 1880s, the Ashio complex began to prosper after its long eighteenth-century lull. (In 1883, Ashio produced 647 metric tons of copper. After the discovery of new veins in 1884, that number more than tripled to 2,286.)[35] In 1884, Ashio accounted for 26 percent of Japan's total copper production. One year later, Ashio produced ninety times the copper (over nine millions pounds) than it had a decade earlier, when Furukawa had originally purchased the operation. This is a pretty good return. By the turn of the century, Furukawa controlled about 40 percent of Japan's total copper production—and hence the key to his country's energy distribution, electrification, and foreign currency acquisition—as well as a considerable number of coal mines.[36] Indeed, this is why he was famously known as the Mining King of East Asia.

Engineers wasted little time in mechanizing conveyance at Ashio by building rails; they also improved the mine's drainage system in the deepest tunnels and provided oil lamps to replace the pine torches used in the Tokugawa years. Over the course of the 1880s and 1890s, a series of technological advances sought to increase production and confine the mine spatially: to transform the Ashio extraction and production complex into one holistic machine with a variety of organic and inorganic parts all functioning harmoniously toward the same goal of producing modernity's king metal. Underground "raccoon-dog diggers" extracted ore that they placed on trams; once ore reached the surface, workers on an assembly line dressed the ore; railway lines then hauled the dressed ore to smelters; and then railways transported the metal to ports to be shipped overseas or to domestic processing facilities (fig. 3.6). Almost everything at the site functioned as a part of this hybrid system.

But this hybrid machine sprung biotechnical leaks, because mining

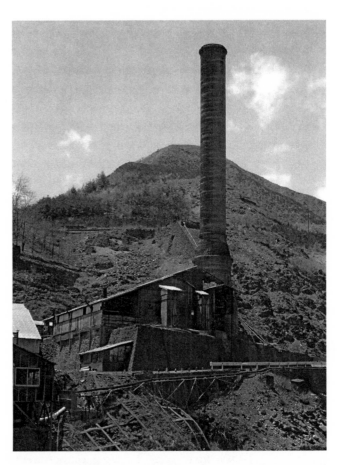

FIG. 3.6 The smokestack at the Ashio smelter. The hillsides around the smelting facilities are still denuded and scarred by erosion. The smokestack was built in 1919. Its height is 46 meters, or 151 feet. The diameter at the base is 5.7 meters, or 19 feet, and the diameter at the top is 3.8 meters, or 12.5 feet. Photograph by author.

is messy business: opening up Earth, particularly deposits far beneath the surface, released previously contained toxins—a virtual chemistry textbook table of nasty elements and compounds, ranging from arsenic to zinc—which poisoned farmers downstream and caused deforestation. Mine bosses and engineers lost their control of this hybrid system as well, because Tanaka Shōzō (1841–1913), a downstream liberal politician, demanded they make concessions in the form of pollution control, which they did reluctantly in 1897. The first unanticipated consequence of the Ashio enterprise was the birth of Japanese environmentalism. When mining technologies interfaced with surrounding ecosystems, the results always proved unpredictable; but the results proved equally unpredictable when mining technologies and ecosystem processes interfaced with downstream social networks.

Just as government warnings that labeled parathion a "special toxin" led to its use in suicides, the Meiji government's unconditional support of the Ashio mine led to forces that pushed for pollution control. The overriding lesson of the Ashio pollution disaster and problems at other mines scattered throughout Japan remains interconnectedness. Where does one realm end and another begin? Where are the lines that separate miners deep in the bowels of Earth, high-tech smelters on the surface, atmospheric and hydrologic currents, oxidation processes, carefully tended rice paddies, human and nonhuman stomachs, and the bone and liver disorders that killed hundreds of farmers when arsenic, cadmium, and sulfuric acid crippled their already-malnourished bodies? The impact of these mines can only be understood holistically, just as medicine was used holistically to understand illness before the atomizing and reducing tendencies that followed the birth of bacteriology. "The environment was not," writes Linda Nash of nineteenth-century American medicine, "a realm distinct from human society but one that was intimately connected to the human body."[37]

Health surveys in 1899 confirmed this intimate connection. In unpolluted Tochigi Prefecture (where Ashio was located), there were 3.44 births for every one hundred people, and in polluted Tochigi there were 2.80 births for every one hundred people. Conversely, there were 1.92 premature deaths in unpolluted Tochigi for every one hundred people and over double that number (4.12) in polluted Tochigi.[38] Birth rates were down and premature mortality was up. Women also began to experience problems with lactation. When Kuma, a forty-one-year-old wife from Aso Province, gave birth to her eldest son in 1878, she recalled producing "adequate milk." For her fourth son, born in 1893, she failed to lactate. When Seki, a thirty-three-year-old housewife from the same province, gave birth to her eldest son in 1888, she produced "adequate milk." Six years later, when she gave birth to her eldest daughter, she experienced "lactation deficiencies." These sorts of stories abound in the historical record, as do stories of financial losses caused by destroyed fisheries.[39]

What is important for this book is that environmental collapse and health problems in the Watarase River basin nearly paralleled technological innovation and environmental engineering at the Ashio complex. So it is not only human bodies that are embedded in natural systems but technologies as well. Because of this connection, the technologies of "mass extraction" also proved to be, at least for those in the mine's biotechnological path, the technologies of pain infliction. Throughout the 1880s, industrial advancement at Ashio continued apace, and engineers introduced some of the world's most extraordinary machinery to the site. In 1885, after Furukawa purchased additional mines from the government, engineers fired up stream-engine pumps to further improve drainage. In 1888, with help from Siemens Company (which also supplied machines to Minamata), Furukawa had Japan's first hydroelectric station built. Dams represent important parts of any organic machine, as they harness the life, motion, and inorganic as well as organic energies of rivers to service industrial needs. Today, much as the trees, brush, and macaques have reclaimed the forests surrounding the Kodaki site, the Watarase River has, over the past century, reclaimed its unobstructed path through the Ashio processing facilities by grinding and eroding the hydroelectric plant into a smooth, wavy redbrick surface.

Harnessed energy meant electrification, and electrification meant motorized pumps, winches, air compressors, and even telephones; pneumatic drills bored faster, centrifugal fans ventilated more efficiently, and electric lights provided more illumination inside the shafts. Shafts became, for all intents and purposes, entirely human-engineered environments. In 1888, Furukawa signed a lucrative contract with Britain's Jardine Matheson Company, made rich during the opium trade with China, for Ashio's copper, and by 1890 engineers had centralized eight of the forty-eight refining sites into thirteen hydrometallurgical separators and three pyrometallurgical smelters. The 1890s also witnessed the installation of a Bessemer smelter, a 400-horsepower hydroelectric turbine-powered pump, ore lifts, electric lighting systems, and an electric railway between the mine and the refining areas. Also in the 1890s, steam engines replaced the oxen and horses that had once hauled copper over the Hosō Pass and out of the basin. By the beginning of the twentieth century, ten power stations that harnessed energy from the Watarase and other rivers replaced the single unit installed by Siemens Company a decade earlier, and the Ashio complex, in a small mountain community in Tochigi Prefecture, had become one of the most technologically advanced and elaborately engineered pieces of real estate on Earth.[40]

However, the same factors that made the Ashio site so sublime technologically also made it the source of an environmental catastrophe and human pain. Ashio created civilization for some Japanese; it destroyed worlds for others. After work began in the Yokomabu lode in 1884 (remember the spike in metric tons of copper produced after 1884), horrible tree blighting occurred; with the introduction of the electric drills and steam-generated pumps in 1885, massive fish kills occurred; and only three years after engineers installed the first hydrometallurgical separator and three pyrometallurgical smelters, copper poisoned some 4,000 acres of farmland downstream from the mine. As it turns out, these ecological events served as cautionary signals within the engineered landscapes of the Watarase River basin. But other factors contributed to downstream pollution as well. Unlike Tokugawa processing at copper mines, where dressers swept the floors of the smelters for copper in order to prevent any waste, the technologies of mass extraction left copper and other metals in the tailings that miners simply discarded or left in heaps strewn about the site. Rainwater seeped through these heaps much as water does in a drip-style coffeemaker, absorbing dissolved metals. It eventually found its way into the Watarase River in trickles and rivulets, and toxins from the mine rushed downstream in floodwaters to paddy lands and irrigation channels. The same irrigation channels that so cleverly diverted water to nourish paddies served as conduits for the heavy metals and poisons that destroyed them. The employment of massive amounts of energy, whether in the form of labor or the burning of fuels such as wood, charcoal, or coal, paralleled the degree of environmental damage: the toxic archipelago is the result of hard work and technological advancement.

BIOLOGICAL SENTINELS

Farmers noticed toxins in the river quite early. In chapter 1, I discussed how silkworm colonies had been devastated after eating mulberry leaves that Ashio smelters had coated with toxins. Other sentinels sounded the alarm as well. Even as early as the 1870s, water from the Watarase River had turned "bluish white" and locals observed dead fish floating down the river. Much like the situation at Minamata decades later, children reportedly waded into the river to catch dazed eels; these same children, once back home, noticed that red sores festered on their legs. Most likely, the fish kill occurred after the addition of ore-pulverizing machines and steam-engine pumps to the Ashio complex. In June 1887, one author of the *Watarase kawasuji kokon enkaku chō* (Survey of the Past and Present Development of the Watarase River) made the connection between the opening of the Ashio copper mine, "poisoned water" (*dokusui*) leeching from the mine pit, and the collapse of freshwater fish stocks.[41] Declining fisheries signaled a poisoned environment; poisoned environments made people sick. The governor of Tochigi Prefecture, Fujikawa Tamechika (governed 1880–83), had learned that silkworms fed mulberry leaves picked from the polluted region had died and that wells containing contaminated water caused severe diarrhea. However, as it turned out, dead fish and caterpillars were the least of the problems the poor souls living along the Watarase River faced. In the Ashio area watershed, which received some seventy-nine inches (over 2006 millimeters) of rain annually, locally harvested lumber provided one means for engineers to shore up always-dangerous mine shafts and construct lodges and other buildings; trees also provided fuel for steam engines and, even more importantly, copper smelters. These trees came from land Furukawa had purchased for next to nothing from the government as part of the latter's privatization scheme, a policy we will investigate in chapter 6. Soon, loggers, under orders from Ashio managers, had deforested much of the Ashio watershed. Loggers, however, proved only partially responsible for the denuding of the Ashio watershed. Sulfur dioxide discharged during the smelting process bleached tree leaves and severely poisoned their root systems. Erosion then swept away most of the topsoil; as early as 1888 locals reported erosion and flooding.

Acidic deposition (or acid rain) occurred because of hybrid causations and nature's agencies: whatever emissions left the Ashio smelters in the air or water seldom remained the same exact chemicals. They were naturalized, just as parathion or cadmium could be under certain circumstances. The metals emitted with the sulfur dioxide served as potent catalysts for sun-induced photochemical reactions. The sulfur dioxide produced by smelters, once in the environment, naturally transformed into highly toxic sulfuric acid that rained down on farmers and their paddies and mulberry fields. Farm animals such as horses and cows also exhibited signs of poisoning, and inhabitants evacuated Matsuki Village because the village sat downwind from the smelters and had become coated with a poisonous sulfuric dust. Here the agency is a chemical one: after acidic deposition, hydrogen ions (protons) are released from sulfuric and nitric acids and chemically bond with elements in the soil, many the building blocks of life.

Hydrogen ions, for example, can rob the soil of such nutrients as calcium and magnesium, leaving moonscapes in their wake.[42]

As a gas, sulfur dioxide, in even modest doses, is dangerous enough, damaging the respiratory system and causing bronchitis; but sulfur dioxide and its neutralizing products ammonium bisulfate and ammonium sulfate usually take the form of metallic particulates, which in water droplets or on ash represent the most potent of the atmospheric acids. Daily exposure to any more than 100 parts per million (ppm) causes chronic bronchitis in most people.[43] In the Watarase River basin, sulfuric acid was the principal polluter, because most Japanese copper ores are highly sulfuric; sulfide compounds make up 30–40 percent of Japanese copper. Smelting released these compounds into the atmosphere.[44] It is remarkable that silkworms—and the human providers who watched over them—lasted as long as they did.

In the 1890s, in response to growing concerns from farmers and a small handful of local politicians, Ashio engineers blasted slag piles with dynamite, which, whatever their intent, released even higher concentrations of toxins into the Watarase River. In the lower reaches of the basin, heavy metals accumulated in the paddy fields and irrigation channels, and the topsoil became as hard as cement and no longer retained oxygen. Subsequently, the topsoil asphyxiated the rice, wheat, mulberry, and other agricultural crops that managed to survive the polluted air and acidic deposition. Eventually, the Ashio complex poisoned nearly 250,000 acres of some of Japan's best paddy lands. Today, rice grown in the region still contains abnormally high concentrations of cadmium, which, as we shall see in the next chapter, poses unusually painful health risks to people, particularly rural women.[45]

Smelting copper represents one of the numerous anthropogenic sources of inorganic arsenic in the environment. When in the drinking water or inhaled, arsenic can be fatal if enough is consumed. In lesser amounts, it penetrates the placenta and, like the most heinous environmental pollutants, finds its way to the fetus. In the previous chapter, we saw how arsenic, both in the United States and, eventually, in Japan, became the biocide of choice in nineteenth- and early-twentieth-century agriculture. In Japan, one of the most high-profile and grisly incidents involving arsenic poisoning resulted when mothers in western Japan fed their infants arsenic-contaminated Morinaga Powdered Milk that the company produced at its Tokushima plant. Initially, according to a 1956 Ministry of Health and Welfare (Kōseishō) survey, the powdered milk poisoned 12,131 newborns and killed 130; however, in March 1981, it became clear that the damage to human health had been far more widespread: of the 13,389 people who had ingested the powdered milk, 600 had died, 6,093 suffered long-term health difficulties, and 624 were plagued with developmental difficulties or severe retardation.[46] If pain can be "world destroying" for the sufferer, as I postulated in the introduction, it is hard to fathom what could be more world destroying than physical pain that results from mother's milk. But, as we shall see, mother's milk was also one manner in which mercury was transmitted to infants at Minamata. At the most basic interface—a baby's tender mouth and a mother's swollen breast—painfully poisonous toxins were transmitted between mother and child.

In adults, chronic exposure to arsenic leads to a whole host of problems, including damage to the nervous system and liver cirrhosis; lengthy periods of open-air exposure can cause skin and lung cancers. Arsenic, among its other talents as a poison, impairs cell tissue respiration by injuring mitochondrial enzymes. Cellular oxidation failure means that the cell produces less energy and the body begins to slowly break down. It is ironic that labor at Japan's copper and coal mines expended and produced energy while inorganic arsenic inhibited energy production at the building blocks of organic life. Perhaps the only toxicological characteristic arsenic does not have in its arsenal is mutagenic capabilities, and so the horrors of gene mutation would be left to mutagenic metals such as cadmium and radioactivity from Japan's post–atomic bomb nightmare.[47]

In August 1890 and September 1891, the first major flooding washed out paddies in Gunma and Tochigi prefectures and covered once-fertile agricultural lands with a layer of sulfuric silt. In July and September 1896, massive flooding occurred again in the wake of torrential rains, and the Watarase, along with the tributary Tone and Edo rivers, poured over their banks and saturated some 115,000 acres in a monstrous concoction of mine poisons. One reason that the floodwaters contained so much pollutant was that miners, in order to dispose of the waste rock piles surrounding the mine, had started crushing the rock and disposing of it in the Watarase River. On 8 September 1896, miners reportedly dumped well over two million cubic feet of crushed rock in the river. This debris and the toxic stew it created had only one place to go: downstream. The flood killed even more land in the basin by solidifying the soil and thereby asphyxiating plant life. Farmers likened their new industrial landscape to a Buddhist hell and renamed the Watarase the "River of Death." Fisheries crashed, insects no longer chirped, seedlings no longer grew, and grotesque sores developed on the hands and feet of the farmers who labored in the paddies and irrigation channels. Farmers drew on local traditions and assumed that the river deities had become possessed by demons, but the only demons were the Ashio bosses who had ordered that waste be discharged into the river: sulfuric and arsenic poisons, ammonia, cadmium, chlorine, copper, iron, lead, magnesia, nitrates, phosphoric acid, and zinc.[48]

"SOCIETY'S GUARDIAN GOD"

As mentioned, Tanaka Shōzō sprouted from the cracks in Ashio's carefully constructed hybrid system, much like the trees and macaques that, a century later, emerged in the terraced remains of the Kodaki mining village. Like rotten fish, dead silkworms, and the sore-ridden feet of children, his activities proved yet another unanticipated consequence of Ashio's operations. As the situation downstream from Ashio grew worse, Tanaka took the cabinet of Prime Minister Matsukata Masayoshi (1835–1924), architect of the earlier privatization of most Japanese mines, to task on the floor of the National Assembly in 1891 for not obeying the Meiji Constitution and protecting farmers and others from the destruction caused by mines. Though swimming upstream against the civilizing tide of the Meiji years, he boldly called for the immediate closing of the Ashio mine. When the government refused to do so, he led the fight to make it.

Tanaka was born in the Watarase River basin, the area known as the Shimotsuke Plain, and raised by his father, the head of Konaka Village and principal of the Jōrenji Temple school, situated only five miles or so from the Watarase River. Tanaka fought with other children at school and even caught syphilis (by his own account) after being persuaded to visit a brothel by "evil friends." Despite his rocky childhood, in 1859, after domain officials promoted his father to superintendent, Tanaka became village head, only to be dismissed and even imprisoned several years later for political intrigue when he challenged a higher-ranking official. On being released from prison in 1869, following the Meiji Restoration and the toppling of the Tokugawa shogun, Tanaka taught at a humble school housed in a small shrine. He studied for a spell with Oda Takizaburō in Tokyo and then departed for Iwate Prefecture. In 1870, constables arrested Tanaka for the death of a prefectural official with whom Tanaka had often quarreled, and

he spent until April 1874 in the Iwate prison, where he spent his time reading Jean Jacques Rousseau's (1712–78) *Du contrat social* (1762) and Samuel
Smiles's (1812–1904) *Self-Help* (1859). Once released, Tanaka decided that
he wanted to live a life devoted to lofty principles, humility, and public
service.[49]

My favorite picture of Tanaka was taken while he was visiting Yanaka
Village, before its forced depopulation, demolition, and submersion as a
holding reservoir for toxins from the Ashio mine. In the grainy picture,
Tanaka is writing at a desk and appears to have his hair in the style of
a samurai, called a *chonmage,* though it is completely disheveled. But as
such he is an even more compelling figure: selflessly fighting a battle he
knows he will lose. Adding to his rustic air, he wears traditional Japanese rain gear, a long coatlike outfit made from layered miscanthus reed
(*kaya*) or sedge (*suge*), called a *mino* coat in Japanese. I like the picture
because it reminds me that he was a daunting, tough figure in his bold
traditional clothing, quite different from the other political power brokers
of his day: the European- or American-mimicking officials in tails and top
hats, who composed the majority of the Meiji government. It also reminds
me that he could be quite prickly. In March 1881, when Tochigi governor
Fujikawa Tamechika hosted a dinner for newly elected assemblymen (of
whom Tanaka was one), Tanaka turned his chair so that his back faced the
table when he thought the governor treated the assemblymen with disre-
spect. When studying in Tokyo, other students often stared at his country
bumpkin figure. "But for my own part I was sorry for them," he reflected
later. "They were only looking, after all, at a man who had chosen to go his
own way."[50] Go his own way he did, often lambasting political chiefs, such
as the head of the Liberal Party, Itagaki Taisuke (1837–1919), for what he
saw as their unscrupulous behavior and lack of principles. Most famously,
he confronted the rapacious governor of Fukushima Prefecture Mishima
Michitsune (1835–88), who oversaw an ambitious road-building scheme
that required, among other abuses, extracting hard corvée labor from villagers.[51] He was genuinely fearless in his fight to protect the underprivileged
from the hardship and pain demanded by the Meiji state.

On 1 July 1890, his native district of Aso, in Tochigi Prefecture, elected
Tanaka to the National Diet in Japan's first parliamentary elections. On 18
December 1891, Tanaka gave his now-famous speech to the Diet in which
he questioned why the Meiji government had not suspended Ashio's opera-

tions, given the Meiji Constitution's assurances that "the rights of property to all Japanese subjects shall not be violated" and concrete steps would be taken if any mining activities "endangered the public good." His deep, explosive voice resonated from the floor of the Diet:

> The poisonous effluent from the copper mine at Ashio in Kami-Toga District, Tochigi Prefecture, has been allowed to inflict heavy losses and hardship each year since 1888 on villages in every district on either side of the Watarase River, where it flows through Gunma and Tochigi prefectures. The effects of the effluent are steadily worsening. With fields being poisoned, drinking water contaminated, and even the trees and grasses lining the dykes being threatened, no one can tell what disastrous consequences the future may hold.

"Why has the government done nothing for so long?" he asked. "What measures does it propose to compensate for losses already incurred, and to prevent their recurrence?" he queried the minister of agriculture and commerce.[52]

Tanaka demanded an answer from the minister, Mutsu Munemitsu (1844–97), but none was forthcoming. Even after the fall of the Heian court centuries earlier, marriage politics were alive and well: Mutsu's second son had married Furukawa's daughter and had formally been adopted as heir to the Furukawa fortune. This marital arrangement reflected earlier business friendships formed when Furukawa served as manager of the Onogumi Company and Mutsu as the chief of the tax division of the Finance Ministry. When Tanaka eventually received an answer from the chief of the mines division of the Ministry of Agriculture and Commerce (Nōshōmushō), it spoke volumes about Japan's priorities during the Meiji years. The chief published his cool response in a Tokyo newspaper on 10 February 1892: "Suppose for the sake of argument that copper effluent were responsible for the damage to the farmland on either side of the Watarase River—the public benefits that accrue to the country from the Ashio mine far outweigh any losses suffered in the affected areas."[53] This quotation also bears directly on the point about pain and nations made in the introduction of this book: although the Ashio mine caused pain and suffering in the polluted areas, the public benefits that accrued for the nation—the same national landscape that Andō Shōeki had become so acutely aware of in eighteenth-century Hachinohe—outweighed whatever pain was occurring in the Watarase River basin. Local pain, Mutsu Munemitsu could well have written, is an important part of participating in national communities, because it is endured for the national whole. Sacrifices must be made for the nation.

Single-minded support for industrialization during the Meiji years might have been the mantra of the Sumitsu'in (Privy Council, 1888–1947) and cabinet, but not for Tanaka, and he was as outspoken as ever. During the national elections of 15 February 1892, the home minister ordered governors and their police to actively promote and support all oligarchy candidates, and in the clashes that ensued, some twenty-five people died and hundreds were wounded. Thugs ransacked Tanaka's office and beat several staffers, but he still defeated the government candidate, although by just under a hundred votes. In May 1892, when the Diet met, Tanaka turned up the heat on his attack against the government, which could only defiantly respond that the mine planned to install "dust extractors" and "sediment basins," useless technological stopgap measures that prefigured the "Sedifloater" and "Cyclator" hoaxes orchestrated by Chisso at Minamata (chapter 5). The Tochigi government also sponsored an arbitration program with Shimotsuke farmers, and many, already facing grinding economic conditions in the wake of Meiji taxation reforms, bought into it. The arbitration agreements concluded: "As a result of this contractual agreement between us, signed today, the Ashio copper mine pollution incident is now completely closed."[54] The similarities between Ashio's cynical "arbitration agreements" and, as we shall see, Chisso's paltry "sympathy payments" and "solatium agreements" stand out as abuses of Confucian paternalism to underwrite industrial greed.

By 1894, conditions in the Shimotsuke Plain had worsened, and so had the callousness of the Meiji cabinet. The managing director of the Ashio complex and future home minister, Hara Kei, was a protégé of Mutsu Munemitsu and now served as foreign minister. Farmers expected and received little cooperation from Tokyo. When severe flooding devastated the Shimotsuke Plain, farmers rallied at the Unryūji Temple and signed a "spiritual compact" to unite and fight the mine. Farmers petitioned the minister of agriculture and commerce, Enomoto Takeaki (1836–1908), but to no avail, and the finance minister dismissed their petitions for tax remissions as well. He responded with perfect bureaucratic callousness: "The tax laws made no provision for poisoning by industrial effluent as a ground for remission." On 26 February 1897, Tanaka's voice once again thundered from the Diet chamber as he questioned Enomoto's frustrating inaction. Two days later, Tanaka met in the Kanda quarter of Tokyo with other social activists, while armed goons hired by Furukawa tried to intimidate them. At this meeting, several notable figures joined Tanaka, including Christian humanist Uchimura Kanzō (1861–1930) and the journalist Tokutomi Sōhō (1863–1957). Even Tani Tateki (1837–1911), an army veteran and right-leaning member of the House of Peers, visited the Shimotsuke Plain on 19 March 1897 and converted to Tanaka's cause, calling Tanaka "society's guardian god." Later, in the autumn of 1901, Uchimura called the Ashio complex the real enemy of Japan's empire and a nation—even world—destroyer.[55] In a written report he said:

Ashio pollution is a stain on the Japanese Empire. If we do not remove it, there is no glory or honor in all our Empire, for all its 13 infantry divisions and 260,000 tons of warships. Ashio concerns not just one province, but the whole nation, the whole human race. Indeed, it may destroy our nation. . . . The eyes of the Japanese are fixed now upon the west, upon the plains of Manchuria; our warships all head westward. Do they not see that it is not in Manchuria but *here* that the enemy is to be found? Why not station the *Hatsuse* in Lake Chusenji, and send the *Asahi* up the Watarase River, to bombard the Ashio mine from both sides? That is what I would do, if I were made Prime Minster.[56]

Needless to say, Uchimura's campaign for prime minister never gained much momentum, but the intertwining of patriotism, Christian humanism, class consciousness, war, and the merits of empire permeated much of his writing.[57]

On two occasions in March 1897, farmers mobilized at the Unryūji Temple and marched on Tokyo; only fifty farmers participated in the first march, but the second attracted four thousand. Even though he visited the Shimotsuke Plain and saw with his own eyes the devastation caused by Ashio, Minister Enomoto acted slowly, creating a Pollution Investigation Committee. And then, on 28 December 1897, he resigned. The most important outcome of Tanaka's thunderous speeches and farmer marches on Tokyo was the 1897 Third Mine Pollution Prevention Order, which directed Furukawa to install filter beds and sediment basins and to dig moats around existing waste rock heaps so that they did not erode or leach into the Watarase River. Spearheaded by Ōkuma Shigenobu (1838–1922), who served as chief of the Foreign and the Agriculture and Commerce ministries at various times in his career, the Meiji government also ordered reforestation and put a halt to cutting any trees that might have survived. With the 1897 Pollution Prevention Order, miners began to feel increasingly threatened by Tanaka's movement and, like the factory workers at Minamata, feared that environmental measures to save farmers and fishers threatened their jobs. It turned out that miners were not the only ones who hated the order: within four years Tanaka labeled it "an instrument of evil" after damage in the Shimotsuke Plain only increased in severity, even though the amount of pollution produced at Ashio had decreased. It was perhaps the sole pine tree that managed to grow near one of the sedimentation basins that most benefited from the 1897 Pollution Prevention Order. The tree became a symbol of Furukawa's prevention efforts. Miners carefully guarded the tree and provided it with fertilizer in the form of dried squid.[58]

In the fall of 1897, Tanaka toured the Shimotsuke Plain, documenting the drop in land values and the doubling of the mortality rate and chronic eye disease among the inhabitants of 136 villages and towns. He continued to push for the Ashio mine to be closed and likened his campaign to the single-minded focus required in Zen meditation:

> This morning I saw clearly this truth. No matter how clever a man may be, if he has many aims, he will achieve none of them: no matter how foolish or ignorant, if he concentrates on one thing only, he can hardly fail.
>
> My *zazen* [Zen meditation] is "running around." My self training isn't sitting in silence, but by journeying by boat and rickshaw or on horseback along rocky roads. All this is *zazen*. *Zazen* doesn't have to be done only in silence, nor even sitting. Deeds are my *zazen*, and I do it everywhere. . . . Since this cabinet was formed I have achieved nothing. In Tokyo politics I am an imbecile. All I do is go from village to poverty-stricken village along the river bank. A duck waddling among the reeds. . . . I've discovered something. Politics is easy, as easy as dealing with pollution is difficult. Astonishing and terrifying, the ease, the superficiality of politics these days.[59]

Throughout early February 1900 Tanaka continued to lecture in the Diet chamber: Why had the Meiji government ignored petitions adopted by both houses? Why had the deaths of one thousand people from Shimotsuke, which had been shown to be caused by copper pollution, been ignored? Why had authorities concealed the results of physical fitness examinations of military conscripts from the area? Meanwhile, farmers continued to mobilize at the Unryūji Temple—five times in all—to descend on the capital. On 14 February 1900, in what is called the Kawamata Incident, while Tanaka assailed the government from the Diet chamber, at the Tone River heavily armed riot police confronted farmers marching on Tokyo and waving banners fastened to maple branches that read "Namu Amidha Butsu," a populist Buddhist utterance. At the Kawamata Ferry crossing, farmers battled riot police, who had drawn their sabers; eventually, the farmers withdrew to the Unryūji Temple carrying fifteen of their members whom police had injured so badly they could not walk. Exaggerating the Kawamata Incident, Tanaka's voice again rang out from the Diet building: the cabinet was "killing innocent citizens, first with poison, then with police." The cabinet ignored Tanaka's tireless flurry of questions. Furukawa, for his service to the nation, was awarded court rank by the Meiji emperor.[60]

On 23 March 1901, his face as red as "boiled octopus," Tanaka burst out with his most controversial indictment yet: "If the government was to be run by traitors who could decorate Furukawa while allowing him to ravage the fields that gave the nation its very life," he began, but before he could finish, cries from the Diet chamber demanded his eviction. From the text of his speech, it appears that Tanaka had called the emperor a "traitor." As authorities escorted Tanaka from the Diet, his fading voice could be heard threatening that "a decision would have to be taken. . . ." The next day, he spoke again at the Diet, venomously referring to the Ministry of Agriculture and Commerce as a "club of criminals in the pay of Furukawa" and to the Ministry of Home Affairs (Naimushō) as "a pack of hobgoblins." He finished the last speech he ever completed in the Diet chamber cryptically: "Gentlemen, if I have taken it on myself to address you, though many other matters claim your attention, it is because none of us knows what tomorrow will bring."[61]

On more than one occasion, in letters and in public speeches, Tanaka spoke of a curious "brain sickness" that made him do and say the things he did. On 24 March 1901, the day after his outburst when he accused Japan's imperial government of being run by "traitors," he blamed his incoherent speaking on this "brain sickness." In a letter addressed 11 May 1901, Tanaka had explored the nature of his sickness:

I've been running around on behalf of the Kawamata defendants, night and day, and on other pollution business and in trouble night and day, too, from my "brain sickness"—a nameless, elusive thing, this sickness. It has nothing to do with physical wellbeing. . . . Less pleasure, more pain. The pain isn't for myself, though. It's for the evil that has attacked our society. It's so hard to fight, and people don't *realize* how evil it is, either in the country or here in Tokyo. It's this that's eating my life away. I'm a sensitive fellow, you know; no hero. I feel the world's ills before the world feels them, that's all. Whatever you do, please don't think that it's worry about being poor or anything of that sort that's made me ill. . . . My sickness isn't an individual thing: it's the world's sickness. If society recovers, I'll live another ten years. If I can't save the Shimotsuke people from death, this year'll be my last. . . . Remember this prophecy![62]

The original text, crafted by radical journalist Kotoku Shushui (1871–1911) under Tanaka's direction, of the "direct petition" that Tanaka failed to deliver to the emperor on 10 December 1901, spoke of the "mad foolishness" of the presenter of the petition. Even though Tanaka appears to have substituted "exceeding" for "mad" in the final version he brought to the Sakurada Gate, while waiting for the Meiji emperor to pass, Kotoku's original choice of "mad foolishness" says much about the nature of radical ideologies in Japan and those who endorsed them. He later reflected on the direct petition: "Shōzō is no longer of this world," he wrote. "He should have died on the 10th. It was a mistake, an unavoidable mistake that he survived."[63]

These references to "brain sickness," "madness," and being no longer of "this world" hark back to the ideological affliction that possessed other political radicals, such as Yoshida Shōin (1830–59), a patriot in the vanguard of the imperial restoration movement decades earlier. The higher principles so honored by Tanaka remind one of the *magokoro*, or "pure heart," embraced by Yoshida; the "brain sickness" that afflicted Tanaka and the "madness" that gripped Yoshida were the symptoms of stepping outside the normality of mainstream political life to see with unclouded eyes.[64] If Meiji high-speed industrial growth at the expense of human and nonhuman life was civilization—and, hence, the global normalcy of progressive, modern nations—then anybody who questioned it was, to varying degrees, able to see the "world destroyers," or those who promoted the madness of unbridled industrialization. Normalcy is to see factories and mines as icons of modern progress; "brain sickness" is when you see them as world-destroying, pain-giving structures: icons of disfigured fetuses, black lungs, brittle bones, and destroyed fisheries.

When the Watarase River flooded in August and September 1902, fewer toxins at the Ashio site meant that the floods proved, for the first time in decades, life giving. In the wake of these floods, in December 1902, the Pollution Prevention Committee offered a series of recommendations for "flood prevention" in the Shimotsuke area (ignoring pollution altogether), the most radical of which included destroying the villages of Kawabe and Toshima in Saitama Prefecture and Yanaka in Tochigi Prefecture in order to build a huge sediment basin. Leaders in Kawabe and Toshima boldly threatened to withhold military conscripts and taxes if their villages were not exempted; leaders in Yanaka, by contrast, fought in the prefectural assembly through 1903 and 1904, but on 10 December 1904, during a secret meeting with an intimidating police presence, assemblymen submitted to the Tokyo proposal. Yanaka became the next front in the Ashio campaign when Tanaka, after spending a stint in a Tokyo jail for "behavior insulting to an official" and at the ripe old age of sixty-three, moved to the village of about one thousand inhabitants. He reflected on the move:

It's not that I've had to steel myself to face the misery of Yanaka; it's been inevitable that I should come here, the natural thing. Buddha had to take the decision to seclude himself on Mount Dantaloka. A common mortal like me comes to Yanaka because it's here, that's all. But maybe, allowing for the difference between us of the great and the insignificant, what he was after and what I am after are not so different; only he *knew* the truth, while I have only the realities of everyday for guide.[65]

In March 1906, "compulsory purchases" began in Yanaka, with farmers being offered a pittance for their properties. Like most forced relocation efforts, the government gave farmers cheap returns on their property and relocated them to poor-quality farmlands. At Yanaka, "The government was at war with its own people," an older and even-more-ornery Tanaka observed. The Privy Council had appointed Hara Kei chief of the Ministry of Home Affairs, and he led the government charge. On 29 June 1907, the same year workers at the Ashio mine rioted, destroying subterranean huts and surface lodges, over two hundred police and demolition workers descended on Yanaka and began to destroy the entire village. Piece by piece, each residence was taken apart and the lumber moved and guarded so that homeowners could not recover what, officially speaking, had been their property. By 5 July 1907 Hara could report that the dismantling of Yanaka was complete. To commemorate the event, the governor of Tochigi had himself photographed in front of the ruined village that afternoon. Even with the village gone, however, much remained the same on the Shimotsuke Plain: periodic flooding, the slow collapse of river fisheries, and the poisoning of local paddies. But Tanaka had, over the course of decades of conflict, condensed his philosophy to two words that later, though not in his lifetime, developed into a new global epistemology: *chisan, chisui,* or "care for mountains and forests, care for rivers and streams." It was the birth of modern conservationism. Predating the "thinking like a mountain" conservationism of Aldo Leopold (1887–1948) by decades, Tanaka reflected: "To care for mountains, your heart must be as the mountains—to care for rivers, your heart must be as the rivers."[66] He wrote in verse:

If I make
The sea and sky my home,
My home is without possessions.
And having nothing,
All things are mine.

If all men would make
The grassy plains their bed
And the mountains their pillow
They would wake to the glory
Of the dawning sun.[67]

His own pain remained embedded in the natural world around him: "Shōzō shares the life of all natural things," he explained to friends. He was simply a spectator to his own life. "If they die, so must he. When he fell, it was because the rivers and forests of Aso and Ashikaga are dying, and Japan herself [*sic*], too. . . . If those who come to ask after him hope for his recovery, let them first restore the ravaged hills and rivers and forests, and then Shōzō will be well again." Portending things to come, Tanaka never became well again and died on 4 September 1913.[68]

When engineers unleashed toxins and washed them downstream into rice paddies—and in doing so caused crop loss, industrial disease, and human pain—they also unleashed one of the most powerful voices in Japanese history. Tanaka Shōzō, much like Andō Shōeki before him and Ishimure Michiko (b. 1927) after him, was yet another unanticipated result of the industrial and technological systems created during the Meiji years: he was a social system accident. "Shōzō shares the life of all natural things," wrote Tanaka, as heavy metals and sulfuric acid saturated the land of his birth. That is, had these chemicals not pumped through the trophic tiers of his home, he might never have dreamed of the myriad ways in which people are connected to the physical environment: toxins from Ashio highlighted the interconnected nature of all things. He saw the links between the mining activities at Ashio and the health of people living in the Shimotsuke area, because toxins allowed those links to be traced.

In the introduction, I conjectured that a book such as this one, with its focus on industrial pollution, ecological collapse, and human pain, makes such celebrated figures as Fukuzawa Yukichi, who was intellectually complicit in saturating the toxic archipelago, look like idiots, with their pedantic preaching about modernity, conquering nature, and promoting enterprise. By contrast, this book transforms such eccentric local politicians as Tanaka Shōzō into heroic spokespeople for a more balanced, sustainable existence with nature. He knew, as few others in his day did, that people seamlessly interfaced with engineered and naturally occurring landscapes. Tanaka knew that this connection, whether a soft baby's mouth suckling a mother's breast or a farmer's dirty hands transplanting delicate rice plants in carefully tended paddies or a village woman retrieving drinking water from a nearby source, constituted the umbilical cord that inexorably tied people to nature. In the *longue durée*, Tanaka's thought, with its ghostly first-person narration, will emerge as the more valuable to life on Earth. Fukuzawa, by contrast, has come to represent the reckless hubris of nineteenth-century notions of modernity and the industrial age.

4 ENGINEERING PAIN IN THE JINZŪ RIVER BASIN

With the beginning of the Meiji wars (namely, in 1895 and 1905), miners started extracting lead and zinc at a frenzied pace from the Kamioka shafts of the mountainous regions of Toyama and Gifu prefectures. This technological complex, and the engineered environments it birthed, seamlessly connected to the Jinzū River basin, which also fed downstream paddies that, in their own way, were engineered environments as well. Smelting and ore flotation devices that allowed miners and processors to extract ever-higher percentages of their desired metals caused pollution problems in nearby agricultural lands. But these pollution problems, particularly their consequences for human health, were the product of hybrid causation. Naturally occurring oxidization and ionization processes in riparian ecosystems created the toxins that caused human pain; but "it hurts, it hurts disease," or cadmium poisoning, was also the proximate consequence of Meiji state pronouncements regarding being a "good wife and wise mother." Women who were both productive and reproductive tended to suffer disproportionately from cadmium poisoning: obeying meant sacrificing for the state. Similarly, women who sheltered themselves from the sun, in a culturally ingrained habit to preserve their white complexions, deprived themselves of nutrients that could have protected them from industrial disease. The web of causation: mining technologies, engineered environments, natural alchemy, state pronouncements, menopause (which also made women more susceptible), and cultural habits enmeshed and intertwined to create disease and pain downstream from this important wartime mine.

MILITARY ECONOMIES AND THE KAMIOKA ZINC MINE

Surely, of all my years traveling in Japan, the most memorable train that I have ever ridden was the Kamioka Railway "one-man car" that transported me to the Kamioka zinc and lead mine, deep in the mountain recesses of southeastern Toyama and northern Gifu prefectures. Inside the train, a charming replica of a brazier, with a fake burning fire with a kettle warming over it, kept me hypnotically preoccupied as it rocked back and forth. The train jostled and jolted as it wound through the mountains, its diesel engine roaring loudly as the car gained altitude. What I remember most are the lengthy tunnels that broke up the view of the Jinzū and Takahara rivers and the rice-farming villages that adorned their banks. Toyama Prefecture is rice paddy country, with fields filling every fertile nook and cranny: between apartments and supermarkets, near Pachinko parlors, and under freeway overpasses. Farmers worked these fields alongside frog-hunting egrets and crows. The farmers, egrets, and crows all looked about the same size as I clunked and clanked by on the old train. Though rural, the area was not wild, not in a wilderness sense, but it was less inhabited than many parts of Japan. The hillsides were thoroughly covered with commercially planted groves of trees, standing in neat, well-kept rows. When I arrived at the Kamioka mining complex, the first thing I did was take a picture of a prominent sign in front of the processing facilities that said, "Photographs Prohibited." Righteously, like a muckraking journalist who had arrived four decades too late, I snapped several digital images of the mine. But later that afternoon, when I could swear that I was being shadowed by company thugs as I tried to hike the perimeter of the sprawling Kamioka complex, I erased those few images. But then I realized that, if accosted, I could claim to be an idiot foreigner who could not read Japanese. In the end, I took hundreds of images and left the site completely unscathed.

The Kamioka zinc and lead mine is another site where industrial technologies interfaced with engineered, hybrid environments to touch nerves that cause human pain. The same hybrid causations at work at Ashio, which we examined in the previous chapter, were also at work at the Kamioka zinc mine. The story of the Kamioka complex, however, is less about labor than it is about highly productive and decisively destructive technologies, in particular flotation separation machines that sorted ore so minutely that poisons and dangerous metals such as cadmium, measured in either hundredths of a millimeter in separation machines or in parts per million in the Jinzū River by health investigators, flowed downstream, entered paddy fields, and penetrated the stalks of rice plants and, eventually, the bodies of consumers. Whether the chlorinated hydrocarbons that laced agricultural crops in the 1950s or the acid rain and toxic floods that poisoned rice paddies in the Watarase River basin or the cadmium-laced rice harvested downstream from the Kamioka mines, it is the interface between human labor, advanced technologies, engineering, idiosyncratic cultural systems, and human consumers that causes industrial disease.

The hybrid interface at the Kamioka complex is of particular interest because of the natural processes involved, similar to the atmospheric photochemical processes that created acid rain near Ashio. In the case of Kamioka, such natural processes transformed relatively benign metallic cadmium into an oxidized, metallic ion that plants and other organisms easily absorbed. Miners separated zinc from silver ore through flotation technologies that required that ore be pulverized into fine particles that could pass through specialized mesh sieves. Even though miners extracted the majority of heavy metals from this dust, mine tailings that were flushed down the Takahara River and eventually into the Jinzū River basin and its network of irrigation channels still contained high quantities of heavy metals and other toxins. Hundreds of metric tons of pulverized cadmium and other heavy metals washed down the Jinzū River every year. Cadmium was the most dangerous of these metals, because once the particulate matter flowed downstream, it quickly oxidized in the sunlight and became more "bioavailable." In effect, the cadmium dust produced through such high levels of mechanized technologies was naturalized into the Jinzū ecosystem once it was released into the environment, oxidized, and then absorbed into the bodies of organisms. Once again, here is nature's agency at work: history is far more than the sum of its human parts.

Finally, these technological and natural processes interfaced with cultural systems to socially construct pain in the Jinzū River basin. Overwhelmingly, women suffered from cadmium-induced forms of osteomalacia and osteoporosis, because of gendered definitions of beauty and

Meiji state expectations that a woman be a "good wife and wise mother." Because Japanese defined beautiful women as having snowy white skin (and defined subjects in their empire by their dark complexions), rural women protected themselves with layers of clothing in order to avoid the sun, depriving themselves of valuable vitamin D, which could have alleviated their vulnerability to industrial disease. And so, just as Japanese aesthetics regarding silk clothing shaped the evolution of biotechnologies such as silkworms, or Buddhist burial practices shaped epidemics of Japanese B encephalitis, aesthetics related to beautiful skin weakened women's resistance to industrial disease.

Kamioka is situated at the uppermost reaches of the Jinzū River basin (fig. 4.1). In the late sixteenth and early seventeenth centuries, when miners discovered copper there, Hida Province, the ancient name for the area around the mine, was seized by the Tokugawa family, much as the Ashio mine had been, in its mostly successful bid to secure the realm's natural resources. Relatively small-scale copper and silver mining continued at the site until the Meiji Restoration of 1868. With the 1873 Japan Mining Law (Nihon kōhō), the government approved some thirty-five mines within the Kamioka area, even though hundreds of "raccoon-dog" holes, remnants of preindustrial techniques, remained scattered in the mountains. The Mitsui Group (an ancestor of the modern Mitsui Metal Mining Industry, or Mitsui Kinzoku Kōgyō) oversaw the Kamioka mines during the Meiji years.[1] The Mitsui Group took advantage of miners' debts from before the era of "enlightened politics" to secure its workforce and, under the patronage of Inoue Kaoru (1835–1915), the foreign minister who was the architect of Japan's early intrusion into Korea, began training miners in modern extraction techniques. In the early Meiji years, the Mitsui Group adeptly manipulated financial and political institutions all the way up to the office of the Toyama governor to buy up mining properties throughout the region. In 1887, for example, the Mitsui Group bought the Urushiyama mine and, two years later, purchased the Mozumi mine. In 1889, the Meiji government began selling all state-owned mines as part of a privatization scheme, the brainchild of Matsukata Masayoshi (1835–1924), the finance minister: the sales both generated badly needed income and placated an emerging class of investors.[2] During this period, the Mitsui Group purchased all the properties (by 1933, some 8,422 acres) that became the Kamioka mine complex.[3] As Mitsui corporate histories trumpet, not incorrectly: "Mining for coal and metals is a basic industry of modern economic society," and after the Meiji Restoration, Japan pursued the goal of becoming a "modern economic society" with little concern for the environmental or human consequences.[4]

Prior to the 1880s, silver, copper, and lead remained the principal ores extracted from the Kamioka complex. Early on, zinc, often mixed with the lead ore, proved more of a hindrance than economically valuable. Often miners picked out the zinc by hand and then discarded it into nearby ravines in the form of tailings. Given the technologies of this early period, smelting zinc ore mixed with lead proved particularly challenging. But economic reforms in the late nineteenth century provided the Mitsui Group with incentives to capture more zinc and lead. In 1897, the Meiji government abandoned the national currency system and went on the gold standard.[5] Consequently, the price of silver plummeted, and silver mines throughout Japan, such as those at Kamioka, watched their profits decline. But just as Hideyoshi's war in Kyushu and the Tokugawa unifica-

FIG. 4.1 The Tochibora area of the Kamioka mining complex, along the banks of the Takahara River. Photograph by author.

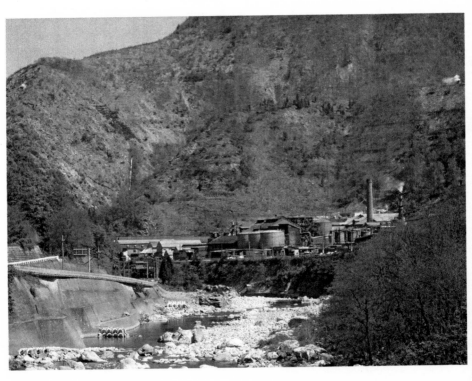

tion campaigns represented boons for copper mines, the Russo-Japanese War of 1905 signaled rising prices for lead and zinc, which are important metals in modern warfare. Presumably, given enough hatred and strength, one could smash in the head of an enemy with a hardy piece of lead ore; but, for killing, lead works much better if subjected to layers of processing. Lead ore is processed into bullets and batteries, while zinc galvanizes steel sheets, tubes, and barbed wire, making them resistant to oxidization, which is important on battleships. Zinc also constitutes about 30 percent of brass (copper being the other component), which was used in the mountings and fittings of machinery ranging from artillery to airplanes. Shrapnel cases were also made of brass and thus required zinc. One British "eighteen pounder," with a 3.3-inch shrapnel, required just under four pounds of copper and two pounds of zinc. With millions of these armaments shot during World War I, the amount of copper and zinc required for shrapnel cases measured in the millions of pounds.[6]

Metal extracted from a handful of mines, and the technologies it fashioned, built Japanese civilization and its ability to wage war and build empire.[7] But because of the pain it produced, it also proved a "world destroyer," to recall the discussion in the introduction. In an abstract way, the calloused hands of a miner evidence our connection to nature just as a body that has been torn open by bullets does: though one represents an honest day's work and the other does not, both are connections to nature refashioned.

Armed with new technologies designed to separate zinc from lead ore, the Kamioka complex shifted its priorities to lead mining (see table 7). The mine supplied Japan's military buildup and empire-building projects in the region just north of the Korean Peninsula. As Michael Lewis demonstrates, participation in empire-building projects promised to transform Toyama Prefecture from the "backside of Japan" to a "centrally important place, no longer apart from the nation but irrevocably a part of it."[8] During World War I, when Belgium and Germany (two important producers of zinc) suffered production declines, Kamioka nearly doubled its output. Just as Ashio became a giant in Japan's copper production, by 1905 the Kamioka mines accounted for an astonishing two-thirds of the zinc being produced in Japan (see table 7). In the name of "rationalizing" Kamioka to increase profits, new technologies replaced miners so that more zinc could be recovered from the site.

The "Potter method" enabled the Mitsui Group to extract much more

TABLE 7 Silver and Lead Output and National Percentage of the Kamioka Complex, 1889–1912

Year	Silver		Lead	
	Kamioka complex	National percentage	Kamioka complex	National percentage
1889	0.454 t	1.1	224 t	37.2
1890	0.558 t	1.1	156 t	20.1
1891	0.734 t	1.3	150 t	18.5
1892	6.075 t	10.1	225 t	24.7
1893	7.627 t	11.0	123 t	11.0
1894	6.264 t	8.7	231 t	16.2
1895	7.504 t	10.4	381 t	19.6
1896	7.873 t	13.4	410 t	21.0
1897	6.181 t	11.4	268 t	34.8
1898	5.779 t	9.6	586 t	34.4
1899	4.395 t	7.8	602 t	30.3
1900	4.338 t	7.3	605 t	32.7
1901	4.508 t	8.2	599 t	33.2
1902	4.968 t	8.6	1,042 t	63.4
1903	4.829 t	8.2	1,274 t	73.9
1904	4.752 t	7.8	1,292 t	71.7
1905	4.221 t	5.1	1,918 t	66.8
1906	4.481 t	5.8	1,934 t	68.8
1907	4.633 t	5.1	2,027 t	65.8
1908	5.380 t	4.5	2,227 t	76.5
1909	5.238 t	4.1	2,444 t	71.3
1910	5.533 t	3.9	2,640 t	67.6
1911	6.021 t	4.4	2,962 t	71.8
1912	6.652 t	4.4	2,941 t	78.8

Source: Kurachi Mitsuo, Tonegawa Haruo, and Hata Akio, eds., *Mitsui shihon to itai itai byō* (Mitsui Capital and "It Hurts, It Hurts Disease") (Tokyo: Ōtsuki Shoten, 1979), 41.

Note: t = metric ton (or 1.1023 U.S. tons).

zinc from the lead ore it dug from the surrounding mines. Whereas earlier techniques involved separating zinc by hand or by more primitive gravitational technologies, the Potter method (named after the English engineer Charles Vincent Potter; 1859–1908) involved mixing finely ground ore with a liquid. When agitated, the liquid turned into a frothy mineral concentrate that miners skimmed from the surface of thousands of flotation cells or tubs. The valuable zinc was easily separated from this frothy concentrate. In November 1901, Potter obtained a patent for the process using hot acid, and between 1903 and 1905 he deployed the process in the Broken Hill District in Australia to recover higher quantities of zinc.[9] The Potter method is only one variation on flotation technologies, which became the mainstay of Kamioka engineers and refinery workers. Even though the premise of flotation technologies is rather simple, it represents one of the most important technological developments in ore recovery. Flotation technologies depend on the tendency of certain oils and other liquids to stick to desired minerals more than to waste rock (fig. 4.2). The key to the process is grinding the ore so finely that when it is immersed in the liquid and agitated with pumped air, the oil adheres to the desired minerals and floats to the surface while the waste rock sinks to the bottom of the flotation cells.

With earlier gravitational methods, miners pulverized ore to about 1 millimeter (mm) in size. With the introduction of the Potter method to Japan in 1909, in order to float the ore properly miners forced the ore through a sieve that had about fifty holes per square inch, which reduced the pulverized minerals to about 0.3 mm in size. Throughout the early twentieth century, a steady stream of new flotation technology patents relied on roughly the same process as the Potter method, but they did require ever more minutely particularized ore. Incremental technological improvement can be measured by the decreasing size of pulverized minerals. In 1928, for example, Kamioka adopted an eighty-hole mesh, which produced mineral pieces that were about 0.18 mm. By 1955, the 200-hole mesh that miners used produced ore pieces that were 0.07 mm. The flotation process required a high degree of accuracy because particles that failed to conform to, for example, the 0.07 mm size adhered poorly to the chemical reagent in the flotation cells and, subsequently, proved economically unviable. Improvements on the Potter method translated into improved zinc yields, even as the ore grade declined precipitously (see tables 8–10).

The best way to illustrate how industrial technologies improved mining productivity, as well as contributed to the metric tons of metallic waste

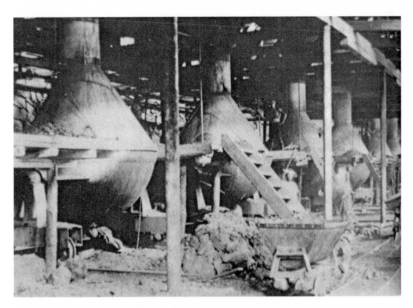

FIG. 4.2 Ore-processing facilities at the Kamioka mine. *Source:* Mitsui Kinzoku Kōgyō Kabushikigaisha Shūshi Iinkai Jimukyoku, ed., *Kamioka kōzan shashinshū* (Photograph Collection of the Kamioka Mine) (Tokyo: Mitsui Kinzoku Kōgyō Kabushikigaisha, 1975).

TABLE 8 Estimated Amount of Wasted Zinc and Cadmium from Concentration Process, Kamioka Complex, 1906–12

		Estimated waste amount	
Year	Zinc production	Zinc	Cadmium
1906	1,833 t	4,914 t	24.6 t
1907	5,772 t	5,437 t	27.2 t
1908	8,878 t	6,841 t	33.7 t
1909	10,553 t	7,137 t	35.7 t
1910	11,183 t	7,637 t	38.2 t
1911	15,397 t	5,804 t	29.0 t
1912	19,656 t	4,734 t	23.7 t
Total	73,272 t	42,504 t	212.1 t

Source: Kurachi Mitsuo, Tonegawa Haruo, and Hata Akio, eds., *Mitsui shihon to itai itai byō* (Mitsui Capital and "It Hurts, It Hurts Disease") (Tokyo: Ōtsuki Shoten, 1979), 48.

Note: t = metric ton (or 1.1023 U.S. tons).

being discharged into the Jinzū River basin, is with some quantitative data. Sphalerite is the most common zinc ore and contains iron and, in certain locations, cadmium and manganese. Between 1913 and 1930, refinery workers recovered 69.2 percent of the zinc from varying grades of sphalerite ore; between 1931 and 1945, by contrast, workers extracted 83.05 percent of the zinc (a 13.85 percent increase). Refinery workers discarded the remaining zinc, lead, and other heavy metals and toxins from the mine in the form of tailings. Between 1913 and 1930, miners discharged 62,877 metric tons (t) of zinc and 314.6 t of cadmium; between 1931 and 1945, although the extraction percentage had increased, so too had the amount of waste, to 64,131 t of zinc and 319 t of cadmium (a 1,254 t and 4 t increase, respectively). Finally, between 1955 and 1973, refinery workers discharged some 814 t of cadmium into the Jinzū River basin. Better zinc yields and hence higher Mitsui profits meant a more thoroughly cadmium-saturated landscape. At the same time that industrial flotation technologies increased yields, the pulverization process ensured that higher levels and more finely ground metallic waste inundated Japan's toxic archipelago.

EMPIRE AND POLLUTION

It was not only technologies that made the tailings from the Kamioka complex toxic but the changing nature of mine and refinery labor as well. Remember my earlier statement: polluting Japan has required an enormous amount of work (fig. 4.3). As the wartime government conscripted highly skilled miners to battlefields in China and the Pacific theater more broadly, Korean prisoners and other unskilled laborers, such as students or members of the Patriotic Labor Corps and Women's Volunteer Corps, steadily replaced them. Take some labor demographic figures: by 1943, 46 percent of the workers at the Kamioka complex—some 2,759 out of a total of 5,924 workers—were Korean prisoners or students. (The percentage of Koreans laboring in the "mining section" was even higher, at 60.2 percent.) Some 919 Allied prisoners also labored at the Kamioka complex during the Pacific War, after a camp was constructed in the township of Kamioka in 1943.[10] Of course, these Korean and Allied prisoners could be excused if they were less than enthusiastic about their new jobs; but the environmental consequences of their lack of enthusiasm and skill were eye-popping (see table 10). In 1941, the year Japan bombed Pearl Harbor, the percentage

TABLE 9 Wasted Zinc and Cadmium Estimates from Kamioka Concentration Process, 1913–30

| | KAMA MINE CONCENTRATOR | | | | MOZUMI MINE CONCENTRATOR | | | | TOTAL | | |
| | Raw ore | | | | Raw ore | | | | | | |
Year	Processed ore	Grade	Retrieved percentage	Wasted zinc	Processed ore	Grade	Retrieved Percentage	Wasted zinc	Processed ore	Wasted zinc	Wasted cadmium
1913	82,875 t	14.9%	66.2	4,174 t					82,875 t	4,174 t	20.9 t
1914	90,272 t	14.7%	70.1	3,968 t					90,272 t	3,968 t	19.8 t
1915	90,375 t	14.9%	69.4	4,121 t					90,375 t	4,121 t	20.6 t
1916	89,470 t	14.7%	70.5	3,880 t					89,470 t	3,880 t	19.4 t
1917	85,725 t	14.6%	71.9	3,517 t					85,725 t	3,517 t	17.6 t
1918	74,804 t	14.2%	71.8	2,995 t					74,804 t	2,995 t	15.0 t
1919	87,610 t	13.5%	70.7	3,465 t					87,610 t	3,465 t	17.3 t
1920	90,799 t	12.8%	71.0	3,370 t					90,799 t	3,370 t	16.9 t
1921	90,252 t	12.5%	67.8	3,632 t					90,252 t	3,632 t	18.2 t
1922	89,389 t	12.0%	71.0	3,111 t					89,389 t	3,111 t	15.6 t
1923	90,948 t	11.6%	71.8	2,975 t					90,948 t	2,975 t	14.9 t
1924	96,075 t	9.9%	67.1	3,129 t					96,075 t	3,129 t	15.6 t
1925	96,370 t	9.3%	62.3	3,379 t					96,370 t	3,379 t	16.9 t
1926	100,520 t	9.0%	62.3	3,411 t					100,520 t	3,411 t	17.1 t
1927	118,110 t	8.4%	62.1	3,760 t					118,110 t	3,760 t	18.8 t
1928	136,565 t	7.8%	64.6	3,771 t					136,565 t	3,771 t	18.9 t
1929	155,139 t	7.1%	76.3	2,611 t	28,923 t	10.3%	80.8	572 t	184,062 t	3,183 t	15.9 t
1930	171,749 t	6.9%	78.9	2,500 t	28,470 t	9.5%	80.2	536 t	200,219 t	3,036 t	15.2 t
Total				61,769 t						62,877 t	314.6 t

Source: Kurachi Mitsuo, Tonegawa Haruo, and Hata Akio, eds., Mitsui shihon to itai itai byō (Mitsui Capital and "It Hurts, It Hurts Disease") (Tokyo: Ōtsuki Shoten, 1979), 61.

Note: t = metric ton (or 1.1023 U.S. tons).

TABLE 10 Wasted Zinc and Cadmium Estimates from Kamioka Concentration Process, 1931–45

Year	KAMA MINE CONCENTRATOR Raw ore				MOZUMI MINE CONCENTRATOR Raw ore				TOTAL		
	Processed ore	Grade	Retrieved percentage	Wasted zinc	Processed ore	Grade	Retrieved Percentage	Wasted zinc	Processed ore	Wasted zinc	Wasted cadmium
1931	175,092 t	6.7%	78.8	2,487 t	29,560 t	9.5%	78.2	612 t	204,652 t	3,099 t	15 t
1932	180,006 t	6.7%	78.5	2,593 t	30,785 t	9.4%	79.9	582 t	210,791 t	3,175 t	16 t
1933	201,707 t	6.6%	80.3	2,623 t	35,350 t	8.8%	78.8	659 t	237,057 t	3,292 t	16 t
1934	207,528 t	6.6%	82.3	2,424 t	35,240 t	8.1%	82.5	500 t	242,879 t	2,924 t	15 t
1935	208,615 t	6.6%	85.3	2,024 t	35,100 t	8.0%	84.6	432 t	243,715 t	2,456 t	12 t
1936	270,009 t	6.1%	85.5	2,388 t	32,460 t	8.2%	84.2	421 t	302,469 t	2,809 t	14 t
1937	330,135 t	5.9%	86.2	2,688 t	36,120 t	7.5%	80.2	536 t	366,255 t	3,224 t	16 t
1938	441,100 t	5.8%	87.6	3,172 t	36,470 t	7.1%	79.8	523 t	477,570 t	3,695 t	18 t
1939	451,407 t	5.6%	83.0	4,297 t	38,660 t	7.4%	83.0	486 t	490,067 t	4,783 t	24 t
1940	751,820 t	5.1%	84.0	6,135 t	55,740 t	7.5%	84.0	669 t	807,560 t	6,804 t	34 t
1941	700,415 t	4.7%	89.0	3,621 t	44,570 t	6.7%	89.0	328 t	744,985 t	3,949 t	20 t
1942	729,810 t	4.7%	87.0	4,459 t	51,538 t	7.1%	87.0	476 t	781,348 t	4,905 t	24 t
1943	850,532 t	5.0%	88.0	5,103 t	68,680 t	7.6%	88.0	626 t	919,212 t	5,729 t	29 t
1944	884,891 t	5.2%	80.0	9,203 t	63,700 t	6.8%	80.0	866 t	948,591 t	10,069 t	50 t
1945	322,585 t	4.1%	79.0	2,777 t	31,570 t	6.8%	79.0	451 t	354,155 t	3,228 t	16 t
Total	6,705,652 t			55,994 t	625,543 t			8,167 t	7,331,195 t	64,131 t	319 t

Source: Kurachi Mitsuo, Tonegawa Haruo, and Hata Akio, eds., *Mitsui shihon to itai itai byō* (Mitsui Capital and "It Hurts, It Hurts Disease") (Tokyo: Ōtsuki Shoten, 1979), 106.

Note: t = metric ton (or 1.1023 U.S. tons).

of zinc recovered at the Kama and Mozumi concentrators was 89 percent, while the amounts of zinc and cadmium discharged as waste were 3,949 t and 20 t, respectively. However, by 1944, with Japan's military irreparably broken and skilled miners being drafted to the front, the yield percentage had decreased to 80 percent, and waste amounts had skyrocketed several-fold to 10,069 t for zinc and 50 t for cadmium. (That is, dislocated and poorly trained labor led to a 9 percent drop in zinc recovery and an increase of waste on the order of 6,120 t and 30 t, respectively.) Basically, the Kamioka mines went back in time ten years. In other words, the best recipe for the creation of high quantities of such pollutants as heavy metals and other poisons was also the most economically profitable during the war years: advanced technologies and cheap, unskilled prison labor. The lesson: creating monstrous environmental disasters requires the perfect storm of ecological and historical conditions. Environmental toxicology is a condition of history.

One other technological advancement led to the discharge of more pollutants from the Kamioka complex. In 1927–28, engineers introduced new

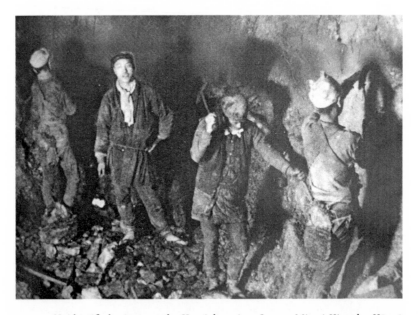

FIG. 4.3 Unidentified miners at the Kamioka mine. *Source:* Mitsui Kinzoku Kōgyō Kabushikigaisha Shūshi Iinkai Jimukyoku, ed., *Kamioka kōzan shashinshū* (Photograph Collection of the Kamioka Mine) (Tokyo: Mitsui Kinzoku Kōgyō Kabushiki-gaisha, 1975).

technologies that extracted desired minerals from the slime created by the pulverization of ore that refinery workers had discarded. This process, however, led to even more finely ground ore dust being discharged into the Takahara River, a tributary of the Jinzū River. Because the ore dust was so finely pulverized, it easily oxidized and created metallic ions. In turn, downstream agricultural crops easily absorbed these naturalized metallic ions.

Oxidation is an ionization process whereby oxygen is added to a compound, with a corresponding loss of electrons. Ionization is the process whereby neutral atoms or molecules convert into ions, which are electrically charged particles. Heat or radiation, such as that emanating from the sun, can cause the conversion. Aiding the conversion can be a solvent such as water, with which the ionic substance, in this case cadmium, molecularly associates itself. In effect, there is an atomic or molecular reconfiguration that partially disguises the substance as either oxygen or water—both vital life-giving substances—and, hence, allows it to be more easily absorbed into a given organism. And herein lies nature's agency once again: the heavy metal cadmium morphed from essentially inorganic to organic matter, and its new composition meant that it easily penetrated plant and animal tissue. The metal became more "bioavailable."

Dams constructed by Hokuriku Electric Power in 1954–55 did little to settle the particulate matter or stem the oxidization process. With hundreds of metric tons of ionizing cadmium and other metals being washed down the Takahara River and into the Jinzū River basin, it should not be surprising that people living downstream suffered industrial disease. But even in the Tokugawa years, villagers had reported problems with irrigation water. In 1694, for example, Zuiganji Temple documents tell of farmers complaining of "bad water" originating from the Kamioka silver mine. Farmers in Kama, Tono, and Higashimachi villages voiced similar complaints regarding tainted irrigation and drinking water emanating from the complex throughout the first half of the nineteenth century. Immediately after the Meiji Restoration, farmers in Kama Village complained in 1872 of "ore-muddied water," and throughout the latter half of the nineteenth century, they complained to local officials of "bad water" with damaging effects on crops and human health.[11] Because of the relative lack of technological sophistication at the mine, "bad water" was probably confined to areas close to the Kamioka complex: engineers had yet to design the technologies that could pulverize ore so finely that it seamlessly entered the bodies of plants and animals. When not sorting ore by hand, for example, pre-1906 methods included the *zaruba* method, in which a bamboo sifter was shaken while water was poured through it; the *neko nagashi* method, in which water ran through a wooden gutter and the heavier ore settled at the bottom of the gutter; and, later, the "Duncan gravitational method," which sorted only particles larger than 8 mm and so did not leave as finely ground tailings as flotation technologies.

After Mitsui assumed control of the mine in 1873, the ten mining wards that were the Kamioka complex constituted 187 mine shafts, 108 smelting sites (where miners smelted lead from silver and copper ore), and 168 roasting areas (where miners used ore-burning furnaces to burn off sulfur). Similar to the situation at the Ashio complex, one dangerous source of pollution emitted from the smelting and roasting furnaces was sulfur. At the Kamioka mines, one roasting furnace (made from stone masonry and about 1.5 meters tall and 1.2 meters in diameter) dressed over eight pounds (300 Japanese *kan*) of ore and burned eighteen Japanese legal feet of wood (one *shaku*, or about one linear foot) in a little over one week. From such roasting furnaces, ore with a sulfur content of about 20 percent emitted about 5–6 percent sulfur dioxide into the atmosphere, which, as we saw with the environments around Ashio, transformed into sulfuric acid through atmospheric photochemical processes. After the introduction of reflecting technologies, such as the "White revolving furnace," ore with high sulfur content taken from the Mozumi and Kama sites of the Kamioka complex could be smelted, releasing even more sulfur dioxide into the atmosphere. Nonetheless, at Kamioka, the principal polluter was always cadmium in the food chain, not sulfur dioxide in the atmosphere (see table 11).

CADMIUM AND PAIN

Over time, physicians began to see the results of the technologies of mass destruction, of the labor generated by mass relocation, and of natural agencies. In 1946, the physician Hagino Noboru (b. 1915), after returning from the war, reopened his small practice in the town of Fuchu in Toyama Prefecture. No doubt he had seen many gruesome and quite-painful wounds as a military physician. But in August 1955, the disease he encountered was formally named *itai itai byō*, or "it hurts, it hurts disease," because of the agony it caused its victims. Even before the naming of the disease, as early as 1947, physicians had constructed a social profile of the disease: farming women between the ages of forty and seventy who had experienced multiple child deliveries constituted the overwhelming majority of the victims. In the 1940s, physicians suspected the relatively common disease, osteomalacia (a softening of bones caused by a vitamin D deficiency or the inability to metabolize this vitamin), as the culprit. Even in the 1940s, however, farmers suspected that polluted water from the Kamioka mine complex was to blame. Along with osteomalacia and osteoporosis (thinning of bone tissue and a loss of bone density over time), symptoms of the disease included excruciatingly severe pain in the inguinal (near the groin) and lumbar (back area between hipbones and ribs) regions, a ducklike gait, proteinuria (high levels of protein in the urine, usually the result of kidney disorder), and glycosuria (high levels of sugar in the urine).[12]

Later studies proved Toyama farmers to be correct. These farmers, we should recall, were environmental engineers in their own right, and they knew nature through laboring at their own rice paddies and silkworm nurseries, just as miners knew nature through their labor underground. Public health officials eventually told the farmers something they already knew: the Kamioka mines were poisoning women. In a report published in 1970, Yamagata Noboru and Shigematsu Itsuzō, from the Institute of Public Health in Tokyo (Kokuritsu Kōshū Eisei'in), outlined the symptoms and causes of "it hurts, it hurts disease." Their conclusion: women proved particularly susceptible, and catalyzing factors included pregnancy, lactation, aging, calcium deficiencies (more a problem for women than men), "unbalanced internal secretion," and having lived in the Jinzū River basin for more than thirty years. Consider this statistic: at the end of March 1968, of the "number of patients to be treated," physicians suspected that one man had the disease, while seventy-two women either had the disease or were suspected of having it. Yamagata and Shigematsu also examined data related to the cadmium content of the Jinzū River and its tributaries. Water tested upstream from the Kamioka complex contained trace or nondetectable amounts of cadmium; however, water downstream from the mine contained a maximum value of 9 ng/g (ng/g = nanograms of constituent per gram of soil or water or tissue; or parts per billion, ppb). This is about 9 ounces of cadmium for every 7.5 million gallons of water. Tests of drainage water emanating from the Kamioka complex fluctuated wildly between 5 ng/g and over 4,000 ng/g (4,000 ppb). To place these numbers in perspective, the U.S. Environmental Protection Agency (EPA) has set a "maxi-

TABLE 11 Cadmium Waste from Kamioka Complex Zinc Smelting, 1955–73

	ZINC ROASTING AMOUNT Zinc electrolysis amount				CADMIUM SMELTING AMOUNT				
Year	1. Ore smelted (t/month)	2. Cadmium grade	3. Retrieved percentage	4. Cadmium waste (t/month)	1. Residue (leavings) (t/month)	2. Cadmium grade	3. Retrieved percentage	4. Cadmium waste (t/month)	Yearly total
1955	2,880	0.0032	0.1924	1.773	19.200	0.3030	0.0839	0.488	27.30
1956	3,190	0.0028	0.0890	0.795	25.142	0.2875	0.0875	0.632	34.62
	2,584	0.0033	0.1710	1.458					
1957	6,295	0.0036	—	—	25.383	0.3465	0.0800	0.704	25.63
	2,945	0.0034	0.1430	1.431					
1958	3,632	0.0029	—	—	36.100	0.2560	0.0500	0.462	12.32
	2,992	0.0032	0.0590	0.564					
1959	3,531	0.0034	0.0200	0.240	35.120	0.2860	0.0500	0.502	24.70
	3,243	0.0035	0.1160	1.317					
1960	3,658	0.0029	0.0180	0.190	40.200	0.2530	0.0500	0.509	21.54
	3,290	0.0034	0.0980	1.096					
1961	4,794	0.0031	0.0050	0.074	45.700	0.3020	0.0500	0.690	28.73
	3,913	0.0035	0.1190	1.629					
1962	4,990	0.0031	0.0050	0.077	47.200	0.2660	0.0490	0.615	23.21
	4,045	0.0035	0.1090	1.543					
1963	4,910	0.0031	0.0200	0.304	52.100	0.2730	0.0500	0.711	33.56
	4,587	0.0035	0.1110	1.782					

Year									
1964	7,512	0.0031	0.0200	0.465	61.400	0.2840	0.0520	0.907	41.76
	6,560	*0.0021*	*0.1530*	*2.108*					
1965	7,746	0.0031	0.0200	0.480	72.100	0.2920	0.0500	1.053	52.89
	7,023	*0.0035*	*0.1170*	*2.875*					
1966	8,584	0.0030	0.0200	0.515	72.400	0.2990	0.0500	1.082	51.80
	7,269	*0.0034*	*0.1100*	*2.719*					
1967	9,286	0.003	0.0200	0.557	77.000	0.3150	0.0500	1.213	56.47
	7,766	*0.003*	*0.1260*	*2.935*					
1968	9,139	0.003	0.0200	0.548	72.900	0.3290	0.0500	1.199	64.32
	8,028	*0.003*	*0.1500*	*3.613*					
1969	9,422	0.003	0.0200	0.565	68.700	0.3490	0.0500	1.199	63.47
	7,835	*0.003*	*0.1500*	*3.525*					
1970	9,282	0.003	0.0700	1.949	64.500	0.3730	0.0500	1.203	83.17
	7,823	*0.0035*	*0.1380*	*3.779*					
1971	8,108	0.003	0.0140	0.341	57.300	0.3630	0.0480	0.998	57.20
	6,896	*0.0035*	*0.1420*	*3.427*					
1972	9,580	0.0032	0.0110	0.337	52.800	0.4750	0.0460	1.154	57.02
	7,348	*0.0035*	*0.1270*	*3.266*					
1973	9,030	0.0032	0.0060	0.173	54.800	0.4420	0.0200	0.484	54.99
	7,380	*0.0035*	*0.1520*	*3.926*					
									814.53

Source: Kurachi Mitsuo, Tonegawa Haruo, and Hata Akio, eds., *Mitsui shihon to itai itai byō* (Mitsui Capital and "It Hurts, It Hurts Disease") (Tokyo: Ōtsuki Shoten, 1979), 157.

Note: t = metric ton (or 1.1023 U.S. tons).

mum contaminant level goal" for cadmium in drinking water at 5 ng/g.[13]

In 1959, two other public health officials performed tests on polished rice. In the endemic area, they discovered cadmium levels of 120–350 µg/g, as opposed to levels of 21 µg/g in the control area (µg/g = micrograms of constituent per gram of soil or water or tissue; or parts per million). Shedding light on how the oxidized emissions from the mine—nature's agency in the form of metallic ions—contaminated the rice, tests on the root systems of rice plants revealed fluctuating figures as high as 690–1,300 µg/g in the endemic area, as opposed to 35 µg/g in the control area. In 1964, Moritsugu Masumi and Kobayashi Jun tested polished rice samples from every Japanese prefecture for cadmium content. Of those samples, a zinc-poisoned mining area in Gunma Prefecture provided the highest, at 1.195 µg/g, while an agricultural experimental station in Tokyo came in second at 0.472 µg/g and 0.421 µg/g. The Toyama agricultural experimental station came in a close third at 0.413 µg/g cadmium content. For the entire prefecture, Toyama (0.189 µg/g) was second only to Tokyo (0.218 µg/g). Of the 203 rice samples taken from throughout the country, the average was 0.066 µg/g. Hence, Toyama Prefecture stood dangerously above the already high national average. Finally, one gets a sense of just how toxic the Jinzū River basin had become when considering samples from specifically mine-polluted areas. Downstream from the Ashio complex on the Watarase River, Moritsugu and Kobayashi measured a cadmium level of 0.243 µg/g, while downstream from the Annaka zinc refinery in the Usui River basin in Gunma Prefecture, they measured a cadmium level of 0.393 µg/g. In the Jinzū River basin, however, the researchers reported 0.683 µg/g.[14]

As a result of these and other alarming studies, in 1968 the Ministry of Health and Welfare (Kōseishō; established in 1938) concluded that chronic cadmium exposure caused the painful disease. In a 1969 study, the ministry extrapolated from earlier tests to generate numbers regarding the daily cadmium consumption of those living in the endemic area. The government estimated that, if the average Japanese person ate 335 grams of rice per day, then his or her daily cadmium intake would be 60 µg/g. If figures produced by Moritsugu and Kobayashi for the endemic region held, this meant that the average cadmium intake of people living along the Jinzū River was 600 µg/g—ten times the national average. During the Pacific War, the Ministry of Health and Welfare estimated that the average concentration in drinking water had been 500 ng/g, or a hundred times the EPA's recommendations. In other words, tests conducted in the 1950s and 1960s identified the interface between the Kamioka complex, the Jinzū River basin ecosystem, engineered rice paddies, and human bodies.

To review, starting in 1909 with the Potter method, flotation technologies at Kamioka had been used that, over the decades, required ever finer pulverized ore. Mining waste washed into the Takahara River and, because it was so finely pulverized, delivered increasingly oxidized cadmium to irrigation systems. Irrigation systems brought water to the roots of rice plants and, ultimately, into the grains of rice that entered the mouths and bodies of farmers living in the affected area. This vector, in turn, introduced poisons to their bodies that caused irreparable harm and painful disease. A bufferless web had emerged among the technologies at the Kamioka complex, the Jinzū River basin ecosystem, and the bodies of the people who called the area home.

POPULATION

"Sick-building syndrome" is an elusive postindustrial illness that, since the 1980s, has sickened women in the United States who work in modern, airtight buildings with efficient, open floor plans. In her exploration of this syndrome, Michelle Murphy traces the gendered "assemblages" (or the "material and yet relational way things came to matter") that led to certain chemical exposures. New kinds of building materials ranging from plastics and adhesives to synthetic carpets and particle board emitted chemicals in air-conditioned and dehumidified spaces designed to protect computers and copy machines. Working in such a potentially toxic environment is specific to the information age. This is "indoor pollution," which, over time, sickened women's bodies with a variety of mysterious symptoms for which it remains hard to identify one causative agent. But chemicals and architecture are not alone among the "assemblages" because gender also shaped the manner in which women were exposed to indoor chemicals. By the twentieth century, writes Murphy, office buildings "had become sites for the articulation of a gendered division of labor and a landscape of privilege in which most menial office work was designated a kind of 'women's work.'" Murphy deploys the term "assemblages" to describe the "historically specific patterns through which building and bodies were connected," noting that these relationships have different histories. Hence, both female bodies and postindustrial buildings proved to be assemblages, ones that contributed to the nature of sick-building syndrome. That is, assemblages—or what we might view as intertwining histories or webs of causation—provided the occupational exposure that, for all its mystery, seriously sickened women.[15]

Similarly, Gregg Mitman, in his history of asthma, argues that health officials had pieced together a causal web for asthma in the twentieth-century United States, one that included cockroach allergens, genetic differences, social class, inhalation of dust mites, air pollution, and, as one might expect, inadequate access to proper health care. In cities such as New Orleans, for example, the legacies of racial, environmental, and economic inequalities structured the nature of the epidemic. Of course, this assertion closely resembles the hybrid causations model used in this book, where natural forces intertwine with historical forces to cause disease. Mitman investigates all these causative agents and others; however, the root of the problem, he insists, was a historical one. "America's urban asthma epidemic," Mitman writes, "long in the making, is a product of the ecology of injustice that structured urban life."[16] Modifying Mitman's language, we might argue that "it hurts, it hurts disease" in Japan was the product of the ecology of gender discrimination and rural poverty that structured Japanese society in the late nineteenth and early twentieth centuries. Downstream from the Kamioka mines, what placed rural women in danger of cadmium poisoning was a cluster of historical forces, ranging from Meiji pronouncements regarding ideal female behavior to the imperial ethnography of skin complexion.

Though distinct, Murphy's and Mitman's approaches are helpful for understanding the outbreak of "it hurts, it hurts disease" in the Jinzū River basin. In our case, though, the assemblages and ecologies under consideration look a little different: the Japanese state's policies promoting childbirth, menopausal physiologies, and idealized definitions of female beauty provided the causative factors necessary for the disease. Moreover, the assemblage of gender history caused, not occupational exposure, but rather physiological susceptibility to the cadmium poisoning.[17] Those rural women who honored modern Japan's principal definition of ideal female behavior—nicely captured in educator Nakamura Masanao's (1832–91) slogan *ryōsai kenbo*, or "good wife, wise mother"—proved most susceptible to the painful effects of industrial disease.[18] Starting about 1890, the Meiji government had rallied women to serve as the moral foundation of the modern nation. As historians Sharon Nolte and Sally Hastings have written, "State propaganda exhorted women to contribute to the nation through their hard work, their frugality, their efficient management, their care of the old, young, and ill, and their responsible upbringing of children."[19] Confucian ideology provided much of the underpinning for the "good wife, wise mother" slogan. It stressed primogeniture, ancestor worship, social and political patriarchy, patrilocal cohabitation practices, and the general subordination of women. By the turn of the century, the Meiji government had eulogized women as the bedrock of Japan's emerging *kazoku kokka*, or "family state." As Sheldon Garon writes, these good wives and wise mothers emerged as central to the "nation's strength, prosperity, and moral well-being."[20]

To be sure, in the Tokugawa period (1600–1868) it was considered women's duty to bear many children to strengthen warlord households; after 1898, however, and the adoption of a new Japanese Civil Code, women again were urged to produce many children, only this time for the family and Japan's burgeoning empire.[21] Despite women's important social roles, however, Meiji oligarchs, in legal actions taken in 1890 and 1900, summarily banned women from participating in political gatherings of any kind. To my mind, Nolte and Hastings phrased it perfectly when they wrote: "The Japanese state denied political rights to women because the state's claims on the home preempted women's claims on the state."[22]

Besides being called upon to supply children, women shouldered an enormous portion of Japan's industrial burden. "Factory girls" provided one type of labor during Japan's first economic miracle.[23] In the next chapter we shall see how women suffered as the mothers of badly deformed children, the offspring of mercury poisoning in the environment surrounding Minamata. Women downstream from the Kamioka mines suffered disproportionately from cadmium poisoning as well, particularly those women who labored in the paddies and gave birth to children, just as the Meiji government had instructed them to do. Surely, Japanese women near Minamata and downstream from the Kamioka mines knew the state through pain. Women were rewarded for their obedience to the nation with industrial disease for a complex set of reasons related to female physiology and cultural practices. Just as Japanese B encephalitis spread as a result of a convergence of Buddhist burial practices, mosquito ecologies, and industrial pig farming, so too did the spread of "it hurts, it hurts disease" depend on a convergence of wartime economic needs, technological advancement, dislocated labor, environmental toxicology, Japanese family values, rural behavior, and the ethnographic aesthetics of empire.

Women who gave birth to children to continue their husband's family, to labor in Japan's factories, or to serve in Japan's Imperial Army and Navy weakened their femurs and sternums, which made them more susceptible to "it hurts, it hurts disease" than men. Weighed down by the state's expectations, they became virtual repositories of heavy metals. The autopsy of one "extremely severe patient" revealed cadmium levels in the femur and sternum of 15,000 µg/g and 10,000 µg/g, respectively.[24] In 1968, when Toyama Prefecture health authorities registered those who suffered from cadmium poisoning, 184 were women and 33 were men. (That is, 85 percent of the prefecture's victims were women.) Of those women, 78 percent were between the ages of sixty and seventy-nine years, which means that they would have been postmenopausal and born between 1889 and 1908.[25] These were the years during which the Meiji government pushed the "good wife, wise mother" slogan most aggressively. Though only circumstantial evidence, it strongly suggests that it was the generation of good wives and wise mothers of Japan's late Meiji period who suffered pain the most in the Jinzū River basin.

Here are some other social drivers that determined cadmium poisoning in the Jinzū River basin. By the late Meiji period, for many affluent urban women the "core of women's familial and social obligations" had become household management and birthing children. However, less-affluent rural women continued to split their time between household divisions of labor reminiscent of the Tokugawa years. That is, they not only managed their households but also engaged in agricultural labor and birthed children.[26] The 1982 book *The Women of Suye Mura*, which carefully documents the sexual and working lives of Japanese women in a village, bears out this assertion.[27] In a 1967 investigation, researchers determined that 96 percent of female victims of cadmium poisoning had lived in the Jinzū River basin for "40 years or more," that 83 percent of them had "worked in agriculture," and that 56 percent had had "six or more pregnancies."[28]

In the 1967 investigation, one statistic really jumps out: 56 percent of the female victims of "it hurts, it hurts disease" had "six or more pregnancies." Historically speaking, "six or more pregnancies" is a higher number of pregnancies for individual Japanese women than in previous decades. To demonstrate this, we now turn to the slippery topic of pregnancies, family size, and population for a moment. To show that women living in the Jinzū River basin experienced an increase in pregnancies and family size, we need to establish that family size increased after the advent of the Meiji state. Unfortunately, this will not determine the precise motivations behind increased individual pregnancies, nor will it take into account such variables as infanticide rates.[29]

The evidence for increased family size is overwhelming. Between 1721 and 1846, Japan's total population hovered around 26 million; the Hokuriku region (which includes Toyama, Ishikawa, Fukui, and Niigata prefectures) may have seen a negligible 0.13 percent increase in population during this time period. Thomas Smith concluded, "It is clear that there was no growth of the national population between 1721 and 1846."[30] By contrast, Akira Hayami estimated that Japan's 1700 population might have been as high as 30 million, but then stagnated throughout the eighteenth century. On the eve of the Meiji Restoration, Japan's population stood at 35 million, with some of that growth having occurred in the Hokuriku region (perhaps by as much as 10–20 percent, depending on the year). Japan's population was 45 million by 1900.[31] In sum, there was little or no population change in the latter half of the Tokugawa period, but then exponential growth after the Meiji Restoration. We can only assume that an increase in the pregnancy rate occurred because of a bundle of nineteenth-century factors, ranging from better medicine and higher standards of living to Meiji slogans designed to have just that effect.

Given the stagnant eighteenth-century population, it makes sense that fertility rates and individual family sizes remained modest in the Tokugawa period. Laurel Cornell notes that stagnant population growth in the eighteenth century was a product of a constellation of factors, including mortality (famine and disease), fertility (infanticide), and temporary migration for labor (called *dekasegi*), which separated couples and, hence, reduced coital frequency.[32] The cumulative effect was little to no population growth. In central Japan, between 1716 and 1823, Smith concluded that the average family size was 4.4 souls. Even among large landholders (defined by Smith as families possessing over eighteen *koku*; a *koku* is a piece of land that could produce about five bushels of rice per year) the mean family size was just 5.3.[33] The Tokugawa shoguns expressed little interest in increasing family sizes, though some domain lords pursued policies designed to increase their populations. The Tokugawa shoguns, for example, did not establish any formal strictures against abortion until 1842, a policy that was principally enforced in Edo (the Tokugawa capital). In the countryside, a 1767 recommendation encouraged neighbors to watch out for infanticide, but it remains difficult to determine the degree to which they actually did. But domain lords did take some interest in increasing populations, because of the economic and agricultural stagnation caused by population decline. Both translated into decreased tax revenues. In Kasama Domain, for example, the domain lord ordered Confucian vassals to lecture farmers on the immorality of infanticide and abortion according to Buddhist precepts. In Sendai Domain, villages set aside economic resources for infant care, in order to curtail infanticide and abortion rates. This policy was institutionalized in 1796 and was underwritten by a revolution in the manner in which Japanese physicians (as we shall see in the next chapter) came to view reproductive medicine. Pointing to these seventeenth- through nineteenth-century Japanese demographic trends, Ochiai Emiko has concluded that the population growth that occurred in the latter half of the nineteenth century—the period we are most concerned with here—was the result of the "centralized control over individual lives" that was wielded by the Meiji state. She continues: "A program to induce population growth itself was an aspect of this major reconstruction of society."[34] A critical part of that program to "induce population growth" was the "good wife, wise mother" campaign that was responsible for high pregnancies in Toyama and, hence, for leaving women vulnerable to "it hurts, it hurts disease."

However, cadmium poisoning was also the product of other determiners in Japanese society: the imperial ethnography of skin complexion, the fetish of whiteness, and religious notions of purity all interplayed to shape "it hurts, it hurts disease." In his pathbreaking investigation of the role of race in the Pacific War, John Dower argues that, in the United States, when it came to constructing racial stereotypes, biological conceptions of race linked "Japs" to other primates and even insects. I mentioned one example of these racist cultural stereotypes in chapter 1: American propagandists' labeling of Japanese as "Louseous Japanicas" to justify their extermination. Though the United States tapped into pervasive beliefs in the supremacy of "white people," Japanese, though purveyors of the concept of a "pan-Asian" brotherhood when convenient, only rarely articulated notions of "yellow supremacy" or "colored supremacy."[35] So, even though as early as 1884, Sugita Teiichi (1851–1920), in "Kō-A-saku" (Policy for Enlightening Asia), spoke of the "Yellow race" as being "devoured by the white," the concept of a "Yellow race" was purely a response to Western imperialism.[36] It turns out that Japanese, too, revered "whiteness" and sought to distance themselves from the "colored" Chinese and South Asians they oppressed within their empire, while still sometimes speaking of "pan-Asianism."

Reverence for whiteness can be traced far into Japan's ancient past. It is evidenced, for example, in ancient courtiers' practice of liberally caking their faces and necks with white paint and in the purity symbolism inherent in white Shinto robes and other regalia. In Japan, whiteness symbolized high social status, human beauty, pure complexion, and lightness, such as that which emanated from the sun. The tutelary deity of the imperial household—Amaterasu Ōmikami, the Sun Goddess—was associated with whiteness as well. Ancient courtiers, such as Sei Shōnagon, scorned people with dark skins as laborers. As Dower remarks, "Dark-skinned people were the laboring class, who worked in the sun."[37]

With notable exceptions, these attitudes toward pure white complexions have carried over into modern times, as any informal perusal of a Japanese cosmetic counter can attest. "Whitening" formulas abound. Unfortunately, limiting sun exposure and, hence, an important natural source of vitamin D proved one consequence of wearing clothing to protect from wind and sunburn. Vitamin D promotes the intestinal absorption and metabolism of calcium, which is critical in preventing osteomalacia and osteoporosis; the vitamin can be acquired by eating fish, eggs, and dairy products, but the skin also produces it when exposed to the sun. Here is the crux of the matter: if rural women painstakingly limited their exposure to the sun (and hence vitamin D) to maintain a white complexion, and if these same women ate few dairy products because of the traditional nature of their diet and just plain old-fashioned poverty, they certainly would have proven more susceptible to the effects of cadmium poisoning than men, who more often exposed their skin to sunlight and, hence, received vitamin D.

Of course, there were probably other proximate causes and mitigating factors: men might have had a diet with higher protein content, particularly while away in the army or school. This experience would not only have removed them from the endemic region but also would have provided them with more vitamin D. For the most part, however, men and women in the Jinzū River basin ate the same food, drank the same water, lived in the same homes, and tended the same paddies, and so we are left to identify those lifestyle habits and practices that differentiated women from men: gendered habits and practices. Just as Buddhist burial practices shaped the nature of Japanese B encephalitis epidemics, definitions of feminine beauty and, possibly, gendered access to diet shaped cadmium poisoning downstream from the Kamioka zinc mines.

In 1968, the Ministry of Health and Welfare had determined that "it hurts, it hurts disease" was pollution related. That same year, Toyama Prefecture established a relief system for "it hurts, it hurts" patients, which registered those souls suffering from the disease as well as provided medical care. On 9 March 1968, eight patients and the successors of six victims of the disease filed suit against the Mitsui Group, basing their lawsuit on a property liability article in the mining law of 1950. On 30 June 1971, the Toyama District Court awarded the plaintiffs ¥57 million in damages. Not surprisingly, Mitsui appealed the decision to the Nagoya High Court; however, the decision was upheld on 9 August 1972. Mitsui, not incorrectly, argued that factors other than cadmium poisoning, such as calcium deficiencies and generally poor nutrition, caused the disease; the epidemiological evidence swayed the Nagoya High Court, however, which, along with upholding the earlier decision, actually increased significantly the amount of damages. For our purposes, the Nagoya High Court's reliance on the web of causation, traced by the science of epidemiology, is an important one, because it demonstrates that the Japanese courts were beginning to understand the complexities—the hybrid causations—of environmental pollution and its deleterious effect on human health.[38]

So far the four chapters of this book have demonstrated the pitfalls of dividing historical analysis between artificial processes and natural ones. Instead, they have deployed a kind of intellectual fusion, wherein their analytical power lies in their utilization of different disciplinary strengths. Environmental problems and ensuing ecological collapse require this sustained, interdisciplinary attention, because their ultimate causations, and even proximate causations, remain so multifaceted and complicated.

In chapter 1, we saw that Buddhist burial practices, which involved hundreds of cisterns and flower receptacles in cemeteries, provided fertile breeding grounds near urban areas for mosquitoes that carried Japanese B encephalitis. Pigs, after Japan's nineteenth-century industrialization, lived near cities and served as "amplifying hosts," morphing the virus into a potentially deadly one. Encephalitis epidemics could never have occurred without these pigs, and placing them in large (and no doubt reeking) piggeries near cities was the product of modern agricultural reforms. Here, seamless interfaces among religious values, insect ecologies, and industrial agriculture caused twentieth-century outbreaks of infectious, highly painful, and neurologically debilitating disease.

Chapter 2 demonstrated how insects, because of the historical and unstable personalities that inhabited them, could also cause famine: insect predation was the product of ghosts and Buddhist transmigration rather than an adaptive mechanism for insect survival. Because spirit possession explained famine, the Tokugawa response was to cast spells and call on Japan's most powerful deities at temples and shrines; only they could take on the disgruntled spirits of centuries past. Later, after the advent of the chemical industry, parathion took the place of spells, but it proved just as enduring as the hatred in Sanemori's calloused heart. Just as Sanemori's bitter soul appeared to become more and more potent over time, parathion's potency amplified under certain natural agencies. It also induced hereditary resistances in insect populations, redirecting the path of evolution on Earth. As I insisted earlier: humans do not just write their history on paper or paint it on canvas but inscribe it onto the landscape and bodies of living organisms every day.

Chapter 3 and the current chapter explored two of Japan's most important mines. They traced the seamless interface among industrialization, wartime economies, advanced technologies, changing labor dynamics, the oxidation, ionization, and photochemical reactions that naturalized chemical emissions from mines, and the social and cultural drivers that shaped the nature of industrial disease. The Meiji "good wife, wise mother" campaign and imperial ethnographies related to skin complexion contributed to the manner in which cadmium poisoned rural communities in the Jinzū River basin. Human bodies are human bodies, no matter the country; and cadmium is cadmium: these are the normative aspects of the story that transcend society and culture. But together they tell only half the story. We have to search for factors other than human physiology, such as menopause or biochemistry, that drove the disproportionate dispersal of "it hurts, it hurts disease" to female bodies. Obviously, the adherence of women to the Meiji ideals of a "good wife, wise mother" set them up for painful disease, as did their efforts to whiten their complexions to fit the ideals of Japanese definitions of feminine beauty. The consequence for them was pain.

Yet, these rural women were lucky in one important regard. At least cadmium did not nefariously penetrate their placentas and disfigure and retard their children: that dubious distinction was left to mercury, the subject of the next chapter. What is worse, I wonder? Suffering the effects of cadmium poisoning in one's own body or the dire effects of mercury poisoning in the body of one's child? The latter represents the pain of helplessness when confronted with a loved one's suffering. But both are painful, which is precisely the point I have been making since the introduction.

5 MERCURY'S OFFSPRING

To this juncture, we have examined how the modern industrial endeavors of insecticide production and application and of copper, zinc, and lead mining introduced poisons to human bodies and caused pain. Both the organophosphate parathion and such heavy metals as cadmium in mining waste entered rice plants through engineered irrigation channels and paddy systems to become part of the food web and, ultimately, a part of bodies. This chapter turns our attention to the marine environments surrounding the Chisso fertilizer and plastics factory in Minamata City. Here organic mercury used as a catalyst in highly advanced chemical production was discharged into the marine ecosystem, where it biomagnified in the food web and poisoned that being at the pinnacle of the global food chain: the human fetus. The Chisso chemical plant and its engineered surroundings are a perfect example of a hybrid metabolism because both depended on the naturally occurring marine environment to function. Just as the Kamioka mines flushed waste into the Jinzū River basin, so too did the Chisso plant flush mercuric waste into its surroundings. The manner in which mercury behaved in the marine ecosystem and within human and nonhuman bodies constitutes the bulk of our story. This is because understanding how industrial disease caused pain in Minamata means understanding the manner in which natural and anthropogenic agencies function in concert. The results of these agencies became the global namesake of mercury poisoning: Minamata disease. It disfigured children and adults and remains the best-known episode discussed in this book.

In the introduction, I promised to imitate a Hmong storyteller's technique by connecting seemingly unrelated incidents in Japanese history. In describing Hmong storytelling, Anne Fadiman writes (in a passage I have already cited) that the "world is full of things that may not seem to be connected but actually are; that no event occurs in isolation; that you can miss a lot by sticking to the point; and that the storyteller is likely to be rather long-winded."[1] No environmental pollution episode explored in this book has as many elements "that may not seem to be connected but actually are" as the outbreak of methylmercury poisoning in Minamata. Therefore, this chapter is divided into two parts. Part I starts with a description and interpretation of the pain suffered by one Minamata disease patient after she underwent an abortion at Kumamoto University Hospital. It then spirals outward to talk about the various connections between this woman's pain and the marine environments in which she lived. To do so, we investigate the histories of Japanese fishing communities, the role of cats in coastal ecologies, bioaccumulation, and the life cycles of two other organisms important for our story: the mussel called *hibarigaimodoki* and the anchovy called *katakuchiiwashi*. Bridging these ecological connections is critical to understanding why this patient suffered the pain she did. Part II will depart from the realm of ecological and historical connections to investigate cultural and medical ones.

PART I

Mercury Poisoning and Pain

After dark, in Kumamoto University Hospital, forty-five-year-old Sakagami Yuki, a fisherwoman from a village near Minamata City, struggled alone to sit upright in her hospital bed. After a life at sea, her once beautiful skin now appeared wrapped too tightly around her emaciated body. The bed creaked loudly and jostled precariously as her slender arms hoisted her thin body upright. Fidgeting, she looked down toward the floor, searching for an oily fish that had slipped from her chopsticks moments earlier. As she scanned the poorly lit floor, the chopsticks clattered noisily against the plate that she clenched in her quaking hands. Different parts of her body often shook uncontrollably: she could only partially govern her movements.

"Come here, darling," she pleaded to the fish. "Don't run away from your mamma." As she spoke, a nervous smile formed on her lips. Still quaking, she positioned her arms beneath her hips and unsteadily eased herself from the hospital bed. It creaked loudly, again. Once down, she began crawling on her hands and knees on the floor. Spotting the fish, she had to use both hands to grab her dinner. "Now, don't you try to escape," she scolded it. "I'll put you out of your misery once and for all." She then stuffed the morsel into her mouth and swallowed it. When she was through, oil and filth from the fish and floor covered her lips and face; she wiped her hands childishly on her hospital gown and then slipped back into bed.

In May 1959, Sakagami recounted this disturbing episode to Ishimure Michiko (b. 1927), who wrote about it in her sobering *Kugai jōdo: Waga Minamatabyō* (Paradise in the Sea of Sorrow: Our Minamata Disease), published in 1972.[2] Sakagami suffered from Minamata disease, or methylmercury poisoning: an industrial disease caused by heavily polluted marine waters that sickened women such as Sakagami and brutally killed, or spared but grotesquely maimed, their unborn children. As we have seen, industrial disease occurs as a result of hybrid causation, because of complex and largely unanticipated interrelationships among advanced technologies, idiosyncratic social practices, and naturally occurring agencies. Indeed, cultural attitudes, such as striving for pure white skin, left rural women vulnerable to vitamin D deficiencies and, hence, osteomalacia in Toyama Prefecture; but naturally occurring processes, such as metallic oxidization and ionization, also made cadmium more bioavailable to human consumers through absorption into rice plants. In the case of Minamata disease, this hybrid causation took on an entirely different form, one analyzed in the pages ahead.

"I must have been mad," Sakagami confided. The episode had actually started when Kumamoto doctors advised her to have an abortion because of complications caused by mercury poisoning, the same toxin that had caused her to lose control of her mind and talk to a cooked fish. "When they pulled it out with their horrible instruments," she explained of her procedure, "my baby writhed in pain, and kicked with its tiny arms and legs." That night, after the abortion, a nurse had brought the fish for her dinner; but she began hallucinating that the fish on the plate was her discharged fetus. "I gasped in horror," she remembered, "convinced that the fish on the tray was the baby the doctors had pulled out of my womb a few hours before." Delirious and determined to mercifully eat her fetus and spare it the chronic pain she experienced daily, she said to it: "You poor little thing, I'll get it over with quickly. I can't bear to look at you, lying on that plate, all smeared with my blood." It was then that she had tried to grip the slippery fish with her chopsticks and it had flopped onto the hospital floor.

In only four years, methylmercury had destroyed enough cells in Sakagami's brain to deprive her of control of herself almost entirely: mercury devours the brains of adults and stops the development of fetal ones. Now confined to Minamata City Hospital, after her abortion Sakagami tried to summon memories of her life with Mohei, her husband of three years, as if a person whose mind mercury had so badly maimed could retrieve those memories easily. "I've spent all my life on the sea," she said in a fading voice. Her life with Mohei and their shared livelihood at sea had represented a kind of tidal motion replete with symbols of fertility. Mohei had launched his new fishing boat (a cherished investment) on the same auspicious day as their wedding. In an earlier era, launching boats and sexuality had intertwined metaphorically. Within the "floating world" of Japanese courtesans, shinzō, or a "newly launched boat," described a young courtesan whose virginity had been taken by a wealthy customer in the pleasure quarters.[3] However, even more pertinently, the word shinzō also meant "new wife" and was associated with family and fertility. Water, in turn, the substance on which boats floated, represented infinite possibility in the Buddhist order. Indeed, aborted fetuses were often called mizuko, or "water children." In coastal communities, the boat served as the principal means by which fishers extracted their harvest from the sea. Referring to the fishing boat, she said, "I took care of it as if it were my own child."

In some respects, boats assumed similar roles in fishing households as children, because they, like children in traditional Confucian linearity, ensured longevity across generations. It should not be surprising that the one thing that troubled Minamata residents most about their disease was that it often terminated their family lines: toxins struck at the core of Japan's social order—the Confucian ie, or family/household, system—by destroying fetuses and leaving women barren. The disease robbed women of the ability to produce offspring, their exclusive roles as creators of male heirs to whom to pass down the family name, to assist with worshiping tutelary ancestors, and to relay knowledge about setting nets, dropping lines, laying traps, and reading tides and currents. The real tragedy of Minamata disease was that, along with killing fishers, it collectively destroyed families by mercilessly devouring the carriers of their fragile futures.[4]

Japan's Fishing Communities

Fishers such as Sakagami could do little about the poisoning of their coastal homes and families. Japanese fishers have always lived outside mainstream political and economic power, whether wielded by emperors, shoguns, Meiji oligarchs, or industrialists. But this situation has deep cultural roots. The *Kojiki* (Record of Ancient Matters; 712) relays a myth wherein the grandson of Amaterasu Ōmikami, the Sun Goddess, sired two children, each representing a different form of earthly bounty and symbolizing competing forms of extraction. The older child was named Umi-sachi-biko (Fortune of the Sea Lad) and represented the marine realm and fishing; the younger was named Yama-sachi-biko (Fortune of the Mountain Lad) and represented the terrestrial realm and hunting. One day, the younger brother, after he finally convinced his older brother to temporarily trade occupations with him, lost the elder brother's fishing hook; the younger brother searched for it and instead discovered the palace of Watatsumi, the Sea Deity, and married her daughter and subdued his brother. Later, the son he sired became, on his enthronement in 660 CE, the father of Jinmu, the legendary first emperor of Japan.[5] Imperial power was tied to the land.

In ancient times, fishers traveled among a wandering world of itinerant souls not connected to the land, which included prostitutes and peddlers, magicians and ironmongers, as well as salt merchants and fortune-tellers. They sometimes traveled by foot on bandit-ridden roads and sometimes sailed up rivers or along the rugged coasts. These "sea-people" (*ama* or *kai-jin* in Japanese) lived itinerant, nomadic lives, but they began to settle in stable coastal villages by the time of the Kamakura shoguns in the thirteenth century. From their settled communities they continued to provide tribute to the court and to the shoguns and produce salt that they then sold to merchants. In the thirteenth through sixteenth centuries, fishers sacrificed some of their itinerant independence when, under the new medieval order, many beaches and littoral environs became fiefdoms; within such coastal villages, inhabitants subsequently began distributing marine fishing territories and net contracts.[6]

As settled Japanese villages increased in size and in number in the seventeenth through nineteenth centuries, the net contracts and fishing territories increased in complexity. Nonetheless, for a variety of political, social, and biological reasons, these preindustrial fishing villages also established ecological balances in their marine and littoral environs that sustained their way of life until Japan's industrial age. Coastal villagers caught fish and extracted salt from nearby waters and gathered shellfish, kelp, and a variety of seafood. Confucianism, Shintoism, and Buddhism shaped the values of these communities. Native Japanese beliefs, referred to as Shinto today, viewed taming nature for human use as coming to grips with the deities (*kami*) that inhabited all "otherworldly" natural spaces, while Buddhist beliefs invested all living things with a soul and saw all animate and, according to some creeds, inanimate things as part of a "continuum of life." In many rural communities, as seen in the first two chapters, insects provided bodies for the souls of former humans. In some instances, fishers saw drifting corpses as deities, and they posthumously anointed the whales they pursued and killed with names and then held festivals to honor the sacrificed cetaceans. Honoring them through ceremonies did not immunize whales from being hunted, killed, and eaten, but it did invest hunting with spiritual meaning, in contrast to the late-nineteenth- and twentieth-century industrial method of unceremoniously extracting the soulless leviathans from the sea and hauling them onto the decks of factory boats to be processed.[7]

It should be mentioned that, since 1983, Japan has claimed to observe the global moratorium on commercial whaling. Nonetheless, under a clause in the 1946 International Whaling Convention, Japan has infamously pursued dubious "scientific whaling" in Antarctic and North Pacific waters. Initially, Japan's scientific whaling activities remained confined to hunting Antarctic minke whales (*Balaenoptera bonaerensis*) and the North Pacific variety (*Balaenoptera acutorostrata*), but in the spring of 2000 the Japanese expanded their "research" program to include Bryde's whales (*Balaenoptera edeni*) and sperm whales (*Physeter macrocephalus*). Despite objections from the International Whaling Commission, the U.S. government, and many other groups, Japan has pushed ahead with the program. In Japan, the Institute of Cetacean Research oversees "scientific whaling," which includes measuring size and weight, determining age and sex, examining stomach contents, and taking tissue samples to check for the bioaccumulation of chemicals and heavy metals. Under the Antarctic program, since 1987 Japanese whalers have taken 400 minke whales annually. Between 1994 and 1999, 100 North Pacific minke whales were killed annually under the sister program. The spring of 2000 expansion of the hunt included an allotment of 50 Bryde's and 10 sperm whales, in addition to the minke whale harvests. In September 2000, despite intense international objections, whalers returned to Japanese ports with 88 whales, including 53 Bryde's and 5 sperm whales.[8]

Some scientists contend that Japan's whale hunts are not confined to the two varieties of minke whales. In December 2000, molecular genetic testing of some 700 "whale products" sold at Japanese markets exposed genetic traces from eight species of baleen whales, as well as sperm whales, beaked whales, orcas, dolphins, porpoises, domestic sheep, and horses. (The sperm whale traces are from products manufactured prior to the formal spring of 2000 expansion of the hunt to include these species.) Overall, traces from these other marine and terrestrial mammals made up about 10 percent of whale products from Japanese markets. Scientists have expressed considerable concern over genetic traces of the Asian gray whale (*Eschrichtius robustus*), for example, which is among the "most endangered population of whales in the world." Scientists also speculated that 43 percent of whale products did not come from legal pelagic hunts in the North Pacific but from "illegal or unregulated exploitation of a protected population in the Sea of Japan."[9] Whatever cultural or political practices had limited Japanese whaling in the eighteenth century had clearly disappeared by the late twentieth century.

In the seventeenth century, however, cultural systems, those identified with Shinto and Buddhist beliefs, did determine the nature of interaction with whales and other marine organisms, but so too did the political and economic systems of coastal villages and their fishing territories. By the time of the Tokugawa shoguns (1600–1868), the sea was no longer an open space but rather an extension of terrestrial landowning patterns. However, this also served to limit overexploitation, which reminds one of California Indians and their ability to resist overexploitation of critical fisheries. Arthur McEvoy writes that, much like preindustrial Japanese, California "Indians carefully circumscribed their harvests with complex systems of legal rights and religious observances." He continues, "Well-defined rights to resources not only limited their use but permitted tribes to monitor the effect of their harvesting at specific sites over time and to adjust their use accordingly."[10] That some coastal households held legal fishing territories—defined marine geographies, or fiefs, that contained and confined their fishing activities—meant that a "tragedy of the commons" type of scenario, at least as described by Garret Hardin, never emerged, even in the context of protoindustrial Japan.[11] That is, Japanese never harbored the capitalist attitude common in open waters today: "Well, if I don't fish these waters empty, somebody else surely will."[12] To thrive, Japanese had to preserve the sustainability of their marine territories for future generations (i.e., Confucian linearity), much as paddy farmers saw to the fertility of their fields through the use of fertilizers or crop rotation. Confucianism, Shintoism, and Buddhism became cultural attributes of sustainability and served as key parts of the highly localized, ecological nature of the Confucian *ie,* or "family/household," system.

Even though pelagic whaling and yellowtail fishing often took these fishers far from their coastal villages, most of them worked the waters near shore, and this was certainly true of people in the villages near Minamata. Nonetheless, as Arne Kalland has pointed out, the limited access to the sea because of fishing territories, gender restrictions (women were prohibited on boats on certain occasions, which meant fewer nets and lines in the water), labor shortages, a limited number of fishing days (for ceremonies, rituals, and weather), and technological inhibitors all ensured that an ecological balance remained relatively intact between coastal populations and littoral fisheries.[13] Interestingly, one terrestrial animal that helped coastal villagers maintain this fragile ecological balance was the domesticated cat. The household cat needs to be seen as part of the highly localized, ecological nature of the Confucian *ie* system, but one that also served as a biological sentinel (much like the silkworm) that alerted people to looming environmental catastrophe after the advent of the industrial age.

Biological Sentinels

I have, on rare occasions, sauntered back to my hotel from bars in downtown Tokyo late at night, when the only other souls around were a handful of other revelers and cats. I mean lots of cats, and of every imaginable size and color. These cats, which often peer stealthily from behind torn garbage bags filled with reeking fish carcasses, spent green tea leaves, and discarded *waribashi* (disposable chopsticks), seldom resemble friendly housecats. More often, they are seriously formidable felines, with ratty coats and scarred faces. They shriek wildly at each other (and you) rather than meow. In Japan, many of these cats inhabit a hybrid space, one that is neither domesticated nor wild: like the Southern California "ecotone" where flocks of feral parakeets live alongside overly acclimated mountain lions.[14] Such formidable felines also inhabited coastal communities, where they performed important duties for which they were perfectly qualified. Rather than munch contently on discarded fish from haughty Tokyo restaurants, they watched over coastal households by hunting rats and mice that could, in a single night, destroy a valuable net.

Cats were members of households, and households constituted not only ideological units of Confucian paternalism and patrilocality but highly localized ecologies, what we might view as patri-ecolocalities or micro-bio-geographies, easily upset by industrial toxins. If canaries guarded mines, alerting miners to toxic gases, then cats guarded coastal households, alerting fishing families to toxins in the marine food web. When Minamata disease first appeared, observers called it the "dancing cat" disease, because cats, an organic part of coastal life, became delirious and wandered and wobbled throughout villages near Minamata City. Eventually, almost all the cats died. Once, cats had been nothing short of ubiquitous: they hunted and killed the rats that destroyed extremely expensive hemp or nylon nets. With the exception of boats, nets were the single largest capital investment of a household; like fishing knowledge and local customs, families passed this technology down through generations. Nishimura Hajime and Okamoto Tatsuaki have determined that over one hundred households in Minamata City (Tsukinoura, Detsuki, Yudō, and other hamlets) raised domesticated animals that, mysteriously, began to die in the 1950s.[15]

Cats started dying even before people did: they were biological sentinels, but few heeded their cautionary sacrifices. They served as sentinels of a deadly toxic environment, much as dying silkworms had in the Shimotsuke Plain (downwind and downstream from the Ashio mining complex). Some Minamata residents remembered it this way: "Then cats started to go mad. We couldn't believe our eyes when we saw them running around and around, or dashing head-on into rocks and trees. . . . In the end they jumped into the sea and drowned. All the cats in the fishing villages around Hyakken died in this way. Then people began to show the same symptoms. The poisoned fish did their job damn well."[16] Nishimura and Okamoto submit that Minamata households raised a combined total of 121 cats, of which 74 had died by 1956. One cat mysteriously died in 1953, and then 18 the next year, 25 the next year, and then 30 the year after that. Evidence suggests that cats had started dying years earlier. Of course, before they died, these cats appeared to be "dancing," because mercury hidden in the fish and seabirds that they fed on had eaten away their brains and nervous systems. Methylmercury destroyed the brains of seabirds and cats much as it did the brains of people and their fetuses.[17]

In *Kugai jōdo*, Ishimure wrote of the deteriorating situation around Minamata. As catches declined as a result of industrial toxins, "Desperate fishermen sold their old fishing gear and borrowed more money in order to buy expensive fashionable nylon nets with which they hoped to catch more fish."[18] They, too, bought into the promise of technological innovation and turned to plastics. By the 1950s, fishers had started replacing their hemp and jute nets with nylon ones, which, unlike natural fibers, were not subject to microbial decay when they broke apart in the water: hence, plastics persisted in the marine environment. Indeed, I have walked many of the beaches of northern Japan, combing for seashells and rare glass net buoys. What I remember most about these walks, though, are the nylon nets and plastic containers that are strewn everywhere.

Plastic is very persistent. Nylon, a synthetic fiber, was developed in the United States by DuPont to replace Japanese silk used for stockings in the years leading up to the Pacific War.[19] But the changing ecologies of Minamata had already deteriorated well beyond the ability of improved plastic net technologies to heal. "Spread out on the beach to dry," lamented Ishimure, "the nylon nets bought at the price of so much sacrifice were soon eaten by rats which, as a result of the death of almost all the cats in the Minamata area, swarmed unmolested everywhere."[20] For the poor fishers of Minamata, the simple luxury of a piece of sliced raw fish, accompanied by a cup or three of strong *shōchū* spirits, had been replaced by a rat-infested otherworld; in their homes, fleas thrived, despite the extensive use of DDT to eradicate them, and vinyl countertops (popular throughout Japan at this time) slowly leached organotin compounds and phthalate (which cause birth defects) into their homes.[21] Just outside, ghostly fishing boats rocked and rotted in barren, toxic waters.

But coastal people knew all this and much more even before lab-coated scientists descended on their homes. They knew that the swirling effluent discharged from the factory was poisonous and that it worked its way from fish to people. Some fishers, for example, moored their boats in Hyakken Bay, near the drainage channel from the factory, because they noticed "all the stuff clinging to the boat's hull would disappear without leaving a trace." Fishers complained that the stench emanating from the Minamata channel resembled a "mass of dead bodies in an advanced state of putrefaction." Near fishing villages, small children waded into the sheltered inlets and bays to catch dying fish and walked onto beaches to catch dazed and dying birds with their hands, just as children did a generation earlier in the copper-poisoned Watarase River. Low tide exposed dying shellfish with shells half open as if they were gasping for air. "The fetid odor of their putrefying flesh mingled with the stench of the waste water from the Chisso factory to form a nauseating emanation," wrote Ishimure.[22]

Bioaccumulation

What fishers had come to understand through their dead cats, even without the help of scientists, was bioaccumulation. In aquatic environments, toxins such as methylmercury and PCBs (polychlorinated biphenyls) concentrate in extraordinarily high levels because of the length of marine food chains and because the buoyancy of water allows aquatic organisms to spend less energy fighting gravity. Subsequently, less energy is lost between links in the chain and more links can be added, meaning higher concentrations of toxins in an organism over time. For this reason, the levels of mercury in the fish pulled from Shiranui waters were in some instances far higher than the mercury content of the water itself. Equally, because human mothers became another link in the food chain, and their fetuses another link still, the mercury that was passed from mothers to their unborn children reached even higher levels. (Remember, fetuses float in a liquid environment, too.) Sadly, the unborn children of Minamata inhabited the highest link in the food chain: they served as the final destination of, and hence as a repository for, Chisso's deadly toxins.[23] In part, these children became the offspring of Chisso chemicals.

Kumamoto University researchers focused on the shellfish of Minamata Bay as possible vectors for transferring heavy metals to human victims. One of the most ubiquitous shellfish was an intertidal mussel called *hibari-gaimodoki* (*Hormomya mutabilis*). If fetuses stood at the top of the food ladder, then mussels—or, more accurately, the plankton they ate—occupied the lower rungs. In 1968, researcher Shoji Kitamura, from Kumamoto University, published results of tests designed to measure the mercuric content of this important source of food for both the human and nonhuman inhabitants of Minamata. Sadly, the exact dates of the study remain unknown, but Kitamura appears to have collected data between May and July 1959. His results revealed that the average mercuric content of the shellfish was about 30 μg/g (or thirty micrograms of constituent per gram of tissue; or thirty parts per million). He discovered the highest amount of mercury in the shellfish off the eastern coast of Koiji Island, which measured 39 μg/g. Interestingly, Kitamura discovered no correlation between levels of mercury in the mussels and levels in the mudflats, mangroves, and rocks they inhabited.[24] But what mercury shellfish harbored easily transferred to other organisms, including people. Separate experiments by Katsuro Irukayama revealed that toxins remained in the muscles and organs of shellfish even after they had been dried or boiled, and that nearly 20 percent of the mercury could be removed from the shellfish through simulated digestion. The results: shellfish proved excellent vectors for delivering industrial toxins to people.[25] Just as cadmium from copper mines poisoned the rice, the staple of paddy farmers in Tochigi Prefecture, mercury from Chisso poisoned the shellfish consumed almost daily by coastal communities. This is why I focused on food and food webs in the introduction.

Even though the shellfish contained dangerously high amounts of mercury, Kitamura actually provided a low estimation of the mercuric content of *hibarigaimodoki*. Other data regarding the mercury levels of this common mussel are available from 1958 through 1963, because other groups, including Chisso researchers, conducted experiments as well. No relationship could be discerned between the levels of mercury in mussels and the seafloor outcroppings they inhabited; but there was a relationship with levels of mercury in the seawater, because plankton, the main source of food for this mussel, absorbed mercury from the water. The mussel then absorbed mercury from the plankton. As expected, the amount of mercury in this mussel was related to the amount of mercury being discharged into Minamata Bay.

Between May and July 1959, about the same time Kitamura collected his data, Chisso decided to divert the waste discharged from acetaldehyde production to the Hachiman sedimentation pools and, ultimately, into the

Minamata River north of Minamata Bay. This diversion served to flush toxins westward into the Shiranui Sea, but not southward into Minamata Bay, meaning that Kitamura's mercury measurements from the bay proved low. The mercury had only washed elsewhere. Other data, some collected by Chisso researchers, measured levels as high as 100 μg/g in late 1958 and early 1959; discrepancies within the data can be explained by the life cycle of the mussels, from reproduction to shell molting, and their changing levels of plankton consumption. After 1960, when effluent was channeled back into Minamata Bay, mercury levels in the mussels shot back up to between 40 and 80 μg/g. Even though *hibarigaimodoki* was not the most popular shellfish consumed by Minamata fishers (oysters were), as sedentary shellfish oysters and mussels live so similarly that one can assume that mercury levels in *hibarigaimodoki* reflect those in oysters as well. The only information related to mercury in oysters is available for the unrepresentative 1959 period, when Chisso temporarily redirected effluent from its acetaldehyde production to the Hachiman pools. But the mercury levels remained dangerously high, nonetheless.[26]

The anchovy *katakuchiiwashi* (*Engraulis japonicus*) also evidences how mercury biomagnified in the marine food web. This small fish spawns in the spring and summer months, and the juveniles stay offshore between April and February of the following year, where they grow and become known to the Japanese as *shirasu*, *kaeri*, and *miseigyo* depending on their length (and specific culinary value). At every interval of the life of these small fish, Japanese harvested them as a source of energy, either for food or for fertilizer. When adult anchovies entered the Shiranui Sea and congregated off Minamata and elsewhere, they became susceptible to the toxins discharged by the factory. Like mussels, observe Nishimura and Okamoto, anchovies principally eat zooplankton (*Acartia clause*) as well as krill (*Euphausiacea*), and they do so by swimming with their mouths open and sifting them out of the water; but anchovies also force water into their gills while swimming, as they are incapable of pumping water into their gills while stationary. Oxygen extracted by the gills and fed to the capillaries was accompanied by the highly soluble methylmercury discharged by the factory. In essence, mercury found its way into the bodies of anchovies via two routes. This made them extremely potent repositories of mercury and prime gateways for this nonmetabolizing toxin to infiltrate the food web.

Once boiled and dried in the sun, anchovies served as an important means by which net owners and net workers transacted with one another. Just as rice, the gold standard under the Tokugawa shoguns, later became the principal vector of cadmium, so anchovies, an important currency between net owners and net workers, became the principal vector of mercury. After fishers dried the anchovies and sold them to a broker, they made a cash payment to the net owner: these small fish mediated complex economic relations in coastal communities. Whether just eaten or boiled and used as stock and flavoring, anchovies transmitted discernible amounts of mercury to both feline and hominid consumers. Near the bottom of the food chain, anchovies were also eaten by a vast variety of other fish that then concentrated high levels of mercury in their bodies through bioaccumulation. But if the introduction of methylmercury into the food chain started with plankton, mussels, and anchovies absorbing it from the water, the food chain ended with fetuses absorbing this highly soluble mercury via the mother through the umbilical cord. Physiologically speaking, fetuses and anchovies absorbed soluble mercury in much the same manner; but because they lived at different points in the food chain, the amount of mercury absorbed by *katakuchiiwashi* proved less than that absorbed by the human fetus. Bioaccumulation is one of the tragic laws of environmental pollution.[27]

From the plankton in Minamata Bay to the anchovies and mussels that ingested them, soluble mercury migrated to the still-developing bodies of fetal human beings through capillaries, much as it did in darting anchovies. Waters near the shore were the first to be polluted at Minamata as poisonous effluent settled there; and the Minamata Canal, which channeled factory toxins into the bay, served as a kind of umbilical cord that linked this technical system to the Shiranui Sea (fig. 5.1). In the 1960s, the sludge at the mouth of the canal had high levels of mercury—2,010 µg/g according to researchers at Kumamoto University—but the umbilical cords of some mothers had high amounts as well. Researchers later became aware of this because some families in Minamata saved umbilical cords as part of a traditional birthing ritual and scientists later tested them at the laboratory. An organic ladder, where the cruel law of bioaccumulation increased toxicity at every rung, stretched from the technological alchemy of acetylene gas being blown over mercuric sulfate to create acetaldehyde in the factory to the fragile process of fetal organogenesis that occurred in the wombs of expectant mothers.

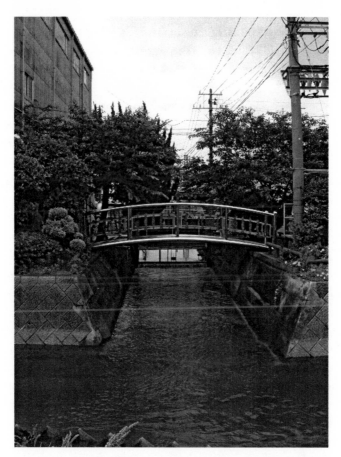

FIG. 5.1 Remnants of the elaborate canal system in Minamata City that transported methylmercury from the Chisso plant to the sea. Photograph by author.

PART II

We now turn our attention to the history of the quest for phosphate and nitrogen, both within Japan and on a global scale. This analysis will connect the "nitrogen problem," as it was labeled in the early twentieth century, to Japan's agricultural needs, European and Japanese imperialism, the ecological footprint of Japan's urban environments, the birth of atmospheric nitrogen fixation technologies, the advent of the plastics industry in Japan, and, ultimately, methylmercury poisoning. Atmospheric nitrogen fixation such as that practiced at the Chisso factory utilized mercury as a catalyst, which was then discarded into the marine environment, ultimately finding its way, as we traced in part I of this chapter, to the pinnacle of the global food ladder, the human fetus. Part II of this chapter explores how methylmercury was produced and how the relationships among women's bodies, fetuses, and the environment were interpreted by Japanese doctors and other health officials. To do this, we will explore elements of preindustrial Japanese medicine, because it was an earlier generation of pluralistic medical practitioners who, more than their modern compartmentalizing counterparts, viewed the body as inextricably embedded in the natural environment. In some respects, the journey of methylmercury to the human fetus only reified a human-nature connection understood for centuries in Japan.

But the first two questions we must tackle are these: How did the Chisso factory arrive at the small, largely impoverished fishing community of Minamata? What were the historical circumstances surrounding its construction and the technological developments that poisoned the surrounding marine environment? As it turns out, even though Minamata disease was the product of local ecological circumstances, the forces that brought Chisso to Minamata were global in scale, and require some discussion.

Phosphate, Nitrogen, and Japan's Industrial Metabolism

Engineer Noguchi Jun (1873–1944) founded Nihon Chisso Hiryō Company (the chemical company referred to as Chisso throughout this chapter) in 1908, during a global push for scientific advancements in electrochemistry, principally for the production of nitrogenous fertilizers and other products. Until Noguchi arrived on the scene, Japan's chemical industry remained confined to the production of sulfuric acid and soda; the Meiji government used the former to print paper money, and industry used the latter to bleach textiles. By the late nineteenth century, the chemical industry had expanded to include the production of matches, which became Japan's leading chemical-industry export. By the early twentieth century, the most powerful chemical firms in Japan sought to develop new kinds of fertilizers to assist with Japan's rapid industrialization. As we learned in chapter 2, Japan's promotion of industrial agriculture after the Meiji Restoration depended on liberal applications of chemical fertilizer.

Along with the chemical industry, Japan's modernizers also sought to transform traditional agricultural practices, and engineers began exploring ways to harness chemistry to boost crops and increase calories in order to fuel more laborers and soldiers. At first, Japanese chemical producers developed "Superphosphates," after learning about them at the New Orleans Exhibition of 1884. In Europe, naturally occurring phosphates for fertilizers represented one of the first energy resources that imperialists sought on a global scale. In November 1802, the indefatigable scientist and explorer Alexander von Humboldt (1769–1859), while in Callao, Peru, wrote about the potential fertilizer properties of guano (a source of phosphorus and nitrogen), and deposits such as these, as Gregory Cushman has written, became one of the major drivers for European and American ambitions in Peru and elsewhere. Between 1840 and 1880, during Peru's "Guano Age," the country exported just under 13 million tons of guano, sparking a "global rush" to colonize even the remotest areas—as long as they were heavily encrusted with bird shit.[28]

After exhausting Peru's deposits, European and American guano prospectors spread elsewhere. After a victorious 1881 war with Bolivia waged over access to phosphate deposits, Chile, employing cheap Chinese laborers who mined guano in horrific conditions, began exporting millions of tons of guano phosphates. Later, Britain (already dependent on agricultural imports) annexed Ocean Island in order to access the energy resource to supply farmers in New Zealand and Australia. Outside labor dug at the phosphate mines, while European supervisors and Fijian police oversaw them. Germany annexed Nauru Island in 1888 and did much the same. By the 1930s, the British Phosphate Commission ensured that one million tons of phosphates left both islands each year to supply the demand for inexpensive fertilizers in the empire. On Ocean Island, miners defoliated and stripped the top fifty feet or so of soil from the small island, leaving in their wake a desolate moonscape. The Polynesian Banaban people tried to stop the rape of their island, but during the Pacific War, the Japanese exiled them to the Caroline Islands; after the war, the British resettled them on Rambi Island.

With the local inhabitants forcibly relocated, the British exploited phosphates with renewed vigor, exporting three million tons a year by the 1960s. When the phosphate mines shut down in the 1980s and 1990s, mining companies had exported about eighty million tons; and British authorities had displaced the inhabitants, paid them a humiliating pittance in compensation, and utterly destroyed the environment of Ocean Island.[29] But for industrial countries, phosphate and nitrogen fertilizers were worth destroying cultures and homes for because in the modern order more productive lands meant fewer farmers and, hence, more people available to labor in mines and factories. John McNeill estimates that, in the twentieth century, the global population would have needed about 30 percent more farmland in cultivation were it not for fertilizers. Starting in the 1950s, about when Chisso entered its peak years, fertilizers also permitted wealthier farmers to outproduce poorer ones, putting the latter out of business on national and global scales. Unfortunately for the environment and fishers who depended on clean rivers, observes McNeill, most nitrogenous fertilizers (by some estimates half) never enter cultivated plants at all and instead drain into rivers and pollute rural waterways.[30] The lesson with chemical fertilizers (as learned in chapter 2) is that not only does producing them pollute but so does using them. Nevertheless, they are one of the keys to industrialization.

Superphosphates (in which sulfuric acid is used as a reagent with phosphates) never really caught on in Japan, because sluggish research and wary farmers hampered its widespread application, even though the capitalist Shibusawa Eiichi (1840–1931), the prominent financier of the Ashio copper mine whom we met in chapter 3, funded their development. Eventually, international events forced Japanese farmers to take a second look at chemical fertilizers. When war broke out between Japan and China in 1894–95, imports of the popular soybean-cake fertilizers from the continent slowed and farmers had to search elsewhere for nitrogen for their fields. War is critical to Japan's environmental history: it fueled hard-rock mining and, as we shall see, coal mining and expanded the nitrogen fixation industry. In the context of Japanese history, much has been written about the human cost of Japan's "total war," but as William Tsutsui observes, little has been written on the extensive environmental cost of total war to the home islands, whether the extensive deforestation, overexploitation of fisheries, worsening air and water quality, or the radioactive aftereffects of Hiroshima and Nagasaki.[31] Even if indirectly, the imperial quest for domination seriously exacerbated most of Japan's environmental headaches.

In the eighteenth and early nineteenth centuries, Japanese farmers had used a variety of naturally occurring fertilizers to improve crop yield. Some, like night soil, manure, plant meal, and rice bran they recycled from farm animals, themselves, their urban neighbors, and their fields. Others, however, such as dried herring and sardines, as well as fish cakes and oils, they extracted from environs as distant as the northern island of Hokkaido and with laborers as exotic as the Ainu. Japanese harnessed the wild lands and exotic peoples of Hokkaido to transport energy to the working lands near their cities. Even such fledgling industrial societies as eighteenth-century Japan harnessed landscapes beyond their immediate homes and forcibly enlisted foreign peoples as inexpensive labor to service the economies of the cities and provide valuable energy, much as the British did with Chinese laborers on Ocean Island and elsewhere.[32] Better crops became particularly important with the rise of cash-crop farming in the seventeenth and eighteenth centuries, when farmers focused more on the bottom line when producing cotton, tobacco, and soybeans because of competitive market prices for their harvests. Bought from wholesalers in Osaka, merchants sold manufactured goods in Japan's many *jōkamachi*, or castle towns, which sprouted up like wild daisies between 1585 and 1630 as a result of the forced removal of the samurai from the countryside. The establishment of castle towns, largely driven by autocrat Toyotomi Hideyoshi's (1536–98) famous "Sword Hunts" (1588), created a formidable ecological footprint, particularly later in the eighteenth century: this urban ecological footprint was, as ecologists dryly define it, "the total area required to meet the demands of its population in terms of consumption and waste assimilation."[33]

Through cash-crop farming, rural inhabitants radically reconfigured rural households to meet the demands of urban ecologies. Whereas fifteenth- and sixteenth-century farmers, if conditions permitted, adopted laborers into their families in traditional Confucian kinship patterns, market prices forced farmers to consider business contracts over kinship and seasonal laborers over family adoption.[34] If savvy farmers knew how to streamline their home businesses, moreover, they also knew—in principle, if not in name—that night soil and other naturally occurring fertilizers provided soil with elements such as nitrogen, phosphorus, and potassium. Powerful merchant guilds sprouted up alongside cash croppers; they collected night soil from cities and sold it to farmers in the countryside.[35] This is part of the urban ecology of eighteenth-century Japanese cities—their "waste assimilation."[36]

The sanitation of seventeenth- and eighteenth-century Japanese cities remains all the more remarkable given that Edo (present-day Tokyo) had a population of probably over one million, while Osaka and Kyoto grew to slightly less than half that size. With one million inhabitants, Edo needed to be supplied with fresh water, so the Tokugawa shoguns placed a retainer in charge of overseeing the construction of the Kanda water system, whereby aqueducts transported water to Edo from Inokashira Pond. Once in the city, an elaborate network of more than forty-one miles of underground pipes, crafted from bamboo and wood, brought water to the private residences of the shogun and powerful lords, as well as to the wells of commoner neighborhoods. Later, when the city needed even more fresh water, aqueducts transported water some twenty-seven miles from the Tama River to the Yotsuya Gate of Edo Castle; pipes distributed water in a descending order of political importance, starting at Edo Castle and ending at commoner wells. In 1878, when an Englishman tested the purity of Edo's water for solids, chlorine, ammonia, and nitrogen, he discovered that near the source, the water supply was nearly pure, but quite understandably, it became less pure the farther it traveled through aqueducts from the source. Given the importance of Japan's *mibunsei*, or status system, in Tokugawa governance, one could characterize this aqueduct system, not as "environmental racism," but rather as "environmental status-ism."[37]

What made seventeenth- and eighteenth-century Japanese cities so much more hygienic than their European or American counterparts was the removal of night soil and waste from their environs, however. In Edo and Osaka, the removal of human excreta, as well as rubbish and other waste, explained the sustainability of even the largest Japanese cities. Generally speaking, the relative absence of domesticated animals, excepting silkworms and packs of tough dogs, made manure scarce and so farmers placed a premium on human waste. Merchants who handled night soil transported so much human excreta from Osaka, for example, that merchants in nearby ports where manure boats docked complained of the stench. Shrugging their shoulders, magistrates could only respond that "it was unavoidable for the manure boats to come into wharves used by the tea and other ships." In Osaka, an elaborate economy evolved around the production, collection, and transportation of excreta. By the eighteenth century, farmers purchased night soil with silver extracted from the mines discussed in the previous two chapters; and tenants relinquished their feces to the owners of their buildings while they retained rights to their urine. Even though urine contains higher levels of nitrogen and potassium than solid waste (and so served as a better fertilizer), the latter's ease of transport made it more valuable. Urine splashes and spills. In Osaka, neighboring farm villages retained rights to buy human waste from most of the city, while "urine jobbers" collected liquid waste and sold it. In Edo, where powerful lords resided in alternating years for surveillance purposes (the *sankin kōtai* in Japanese), farmers bought night soil directly from these residences. The Hitotsubashi lord, for example, sold the night soil from his residence to a farmer named Hanbei, who paid him with either copious numbers of *daikon* radishes or two gold coins.

Garbage also found its way out of these large cities. After 1655, Edo officials ordered that all garbage and rubbish be deposited on Eitai Island in Edo Bay; before this order, it appears that most residents of the city simply dumped their garbage in the nearby rivers. For about a decade after the opening of Eitai Island as a garbage dump, officially designated garbage-pickup sites were used in each ward. Periodically, laborers collected the garbage from these sites, loaded it on boats, and transported it to Eitai Island. But officials established other landfills as well, which, because they eventually created new fields, proved profitable to oversee. Japanese placed a premium on the cleanliness of their cities, and concerns regarding symbolic pollution, originating with early anxieties about the transmission of disease, prompted hygienic practices in individual homes.[38]

After the Meiji Restoration of 1868, Japan's modernizers replaced the pungently odiferous Tokugawa system with the modern fertilizer industry. When the use and importation of traditional fertilizers slowed in the 1890s, farmers experimented with chemicals and quickly discovered improvements. Globally, fertilizers symbolized the great promise of chemistry in the twentieth century, especially technologies that made possible the fixation of atmospheric nitrogen. Farmers had utilized nitrogen in soybean cakes and human excreta, but chemical fertilizers offered twice to three times the amount of nitrogen per application. Modernizers also viewed nitrogen fertilizers as more hygienic. After the Pacific War, reformers targeted the use of night soil in rural villages as feudal and unhygienic: one 1956 booklet on rural lifestyles explained that storing human waste bred flies, mosquitoes, and bacteria, while intestinal parasites, pervasive among farmers, spread through such practices by contaminating the food chain and threatening urban families.[39] The last thing modernizers wanted, as evidenced in chapter 1, was to inadvertently create more breeding habitat for mosquitoes, particularly ones that might carry Japanese B encephalitis.

Noguchi, the founder of Chisso, came of age when the "nitrogen problem" emerged as a national priority in Japan and other industrialized nations. A bright engineering graduate from Tokyo Imperial University,

Noguchi built the Chisso factory in Minamata in 1907 to produce calcium carbide and nitrogenous fertilizers. The next year, Noguchi's fledgling enterprise merged with Sōgi Electric: together they formed the powerful Japan Nitrogenous Fertilizers, Inc. Through savvy entrepreneurship, friendships with bankers and shareholders, and cozy connections to the military, Chisso quickly became a corporate and technological leviathan in Japan and its empire. Once again, similar to the demand for dried-herring fertilizer during the age of the Tokugawa shoguns, or the fertilizer demands of the British Empire, the energy demands of Japan's empire required exploiting landscapes beyond its national borders. In 1929, for example, Chisso built a sprawling fertilizer factory in Hungnam, in northern Korea, transforming that bucolic fishing village into an industrial metropolis of over 180,000 inhabitants. Elsewhere on the Korean Peninsula, in the 1920s and 1930s Chisso oversaw large-scale hydroelectric projects on the Pujon, Changjin, and Honchon rivers, as well as on the Yalu River on the border with the puppet state in Manchuria. Chisso also set up munitions factories in Taiwan and ore mines on Hainan Island in Southeast Asia.

Along with fertilizers, Chisso also produced acetylene, which fueled everything from bicycle lamps to the lamps bolted on the helmets of copper and coal miners; but acetylene also made night fishing possible in Minamata, extending the temporal rhythms of coastal communities, as well as changing their relationship to the estuary and increasing catches of certain fish. Festooned with acetylene lamps, squid boats rocked serenely in the bay like bright lamps being hoisted up and down during some raucous village festival; some fishers called the Chisso factory "the nightless castle," and it often served as a beacon to guide them home after fishing throughout the night. It became a permanent fixture in the landscape whose light was never extinguished and that signaled home.

As Timothy George has carefully documented, it did not take long for Chisso, still under the reins of the ambitious Noguchi, to develop a series of new technological breakthroughs that resonated throughout Minamata and beyond. In the industrial age, human activities mediate and amplify the destruction of the environment through the development of certain technologies and the quest for greater degrees of efficiency and social affluence. This was true of the advanced smelter technologies introduced at the Ashio and Kamioka mines, and it proved true for the Chisso factory as well. In 1909, Noguchi had purchased rights to the German Frank-Caro "calcium cyanamide process," whereby engineers blew steam over calcium cyanamide to produce ammonia and limestone.[40] Then, in 1918, they added sulfuric acid to the ammonia to produce ammonium sulfate and, as a by-product, Portland cement. The factory now produced carbide, ammonium sulfate, and cyanamide, from which they produced fertilizers that contained even more nitrogen. Chisso's mainstay for decades, nitrogen fertilizer increased the ability of farmers to produce food; but Chisso also continued to produce such chemicals as acetic acid, ammonia, and butanol from calcium carbide for a variety of industrial and military applications. In 1932, Hashimoto Hikoshichi, another engineer at Chisso, developed a procedure known as the "reaction liquid circulation method," in which factory workers blew acetylene gas over mercuric sulfate to produce acetaldehyde. This process further increased production, to be sure, but it also led to the dumping of even deadlier toxins into the marine environment.[41]

Hashimoto's exploration of the catalytic qualities of mercury for industrial application tapped into a long and diverse history of interest in the liquid metal in traditional East Asian sciences and, especially, in Taoist alchemy. The industrial applications of the chemical processes that occurred in the Chisso factory may have been new—technological breakthroughs fueled by dreams of personal wealth and the patriotic ambition to solve Japan's perennial nitrogen problem—but scientific interest in mercury was decidedly not. Chinese scientists since the Han dynasty (206 BCE–220 CE) had expressed interest in the chemical properties of organic and inorganic materials; the production of alchemical elixirs of immortality using cinnabar, or red mercuric sulfide, remained principal among their endeavors. Taoists marveled at how cinnabar transformed into silvery liquid mercury and then mercuric oxide when heated properly; the changing colors—from vermilion to silver to vermilion again—became emblematic in Taoist science of the rejuvenating promise of elixirs and the doctrine of change that was inherent in the human condition and all of nature. Subsequently, many Taoist drugs contained high levels of mercury because of its metamorphic qualities; but for this reason many of these same drugs proved seriously poisonous and eventually killed some of those who experimented with them.[42]

The industrial waste produced by the Chisso factory and dumped into Minamata Bay proved several times more toxic than any Taoist elixir, particularly after August 1951, when Chisso engineers replaced manganese with nitric acid as the oxidizer in the production of acetaldehyde. The factory also drew brackish water from the mouth of the Minamata

River for acetaldehyde production and thereby created a highly soluble type of organic mercury as a by-product. This was the soluble mercury that moved so easily through the gills of shellfish and fish, as well as through the umbilical cords of mothers to their fetuses. But fertilizers and lamp oils were not the only products manufactured at Chisso. The company had even bigger consumer fish to fry: plastics.

Plastics

The 1950s also witnessed a boom in the PVC (polyvinyl chloride) plastics market, as well as other related chemicals essential to the mass-consumer society that Japan was becoming after the Allied Occupation (1945–52). A German chemist first created PVC as a solid polymer in 1872; later, known only as "vinyl," PVC compounds opened new vistas in the commercial applicability of plastics.[43] Following its move into plastics in the 1930s, Chisso nearly cornered the industrial production of DOP (dioctyl phthalate), an important ingredient in making celluloid for camera film, insulation for copper electric wires, and other products made from PVC. The irony that Chisso produced plastics for camera film was not lost on the photojournalist W. Eugene Smith (1918–78), who documented the destructive consequences of Minamata disease: his simultaneously horrific and beautiful images of patients stunned the world in the early 1970s.[44] But plastics linger longer than human memories do, even when such images are "captured" on celluloid. Julia Adeney Thomas demonstrates in her analysis of an exhibition of photography shown at the Yokohama Museum of Art that photographs and their exhibition can be as much about historical amnesia as about historical memories.[45] Unlike her exhibitors, plastics exhibit no amnesia; they, unlike the images photographs offer, have little to no problem with time.

But images do better with space: images travel and evoke far more than the plastics from which they are made. One of Smith's most famous photographs, of congenital patient Kamimura Tomoko and her mother bathing together in a small bathtub, inspired Helena María Viramontes, a Chicana author, to write her most anthologized short story, "The Moths." In this story, a young woman finds herself tenderly bathing and caressing the dead body of her grandmother soon after the elderly woman has passed away. It proves a moment of deep reflection.[46] In a later interview, Viramontes explained that, when viewing Smith's photograph, she was "overpowered by the love I saw between this mother and her deformed child. While the child looks into space, the mother shows such love and compassion in bathing the child. I felt the strength of bonding, love and trust between the two. I wanted to capture this feeling in the relationship between the grandmother and her grandchild in 'The Moths.'"[47] Make no mistake: the production of fertilizer and plastics created Minamata disease. But, paradoxically, the production of plastics also created the celluloid that captured one of the disease's most enduring images—dare I say beautiful images—that was displayed around the world, where it spawned artistic reactions as well as passionate outrage and helped fuel the modern environmental movement.

Oblivious to both the hardship the company would cause and the sublime art it would later inspire, Chisso also built an octyl alcohol facility, which produced that chemical from acetaldehyde but which also represented one step in the manufacturing of PVC. Such plastics produced even cheaper, disposable consumer goods that people clamored for; but the real price tag of such goods remained lost on the Japanese public until the 1970s. In Japan, as in the United States and the rest of the world, the development of plastics brought a dazzling array of new products: a democratization of consumerism. The 1930s witnessed the birth of the "Plastic Age," when chemistry's most accomplished offspring and the synthetic "emblem of modernity" served as an icon of human control, of consumer utopia, of displacement from the organic, and of liberation from "nature's imperfections." Jeffrey Meikle argues that chemistry made nature "malleable in the face of human desire."[48]

Chisso publications from 1937 picture some of the consumer goods crafted from what the company proudly called "Chissolite" and "Chissoloid," including telephones, radios, clocks, pencil sharpeners, electric fans, cosmetic containers, electric lamps, and other household stuff that today is utterly ubiquitous. It is not surprising that Chisso became a leader in the production of plastics. Earlier, when Japanese companies such as Chisso had begun producing early synthetics such as celluloid (developed by Celluloid Manufacturing Company in 1871), it sparked demand for the natural resources used for its production. In the early twentieth century, for example, Mitsui, a Japanese corporate colossus we have already met, even stymied European and American competitors by monopolizing access to Formosan camphor in the Japanese colony of Taiwan. Camphor, a crystalline distillate extracted from the camphor laurel tree (*Cinnamomum*

camphora), served as the primary ingredient in celluloid, and after deforestation in China and Japan, by 1900 the laurel trees of Taiwan were the
world's only source.[49]

Even in the economically poor homes near Minamata City, vinyl countertops and flooring, as well as plastic food containers and radios and nylon
nets, became commonplace by the 1940s and 1950s. Rather than represent a
democratization of consumerism, however, the production of plastics near
their homes proved the final blow to communities already suffering from
grinding and relentless poverty in the wake of Japan's frenzied industrialization. But, as we learned previously, the alienation from wealth and
power of fishing communities was nothing new, as our foray into the history of the *kaijin*, or "sea people," has already demonstrated.

To this point, I have introduced the delirious Sakagami Yuki and
explored Minamata's estuarine ecosystem, the bioaccumulation of toxins
in shellfish and fish, fertilizers and the ecological footprint of eighteenth-
century Japanese cities, and the activities within the Chisso factory.
Regarding Chisso, I have examined the facility's alchemic birthing process
and listed the many consumer goods, from fertilizers to plastics, that the
factory birthed. To complete my exploration of Minamata disease, however, I shall now turn to the human body and its complex birthing process:
in particular, the process of fetal organogenesis and how the mercury from
Chisso interfered with this most delicate of biological processes.

Without the interference of toxins, mothers from Minamata birthed
children who continued ancestral families. In light of Japan's enduring
Confucian social values, I have already characterized Japan's paternalistic
households near Minamata as patri-ecolocalities or micro-biogeographies,
because of the manner in which Confucian values influenced environments. Families constituted core ecological units as well as social ones.
What allowed these families to survive was the ability of mothers to birth
healthy children. Indeed, the inability of mothers to birth healthy children
constituted legal grounds for divorce in Japan's ancient (and even not so
ancient) past. The eighth-century Taihō-Yōrō Codes do not mince words
on this point; neither did much of Meiji (1868–1912) law. But Chisso's effluence interceded in the birthing process—somewhat like a secret lover—
and that is why this chapter is titled "Mercury's Offspring." In the villages
around Minamata, it was no longer simply the mother's egg and the father's
seed that created the next generation of life within these patri-ecolocalities, because mercury, too, contributed to create these offspring. Like the

genetic codes of their mothers and fathers, the legacy of mercury (and its history) inscribed itself onto the bodies and the minds of mercury's offspring. Their deformed bodies are a physical manifestation of our shared modern industrial ideals.

Interpreting the Fetus

Of the relationship between human health and the environment, Gregg Mitman observes: "Whether through intimate bodily experience of illness and place, or through abstracted scientific knowledge of ecological communities, conceptions of health have been integral to environmental experience and understanding."[50] But, as Mitman and others argue elsewhere, "environment and human health have long been seen as having separate histories."[51] That is, U.S. historians often embrace narratives that too seldom embed human bodies in landscapes, for reasons that have to do with viewing humans as outside, rather than a part of, nature, even at cellular or molecular levels. But traditional Japanese pluralistic medicine embedded bodies not only in physical landscapes but in moral ones as well. Because traditional Japanese notions of the body, the fetus, and the landscape drove, at least in part, the manner in which human health and environmental toxins were understood—even in the twentieth century and in the context of discovering the causes of Minamata disease—we must dive into the complicated topic of Japanese conceptions of bodies and landscapes.

As Yuki Terazawa has shown, obstetrician Katsuki Gyūzan (1655–1740) viewed bodies, in particular women's bodies and the process of reproduction, through the holistic lens of Chinese medicine.[52] The Chinese text *The Yellow Emperor's Classic of Internal Medicine* (compiled between the third and fifth centuries BCE) established much of the theoretical basis behind early East Asian medicine. It, and a whole host of East Asian practices, came to Japan in the seventh and eighth centuries. The body came to be viewed as a microcosm of the entire universe, and so harmony with one's environment translated into harmony with one's body.[53] "Those who disobey the laws of the universe will give rise to calamities and visitations," explains the *Classic*, "while those who follow the laws of the universe remain free from dangerous illness, for they are the ones who have obtained Tao, the Right Way."[54]

Japanese practiced more "native" medical traditions as well, ones that viewed disease as the product of spirit possession or "pollution" and "defilement" caused by contact with blood, corpses, or people with skin diseases. Early Japanese labeled this condition as "having a spirit polluted by bad poison," and they believed it to be communicable and, more devastating to the Confucian household, hereditary. Treating disease meant purging such pollutants through herbs and baths in hot springs, and the more violent the purging, the better; prevention, through ritual purification, gargling, and bathing, still remains central to Japanese hygienic practices. Just as there could be landscapes of disease, there could also be landscapes of healing or medical geographies, such as those that contained geothermic baths.[55]

Katsuki had studied with Kaibara Ekken (or Ekiken, 1630–1714), a Confucian scholar, and this experience shaped his decidedly Confucian views regarding reproduction and the belief that "essential vitalities" invigorated households through the production of generations of male heirs. In preindustrial Japan, patrilinear continuity, patrilocal places, and the preservation of the household remained hallmarks of the Confucian milieu, and Japanese viewed communicable or hereditary diseases as particularly devastating. Diseases poisoned these Confucian patri-ecolocalities or micro-biogeographies, not just individual bodies. Disease proved socially constructed and socially symptomatic. Much as Minamata disease did, hereditary diseases injured not only the individual but the core values of filial piety and familial continuity. Japanese physicians such as Katsuki considered the etiological basis for many afflictions, including those related to reproduction, to be related to imbalances of yin and yang forces and emotional excesses; but they considered demonic possessions and Buddhist karmic retribution causative agents as well. For example, if women failed to become pregnant, Katsuki blamed their sterility on insufficient blood and, hence, on improper levels of yang. If men possessed the proper "essence" and women proper blood circulation, the child they conceive, he wrote, "will live long without having any accidents and will be blessed with luck, wisdom, and intelligence."[56]

Similarly, the female "heart learning" (shingaku) scholar Rakuhoku Shōko postulated in 1785 that a pregnant woman's attitude, specifically whether or not she obeyed her husband, often determined whether the child would be smart or stupid, good or bad.[57] Tadano Makuzu (1763–1825) spoke of the "humble" attitude of women as well, but she embedded female subordination in the natural, cosmologically rooted differences between men and women. Obedience had less to do with intelligence, she insinuated, than it had to do with yin and yang balances: what she described as competing "lack" and "surplus." She explained: "Women exist for the sake of men; men do not exist for the sake of women. Even if she is more intelligent, how can a woman who thinks she is lacking something triumph over a man who always thinks of himself as having a surplus?" Tadano was no physician, but in *Hitori kangae* (Solitary Thoughts; 1818) she speculated on the role of yin and yang forces in determining male and female sexuality and, in adulthood, constructing gendered emotions and social roles. While Katsuki had explained that balances of yin and yang determined whether fetal development occurred properly, Tadano traced the natural difference in gender temperaments in adults to sexuality and likened intercourse to a violent clash of genitals: "In that in examining our bodies, we become aware of a surplus and or a lack, it is clear that human feelings are rooted in the genitals and spread from there throughout our bodies. When men and women make love, they battle for superiority by rubbing their genitals together. For a husband and a wife who are one this may not be an issue." The product of this "battle for superiority" between men and women (though some married couples apparently were exempt), between those with "surplus" and those with "lack," was the human fetus, and its development was shaped by the social behavior of those involved.[58]

Katsuki did not, however, level blame for sterility exclusively on women's behavior, and he repeatedly warned men that women's blood was not the only factor. He urged couples to time the rhythms of their sexual activity to the Chinese calendar, as fertility and cosmology were interrelated—the body was embedded in not only physical landscapes but temporal ones as well. Besides problems with blood, circulation of *ki* (ether; psychophysical stuff), and "pollution," infertility could also be caused by moral lapses. Sometimes couples failed to conceive children because they engaged in "evil thoughts and conduct." By cultivating virtue, what some called "fetal education," the "charity of the emperor in Heaven will penetrate nature so that the couple will be able to have children and maintain future generations." Katsuki remained concerned about patrilineality and so did not practice abortions; however, one 1668 text from the competing Chūjō School of obstetrics (which focused on herbal remedies) described a concoction made from metallic mercury, palm nuts, and Japanese mint that, when inserted into a pregnant woman's vagina, reportedly induced an abortion.[59]

The Dutch doctor Pompe van Meerdervoort (1829–1908) wrote in the mid-nineteenth century of "famous abortionists" near Nagasaki. Along with using lances, which they "handle quite well," these abortionists sometimes deployed "live mercury" to induce abortions in expectant mothers. Even though the Tokugawa shoguns had prohibited the practice in the mid-seventeenth century (specifically, the Shōhō years: 1644–48), obstetricians and abortionists flourished. Pompe speculated on the ethics of this matter: "It is true that murder was outlawed in the country, but then the victim would be alive first, and an unborn fruit was not considered to be a living individual yet. It belonged to the mother, they [Japanese physicians] said, as part of her body, and she was free to do what she wanted with that body."[60]

Japanese obstetricians thought that "pollution" was generated during the birthing process itself. Many preindustrial Japanese obstetricians believed that fetal poisons could contaminate just-born children, so they encouraged proper ritual purification. Japanese have observed such practices, as classical diaries reveal, from ancient times. In the *Kagero nikki* (Gossamer Years; 970 CE), for example, after a child is born, the father conveniently brushes off the fatigued mother by saying, "I know that you will not want to see me until the defilement has worn off."[61] In the thirteenth century, Lady Nijō provided an even better window into child labor and delivery with rare frankness for her stylized age. She described, for example, the empress, Higashi Nijō, in labor and remarked that, because she was "somewhat advanced in years" and had "suffered complications in her earlier deliveries," the emperor summoned a priest to perform "every possible esoteric rite for her benefit, offering prayers to the Seven Healing Buddhas, the Five Great Guardian Kings, Fugen Bodhisattva, Kongō Dōji, and Aizen-ō." Her memoirs attest to a child labor and delivery atmosphere replete with Buddhist ritual and prayer, Confucian paternalism, and Shinto anxieties regarding "pollutants":

> At signs that the child was about to be born, the prayers grew so fervent they seemed to rise like billows of smoke. The court ladies handed unlined gowns and raw silk gowns under the blinds to the attendants, who presented them to the courtiers. Then imperial guards passed them to the priests reciting the sutras. At the foot of the stairs sat the nobles, hoping the child would be a boy. The masters of divination had set up offeratory tables in the garden and were repeating the purification rite a thousand times. Courtiers passed the purified articles to the ladies, who thrust their sleeves under the blinds to receive them.

At the same time royal attendants and junior imperial guards were bringing out the offeratory horses for His Majesty to inspect before they were distributed to twenty-one shrines. No woman could hope for a more auspicious set of circumstances.[62]

With such ceremonial precautions, it should not be surprising that Higashi Nijō safely delivered a baby girl; the "unfortunate" news was signaled by a rice kettle being rolled down the north side of the palace roof. When Lady Nijō gives birth to her son, along with prayers offered to a dazzling pantheon of Buddhas, Bodhisattvas, and Shinto deities, "bowstrings were twanged to ward off evil spirits." On the occasion of the birth of her second child, "rice water" was brought to sanctify the auspicious moment; and Nijō spent one hundred days at the palace until the period of defilement associated with delivery had passed.[63] Early notions of defilement and mourning remained so important that, for women, having sexual liaisons during periods of defilement or mourning, at least according to some ancient sources, constituted a form of sexual "violation," sometimes being likened even to rape.[64]

Through much of Japanese history, it was the midwife's job to handle pollution created by the birthing process. (In Japanese, midwives were known as *toriagebaba,* or old-women-deliverers.) Normal deliveries meant that women kneeled down and held a rope that suspended from the ceiling. When women assume the proper delivery position, "the fetus," wrote Katsuki, "as if awakened from a dream, separates itself from the afterbirth, and seeks its way out."[65] Women's attitudes, their moral behavior, their conformity to Chinese calendars, and what they ate and drank determined the success of the delivery, the health and intelligence of the child, and the future prosperity of their husband's household.

Katsuki also wrote about fetal development. "In the fourth month," he wrote, "it materializes."[66] To ensure that the fetus developed properly, he recommended that women regulate their circulation of psychophysical stuff by not urinating in improper places, not lifting heavy objects, and not drinking to excess; premature birth and other problems with delivery awaited women who failed to observe these basic moral instructions. Katsuki's writings expose an understanding of the organic ties between the mother and the outside world, as well as between mother and fetus. His age never witnessed the poisonous effects of methylmercury, but the idea that pollutants could disfigure fetuses during the process of organogenesis would not have surprised him because, in principle, the theory conformed to his understanding of connections among the mother, fetus, and pollution emanating from the world external to the placenta. Not all Japanese physicians accepted Katsuki's theories regarding pregnancy and fetal development, however. Kagawa Gen'etsu (1700–1777), for example, another obstetrician, also wrote about fetal development. He argued that the fetus is actually formed 120 days after conception. Kagawa and later practitioners of the Kagawa School introduced the use of surgical instruments, such as an "iron hook" to remove dead fetuses from the bodies of women, well before significant European influence on Japanese medicine.

The late 1850s and early 1860s witnessed the birth of modern medical education in Japan. Slowly, Western-style bacteriology and organ-specific medical practices intertwined with Japan's holistic view of the body and etiology of blood-borne pollutants; and official forms of medical certification replaced the legitimacy of hereditary learning and daily practice. In the late nineteenth and early twentieth centuries, even midwives had to gain certification to practice their craft, and so they too came under the control of the watchful Meiji state. The many Western physicians who taught in Japan embraced a medical philosophy different from that embraced by Katsuki and his colleagues.

It was this Euro-American style of medicine that originally defined the approach of the Kumamoto University research team as it sought an explanation for the "strange disease" that afflicted Sakagami Yuki and others.[67] However, as Kumamoto researchers later understood, the answer to the question of what caused Minamata disease was actually more environmental—that is, embedded in ecological landscapes—than physiological.

Fetal Education

Understanding how methylmercury injured the fetus to create congenital Minamata disease requires some discussion of fetal organogenesis, as understood by today's medicine. I have already projected fetal development back in time to explore traditional Japanese understandings of human creation. Henceforth, with the assistance of ecologist Sandra Steingraber, I will investigate how contemporary science understands human organogenesis and deformities. To put it simply, organogenesis is the formation of body parts: the genesis of limbs and organs that compose human beings and other creatures on Earth.[68] Organogenesis occurs between the sixth and the tenth month. Today, medicine explains that organogenesis occurs through stem-cell migration and induction: as these immature cells migrate throughout the liquid world of the fetus they latch onto more specialized cells, taking on their characteristics. Just as Buddhism saw endless potentiality in the liquid world of the womb, so too do stem cells realize this potentiality through their migratory and metamorphic qualities. That is, they change from unspecific to specific cells to become the building blocks of particular organs. It does not matter what country you come from or what religion you practice, all human beings develop in this manner: the similarities in our biological origins and our ability to be mutated by industrial toxins transcend culture and unite peoples around the globe. This is the physical reality that underlies all forms of cultural construction.

It is during this biologically magical phase of development that the fetus proves vulnerable to toxins that penetrate the placenta. The placenta trades carbon dioxide and other wastes for oxygen, water, minerals, antibodies, and other elements critical for fetal subsistence. Like the brain and testicles, the placenta possesses the ability to block toxins; but chemicals with lipid solubility, such as mercuric effluent (which brackish water from the estuary made soluble), clandestinely penetrate the placenta's protective barrier. Unknowingly, the placenta pumps methylmercury, as it would a molecule of calcium, into the capillaries of the fetus (in a manner similar to how mussels and anchovies extract oxygen from marine water), and in no time the levels of mercury in the umbilical cord exceed those of the mother's own blood. During the fourth through the sixth month of pregnancy, the fetus is most vulnerable to methylmercury: at this critical juncture brain cells migrate to form the brain, and methylmercury disrupts the movement of these critical cells.

The notion that the fetus stands at the top of the food chain is a modern scientific construct and does not necessarily represent how Japanese coastal villagers, even in the 1960s, would have viewed their unborn children. Over the centuries, Buddhism has shaped Japanese attitudes toward fetal development, infants, and, at the other end of the course of the human life, the elderly. Traditionally, Japanese saw young children as possessing lives, to be sure, but ones that precariously float, until about their seventh birthday or so, in an unpredictable liquid realm of potentiality that ebbs and flows between this realm of existence and the next. Likewise, as the elderly advance in age, they too begin to tread in this liquid world, because with Buddhism, no definitive line separates life and death. Evidencing this point are persistent stories of Obasuteyama, where, as legend has it, a villager nearly committed geronticide when he sought to "throw away his grandmother in the mountains," something he could conceivably do, particularly in the context of famine and other hardships, because of her advanced age: she was phasing back into the liquid world. These enduring stories illustrate that, whether rooted in actual practice or not, the liquid nature of the human life cycle pertained not just to childhood but to the other end of the life spectrum as well.[69]

Such attitudes served to shield Japanese emotionally from high infant mortality (from famine and disease) and "family-planning" decisions regarding sex-selected infanticide (principally females) in the early modern period.[70] Indeed, in some rural communities, often people did not even bestow names on children or register their names at local temples (in what were called *shūmon aratame chō* registries) as required by law until the children had passed their fifth birthday, as they knew that many children died before that age. But the souls of these dead children, known as *mizuko*, or water children, continued to inhabit the liquid world of potentiality. Later, in postwar Japan, in a practice known as *mizuko kuyō*, or water-child memorial services, dead fetuses were memorialized with *jizō* statues, often tenderly adorned with children's clothing and recognized in elaborate ceremonies.[71] Water symbolizes potentiality in many Buddhist creeds: it is the source of all possible existences. We should conclude in this manner: infant death and childhood mortality would have shocked neither Minamata fishers nor their ancient ancestors, though it surely saddened them, as it does us all, very deeply.[72]

No doubt the appalling childhood deformities caused by industrial disease did shock them, however, because preindustrial Japanese society appears to have had little experience with monstrous infant deformities. Early Japanese "freak shows" and "menageries," subsumed under the name *misemono*, featured, alongside other caged animals, sadly disfigured people, but such cases appear to have been relatively rare, suggesting that many birth deformities or childhood development disorders may be in part a product of our modern industrial nightmare: birth deformities may be largely unique to *Homo sapiens industrialis*. (Or, just as likely, deformed children might have been the target of infanticide and hence seldom appear in the historical record.) The physician Negishi Yasumori (1737–

1815) famously relayed a few stories about infant irregularities or deformities. One tells of a poor man from Nikkō who bought a large storage chest from a wealthy household in the hope that it would make him wealthy, too. Indeed, the storage chest did make him wealthy, but afterward he sought to sell the chest because it housed a long snake that needed constant attention. Seasonal grasses needed to be packed in the chest; and the serpent required feedings in the mornings and evenings. Once a year, moreover, he had to enter the chest and purify the snake by wiping clean its long, slender body with a cloth. It turns out that the reason the original owner of the chest had sold it was because one year, when his wife gave birth, she gave birth to a snake.[73] In traditional Japan, "snake-baby" folklore is quite common, and although folklorists have interpreted the stories as warnings against tabooed human relations, one might also speculate that any references to strange birth defects reflect just that, the existence of birth defects that Japanese attempted to explain.[74]

If we look back centuries, all the way to 1291, when the courtier Lady Nijō encountered a "dwarf" from Iwami Province at a famous shrine near the ancient capital of Kyoto, we get some indication of how early Japanese explained birth deformities. She remarked: "Talk centered on his deformity; no one could imagine what kind of karma might have caused it." For Lady Nijō, Buddhist notions of karma, in which a person's moral conduct and behavior in a previous life determine his or her form in this one, explained such human deformities, not issues of disease or problems with fetal organogenesis.[75] No doubt, some mothers of deformed babies in Minamata similarly speculated on the grave misconduct by themselves and their children in a former life that condemned them to such hellish suffering.

In a different kind of story, when Negishi's grandson was born, the midwife failed to return by the third day, a critical period in which the baby needed to be bathed and, thereby, purified from the birthing process. Blood and afterbirth, in the Shinto tradition, represented pollution and defilement, and so the infant needed to be cleansed. Ultimately, because of the failure to cleanse the child, on the sixth day his grandson developed lockjaw and died.[76] Japanese obstetricians have long struggled with the defilements and pollutions inherent in the birthing process: in fact, it remained their principal task for centuries.[77] In some limited way, it became their principal task again at Minamata centuries later.

Harada Yoshitaka, a researcher at Kumamoto University, did not know precisely how methylmercury penetrated the placenta, but he did know that many children in the Minamata area, the majority of whom had never eaten fish caught from the waters near the Chisso factory spillway, suffered from severe forms of the industrial disease. That is, they got sick before they were born. Though educated in Euro-American medicine, in reality he practiced a kind of environmental medicine, much as Katsuki did centuries before him. That is to say, rather than spend his time thinly slicing human brains in a laboratory, so that he could fix his anatomizing gaze on their different strata, he collected data on the relationship of coastal families with their environment and social networks; he was interested in piecing together a more holistic picture of what social and environmental conditions caused children to be born with Minamata disease. He transcended the particularizing gaze of modern science and took a page right out of the *Yellow Emperor's Classic* by conducting surveys of the occupations of the parents, determining whether the ailing children were breastfed, questioning whether the parents shared blood relations, and measuring the levels of mercury in the hair of the mothers and children as well as in the blood preserved in dried umbilical cords; he already knew the damage caused to specific organs from autopsies of the most severely deformed children.

Harada discovered what his eighteenth- and nineteenth-century colleagues would have already assumed, that the environment where the mother lived and pollution—not symbolic defilement or moral transgressions but poisonous industrial toxins—caused birth deformities and inhibited mental abilities; that such social factors as occupation, eating habits, and poverty spawned disease. He wrote in a report issued in 1968, "The fetal period is the most critical stage for the growth of the central nervous system and it is the most affected" by toxins introduced through the placenta. Harada continued: "It has been proved by our investigation team that the organic mercury is deposited in the bodies of adults and children by taking the fish and shellfish, caught in Minamata Bay. Infants under breast feeding were positively affected through the placenta at the fetal period, or through mother's milk at the post-natal period." He noted that the levels of mercury both in children's hair and in the blood preserved in umbilical cords were "higher in this district than in the control district."[78]

Just as modern industrialism has produced factory effluence and this ecoepidemic, so too has it produced the compartmentalizing and particularizing mind-set that blinds us to the interconnectedness of things and robs us of our age-old ability to see the interrelated nature of our lives and the environment. The technological promise of microscopy and all the other technologies of the laboratory certainly aided Kumamoto University researchers in their discovery of the physiological effects of Minamata disease; but it was mainly when they stood back and imitated their preindustrial colleagues that they discovered the cause. The linkages between human and environmental health, and of the organic and the machine, came into better focus.

This chapter has demonstrated that an enormity of factors not only caused Minamata disease but crafted the networks that generated the scientific knowledge that unveiled the nature of its etiology: marine ecosystems, phosphate and nitrogen fertilizer production, "dancing cats" and coastal ecologies, nitrogen fixation, urban ecological footprints, plastics and modern consumerism, preindustrial and industrial medicine, and notions of organogenesis. We now must turn full circle, however, in order to tackle once more the issue of pain, because pain in the body signaled the culmination and accumulation of the above historical factors—it was how people, the victims of Minamata disease, knew they were connected to the Chisso factory in an organic way.

The discovery of Minamata disease occurred officially on 1 May 1956. Three years later, on 20 July 1959, researchers at Kumamoto University, including Harada Yoshitaka, announced that they believed mercury discharged by the Chisso factory caused the disease. But the company could have predicted the results contained in the stinging announcement by Kumamoto researchers. On 7 October 1959, company doctor Hosokawa Hajime, after feeding factory effluent to the unfortunate "Cat no. 400," had replicated the disease in the laboratory, and although he alerted company leaders, only on his deathbed did he divulge that he and the company had known that mercury was the culprit. By that time, it was too late for the hundreds of victims.

It did not take long for Chisso to announce that technologies such as a Sedifloater and a Cyclator, designed by the Ebara Infilco Company, would be added to the factory to purify the effluent. Of course, promises of a technological fix, underwritten mostly by empty corporate promises and the sheer complexity of the gadgetry itself, characterized the early responses to the Ashio and Kamioka disasters as well. By early 1960, engineers had installed the gadgets and had them operating; and in a public relations stunt without parallel, company president Yoshioka Kiichi even drank a glass of water directly from the Cyclator, though he was perfectly aware that dangerous toxins from the acetaldehyde production were not being channeled through the purifiers. As attorneys later confirmed, Ebara Infilco engineers never intended the technologies to remove dissolved organic mercury. Not surprisingly, with no real purification technologies on-site, estimates regarding the amount of toxins dumped into the sea depend on who produces them, but between 1930 and the late 1960s, Chisso dumped somewhere between 224 and 600 tons of mercury into Minamata Bay.

In the face of pressure by fishing cooperatives and victims, Chisso began to offer paltry "sympathy payments" and "solatium agreements" to people in the Minamata area, a tactic also employed in the Shimotsuke Plain near the Ashio complex and designed to entice the poorest members of Japanese society. And other inhabitants of Minamata City and the nation at large proved disappointingly hostile to the victims. In short, the "selfish demands" of the victims threatened to close down the Chisso factory, just as Ashio's pollution-control efforts threatened to shut down the mine. Such efforts threatened the livelihoods of many workers who themselves had families to feed. Shutting down the factory was "world destroying," to evoke Elaine Scarry's language from the introduction, even if the intended effect was to ameliorate pain. The initial set of "solutions," reached in 1959, proved ineffective, as the congenital form of Minamata disease continued to appear in poor fishing communities. Almost a decade later, Minamata disease victims took their case to the courts and won hard-fought victories over Chisso. After years of fighting against public prejudices and private power, on 20 March 1973, Judge Saitō Jirō, of the Kumamoto District Court, decided in favor of the victims and accused Chisso of "corporate negligence."[79]

Even though it included "compensation agreements," the victory tasted bittersweet to most. The pain persisted; it continued to destroy worlds, many of them. Images of bedridden victims, with contorted faces, painfully etched grins, empty stares, and permanently clenched, clawlike hands, testify that only shells of human beings remained to receive the yearly gifts from healthy corporate patriarchs who showed up at individual homes in their best summer suits. On 31 March 2000, physicians had certified 2,264 victims as suffering from Minamata disease, and most received compensation under the 1973 agreement; another 10,353 victims received compensation under a 1995 agreement.

To conclude this chapter we will bear witness to a remarkable scene, one that perfectly intertwines industrial disease, human pain, and the nature of Japan's national community. Remember that in the introduction I argued that nations are not entirely invented entities, as is so often asserted, because the dangerous effects of pollution demonstrate that people really do physiologically experience national policies and priorities. Here is testimony to that assertion: on 22 September 1968, Sonoda Sunao, from the Ministry of Health and Welfare, traveled to Minamata as part of an observational visit. He planned to inspect the Yunoko Sanitarium, where Sakagami Yuki, whom we met at the outset of this chapter, had been transferred. Divorced from Mohei, Sakagami now went by her maiden name, Nishikata. She remembered the visit: "Some thirty gentlemen wearing fine suits came in and crowded round my bed, staring at me as if I was some rare animal. I also looked them up and down, trying to guess who the minister was. I didn't mind 'em gaping at me; I'm used to being shown like a freak in a circus." Her delirious episodes had for the most part subsided; no more blood-drenched fish swam in and out of her corroded mind as aborted fetuses. Then one of the men took a photograph of her with a blinding flash, perhaps as evidence of industrial disease or as a personal keepsake. The flash immediately sparked something and the "inside of my head went dark," she later recalled, "and here they came on again. . . ."

Directly in front of the minister, she went into convulsive fits. Three doctors struggled to hold her down, and as tears streamed down her face, she smiled bravely with that same haunting grin common to most Minamata victims. Before Minister Sonoda and his entourage could leave the room lest they confront the real face of *Homo sapiens industrialis*, Sakagami shouted, "Long live the emperor!" And then, as a silence fell over the sanitarium, in a "thin, trembling falsetto" she began to sing Japan's national anthem.[80]

6 HELL AT THE HŌJŌ COLLIERY

In Fukuoka Prefecture, the area around the Onga River, which flows south to north as it carves its way through the ancient provinces of Chikuzen and Buzen, is referred to as the Chikuhō region. In Japan, to say "Chikuhō" is essentially to say "coal," though today one is struck equally by the area's limestone mines, which have conspicuously decapitated entire mountains. There is a good reason to conflate "Chikuhō" and "coal": the region boasts some of Japan's richest coalfields, and its history is steeped in the triumphs and tragedies of coal mining. Coal extracted from Chikuhō fueled Japan's modernization in the nineteenth and early twentieth centuries (the region produced about half of Japan's total coal in the late Meiji era); the region also became home to thousands of forcibly displaced Koreans who were recruited as labor within Japan's expanding empire. These Koreans died in droves in the Chikuhō coalfields. Today, ornate redbrick buildings, towering smokestacks, and slag heaps that loom dramatically over modest farming villages stand as monuments to this tumultuous past. So do ubiquitous street gangs and "Pachinko Pros," who remain mired in poverty despite their gambling skills: with coal shafts filled with groundwater, Chikuhō is now famous for its welfare recipients.

Up to now, this book has explored three keys to Japan's modern industrialization: scientific agriculture and pesticide application, copper, lead, and zinc mining, and the nitrogen fixation technologies that produced fertilizers and plastics. This chapter turns our attention to the coal that, when burned in locomotives, factories, and steamships, produced the calories that fueled Japan's rise to industrial prominence. Our interest, however, is quite specific: this chapter focuses on a 15 December 1914 explosion at the Hōjō colliery that left 687 people dead, as well as a handful of non-human animals. It stands as the largest mining disaster on Japanese soil (though not, as we will see, at a mine under Japanese control).[1] It is of interest because the explosion was the result of hybrid contexts and causations: carefully engineered subterranean environments conducive to extracting thousands of tons of coal interfaced with naturally occurring methane-gas deposits. Miners labored alongside mechanical ventilation and dampening systems, which sought to keep methane and coal dust suppressed; mules and horses pulled ore carts alongside electric lifts called "cages" that lowered miners deep into Earth at ear-popping speeds. The Hōjō mine functioned as a hybrid system comprising biological and mechanical parts; but it was precisely the holistic, integrated nature of these biological and mechanical parts that caused the unanticipated 1914 explosion at the site that killed so many. This chapter contains a systems analysis of the technological risks associated with fueling modern nations.

FUELING MEIJI

When historians teach students about the Meiji years (1868–1912), two slogans are scratched on chalkboards across the country: *bunmei kaika*, "civilization and enlightenment," and *fukoku kyōhei*, "rich country and strong military." The latter of these two slogans relates to Japan's coal-mining history, because both the industry that was to make Japan rich and the military that was to make Japan strong demanded caloric energy, just as an organism does. Recall from the introduction: ecological food chains and food webs are essentially about the transference of energy; and in some respects the politics of nations are, too. In the early Meiji years, energy from coal found its way into steam trains, steamships, and cauldrons for the salt industry. But after the Sino-Japanese War of 1895, coal also fueled industrial development and war. Just as the Sino-Japanese War represented a turning point in the zinc- and lead-mining industry, so too did it signal the birth of Japanese heavy industry and ramped-up extraction of the coal that fueled large factories. This book, in many respects, has been the story of the ecological footprint of Meiji modernization, both its industrial development and its empire-building projects.

The connection between war, industrial development, and resource extraction is not a whimsical one. Many of the prominent German economists who so intrigued Japanese pundits and politicians in the late nineteenth and early twentieth centuries saw a direct relationship between war, or at least preparation for war, and large-scale capitalist expansion. Werner Sombart (1863–1941) was one such economist. In *Krieg und Kapitalismus* (1913), he celebrated cooperation between the "warlord and capitalist," because in order to meet military demand, economic scales of production and management strategies needed to be radically transformed. War stood at the heart of economic innovation, he argued. War centralized and integrated national economies, as well as led to technological advancement, in a manner that few other state endeavors did.[2] Although a Chinese Qin dynasty (221–206 BCE) political ruler first coined the slogan "rich country and strong military," Meiji modernizers resurrected it. Richard Samuels observes that it became "the formal ideological foundation of industrial and technological development during the Meiji period." Ultimately, the slogan served to justify dismantling the Tokugawa decentralized polity and bringing military and industry under the control of the state. The policy initiatives of Ōkuma Shigenobu (1838–1922) exemplified the Meiji tendency to bring the military and industry under central control. When justifying the creation of the Ministry of Industry (Kōbushō; 1870), Ōkuma articulated the need to "encourage all industrialists to work for the benefit of the nation and the people." The new ministry, he reasoned, would foster "richness of the country" (*kokka fukyō*) and meet "the need for military buildup" (*gunkaku hitsuyō*). Important for our discussion, one of the first activities of the ministry was the manufacture of mining technologies and equipment at shipyards located in Yokosuka and Nagasaki. Later, the ministry became part of the sprawling Ministry of Home Affairs (Naimushō, 1873), which oversaw industrial development, civil law, railway administration, and civil engineering. Minister of Home Affairs Okubō Toshimichi (1830–78) fostered an enduring business relationship with Iwasaki Yatarō (1835–85), a shipping company executive who founded Mitsubishi, owner of the Hōjō colliery, in 1870.[3]

But back to the heart of our discussion: industrial production, particularly in heavy industry, paralleled Meiji war-making. Take a few choice industrial names and their founding dates, the important point being that 1905 was the date that the Russo-Japanese War was waged: Hachiman Seitetsu (Hachiman Iron Manufacturing, 1901), Sumitomo Chūkō (Sumitomo Steel Casting, 1901), Kobe Seikō (Kobe Steel Manufacturing, 1905), Nippon Seikō (Japan Steel Manufacturing, 1907), and Nihon Kōkan (Japan Steel Tubing, 1912). The massive furnaces at these prominent industrial sites, which forged munitions along with other industrial products, hungered for high-calorie coal: by 1907, Japanese coal production had increased three-fold when compared with only a decade earlier.[4]

Coal had been mined earlier, of course. In the sixteenth century, domain lords had exploited coal from the Chikuhō region on a modest scale: along with wood charcoal, it was used mainly to heat homes. But the Meiji modernization scheme demanded energy on a heretofore-unseen scale. By 1936, coal served 51.4 percent of Japan's energy needs, providing calories for both industry and private households. Four years later, coal provided a whopping 66.1 percent of Japan's energy needs. As observer Kōno Ekitarō wrote in 1898 in a Chikuhō coal-industry magazine, in the 1870s miners had dug coal like "raccoon-dogs" (a reference to the *tanuki-bori* method discussed in chapters 3 and 4), but by the 1880s engineers had designed "sloping shafts," called *shakō*, that could descend much deeper into Earth.[5] Economically, Japan's coalfields remained under the oligopolistic control of the famous *zaibatsu* firms such as Mitsubishi: their reliance on cronyism (take as an example the relationship between Ōkubo and Iwasaki), cheap labor, and natural resources exploited at home and throughout the empire fueled Japan's prewar economy. Japan has coalfields on the northern and southern islands of Hokkaido and Kyushu. Energy independence meant relying on domestic coal for Meiji industrialization. Later, however, one of the reasons frequently cited by Japanese expansionists for the thrust into Manchuria was access to coal deposits there. It should not surprise us, then, that the largest coal-dust explosion that ever occurred happened in China, in the Japanese puppet state of Manzhouguo (Manshūkoku in Japanese) at the Benxihu colliery (Honkeiko) on 26 April 1942. Later in the chapter, we will investigate this disaster for comparison with the Hōjō colliery explosion.

In the 1880s, the Meiji government sold Japan's coal mines to such *zaibatsu* firms as Mitsui, Mitsubishi, and Sumitomo, which used the income to invest in other businesses. That is, these *zaibatsu* firms exploited mines to supply capital for other divisions of these massive conglomerates; in turn, they invested precious little in technological mechanization or labor. What this meant was that Japan's coal mines were, to put it mildly, tough places to make a living. At times, as much as 80 percent of the profits of the Mitsubishi conglomerate came from the mining division. *Zaibatsu* mines controlled Japan's coal output throughout the pre–Pacific War years. Laura Hein has observed that in the prewar years, "The mines were a cornucopia of wealth for their owners."[6] Later, during the war, firms such as Mitsubishi and Mitsui benefited from the forced labor of workers brought to Japan from Korea and elsewhere: in 1884, convicts made up 53 percent of the 2,340 miners at Miike (also on Kyushu); by 1896, 75 percent of the 1,932 miners were prisoners, although this number later dropped.[7] By 1944, 35,209 Koreans worked in Hokkaido mines, 74,736 worked in Kyushu mines, and 18,245 worked in Honshu mines. Koreans constituted some 31.9 percent of the mining workforce in Japan in the final years of the Pacific War.

With so much riding on Japan's coal mines, villages in the Chikuhō region came to constitute strangely cruel worlds unto themselves: *zaibatsu* territories within the Meiji state. The "lodge system," a reference to the lodges where miners were forced to live, served as the core community structure in the coalfields; elected "headmen" met regularly with company representatives and then relayed important directives to the labor force. In these tightly controlled lodge communities, companies maintained law and order independently of local police through the use of "labor control offices" and their well-known connections to *yakuza* crime syndicates. Not surprisingly, a culture of violence emerged within these communities, particularly as the coal industry began to decline and petroleum became the fuel of choice in the 1950s.[8] Violent as it was, one cannot conclude that the Chikuhō region was a man's world: women had come to constitute about 25 percent of miners by the 1940s. With the 1910 annexation of Korea, miners from that country began to arrive in the Chikuhō region, as did Chinese after the 1931 invasion of Manchuria (the next year Manzhouguo was formally established). Always, the production of coal and the demographics at Japan's mines mirrored war and empire, just as industrial expansion did. As with the increase of the zinc and lead mining at Kamioka, the relationship between war and coal simply cannot be ignored. In 1932 there were some 140,000 coal miners in Japan; but by 1945 that number was 440,000.[9]

War demands calories, as well as the blood of the young and the treasure of the nation. In their own ways, both war and coal fueled industrial expansion: consider industrial expansion the economic footprint of war.

After the Pacific War (1937–45), Japan's Allied occupiers also pushed for coal production. In 1946 the Coal Priority Production legislation was passed, which gave the state more control over the coal industry. To lure miners back to the Chikuhō coalfields, incentives such as free *bentō* lunches and lodging were offered to a population suffering from malnutrition and lack of shelter. Simultaneously, Tanrō, the Union of Coal Miners, was established with the support of the New Deal occupation, and by 1948 some 50 percent of miners boasted membership in the leftist union. With proper legislation, economic incentives, and Korean War procurements in place, the coal industry boomed. In 1951, the industry experienced peak production before entering a spiraling decline with the emergence of oil as the energy source of the future. But just as the rise of the coal industry paralleled war and empire, increasing levels of technological risk paralleled the rise of the coal industry. High accident rates accelerated during this critical boom period: historians estimate that between 1950 and 1960, some 5,000 miners died in the Chikuhō region. Between 1936 and 1970, Mitsubishi lost 1,392 miners: nearly half of those died in the 15 December 1914 incident at the Hōjō colliery.[10]

WOMEN IN COAL MINES

Women were far from immune to mining risks. Well into the Meiji era, women remained ubiquitous presences at coal mines, often working for just over 70 or 80 percent of the wages of their male counterparts. But because women often performed the same arduous labor as men, some mines paid women and men equally. "Women and men did the same kind of work," wrote one female miner. "It's not true that women were weaker physically. We did the same work. . . . There was a woman who used to lift up huge chunks of coal that men could not carry."[11]

In the nineteenth century, the mechanization of ore conveyance demanded increased productivity of miners at ore faces and, therefore, a more stable and dependable workforce: this meant families. Subsequently, foremen recruited families to settle on-site and raise children in the cruel state-within-a-state environs of Japan's coal mines. Even at coal mines, the

Confucian family constituted a patri-ecolocality or micro-biogeography (a notion introduced in the previous chapter), a social unit that shouldered the burden of the technological risk, environmental pollution, and human pain at coal mines. One 1906 announcement from Mitsui Corporation's Tagawa mine, located next door to the Hōjō colliery, explained: "First preference to families consisting of a couple with a child of 12 or 13, all three of whom will be required to work; plus one elderly person to serve as cook" (fig. 6.1). Just as the Tokugawa shoguns mustered Confucian filial piety to promote loyalty, so too did Meiji oligarchs recast the Confucian dictum of "three generations under one roof" to serve the energy needs of rapid industrialization and empire creation after the Sino-Japanese War. In the early twentieth century, the Confucian family emerged as the core social unit of late Meiji society, and it, rather than the individual body, became the site of pain at Japan's coal mines: entire families, some nuclear, others extended, were often incinerated in one coal mine explosion, their surnames obliterated.

By the early twentieth century, the majority of miners at most Kyushu coal shafts were employed as families, at least until convicts or Koreans replaced Japanese miners at many of these sites. Generally, at the mines, men dug at the coal face and women hauled the ore to the surface. Though women could not enter the mines when "defiled" by menstruation for fear of offending deities (usually "mountain deities," or *yama no kami*, whom locals believed to be jealous females), they worked the rest of the time and then, on returning to the lodge, undertook most of the exhausting domestic chores. The polluting nature of women prohibited them from other productive spaces as well. In coastal communities, as we have seen, defilement and pollution excluded women from fishing on certain days; and because the spirit of saké breweries was female, women's entry into breweries sometimes aroused her spite. Just north of Tokyo, for example, women wore talismans on their *obi* belts with stylized images of skeletons and wording that said "for canceling the ban on women" and thereby could enter saké breweries without attracting the deity's jealous wrath.[12] Apparently, sympathetic to capitalism, deities could be placated with enough talismans and market demand.

When Ishimoto Shidzue (also known as Katō Shidzue; 1897–2001), first arrived at the Miike coalfields of Kyushu with her husband as a young bride, she could hardly believe her eyes: "On both sides girls were at work, sorting coal lumps by size," wrote the petite woman of aristocratic upbring-

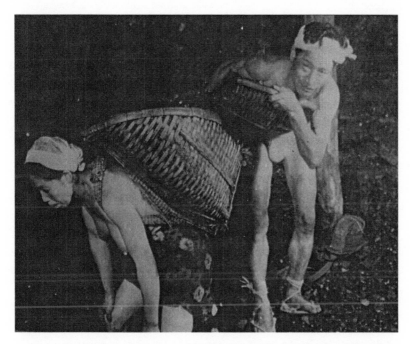

FIG. 6.1 At coal mines such as Tagawa, in north-central Kyushu, mine bosses employed families because they represented a more stable workforce. Here, a woman is hauling coal to the surface in a basket with straps. Photograph courtesy of the Tagawa Coal Mining Museum (Sekitan Hakubutsukan), Tagawa, Japan.

ing. "Black fragments of coal were scattered everywhere." She explained that at Miike there "was no holiday on this industrial battlefield" and that the "miners had to work as long as engines were active" or, presumably, as long as their bodily engines remained active. Once, Shidzue's husband brought her down inside the bowels of the Kattachi shaft. She remembered horses, "worn and feeble, their energy lost by their long stay underground," which miners used to transport ore to the surface before the mechanization of conveyance in the form of trams and railways. Often, these animals never saw the light of day: they were merely four-legged ghosts in this subterranean otherworld. Women too hauled coal, often crawling on their hands and knees "like wiggling worms" in order to pull baskets of coal to underground loading zones where horses, wagons, or trams waited (fig. 6.2). "While carrying coal in baskets from pit to wagons, the girls were often crushed by the sudden overturn of the heavy coal trucks." Shidzue remarked: "Often pregnant women, working until the last moment, gave birth to children in the dark pit." When these mine babies opened their small, glassy eyes, they saw only the artificial light of this engineered world. Family life at the mines was, in her words, a "picture of Hades." Once back at their lodges, "They cooked, washed and nursed like other women whose energies are spent only on such domestic tasks. Naturally they were abnormally nervous and exhausted. They often beat their impatiently hungry children who could not wait for their mothers to cook their meals."[13]

Most women who hauled coal at Kyushu mines were utterly uneducated, often miserably poor, and usually married, but they did, on occasion, make twice the wage of their "factory girl" counterparts at the textile mills. However, a drop in coal prices in the 1920s, the importation of cheap coal from the empire, and legislation limiting the role of women at mines slowly eroded the place of women at many of Kyushu's coal mines. By 1926, the "peak year" for technological innovation at the mines, explosives, drilling tools, and other forms of mechanization had replaced women at many of the mine shafts and surface workplaces.[14] Yet their mere presence, combined with the fact that they sometimes birthed children in subterranean shafts, bolsters my point about the Confucian *ie*, or family/household, being the key to Japan's environmental history. If, as many ecologists suggest, ecological systems are essentially about the transference of energy among organisms, then the core node in Japan's national production and transference of energy was the idealized Confucian family.[15] Within these Confucian families, mercury's offspring were destined to be hideously deformed; Chikuhō's offspring were destined to labor in the coal mines. Sometimes they were even born in them. Whether defending their nets from rats on the beaches of Minamata or trapped in the run-down lodges and dank mine shafts of the Chikuhō region, the Japanese *ie* constituted a patri-ecolocality or micro-biogeography that is the birthplace, nurturing site, and principal victim of Japan's toxic archipelago.

BUDDHISM AND THE SUBTERRANEAN

Ishimoto Shidzue called the bowels of the Miike mine—with ghostly horses and half-naked female figures hauling baskets of coal to the surface to service the hungry machines of war—a "picture of Hades." Indeed, one might speculate that, in terms of the technological risk and sheer pain associated with Japan's coal mines, hell offers the closest approximation to the pain actually inflicted in this subterrestrial world. We can look at Japanese

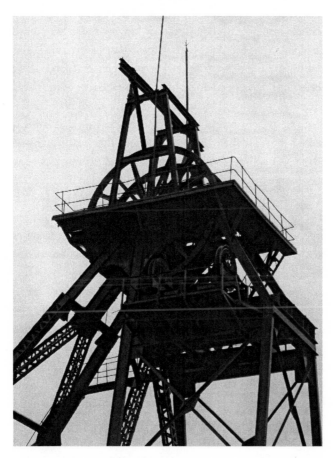

FIG. 6.2 The top of an old cage lift, or head frame, at Tagawa, near the Hōjō coal mine. Photograph by author.

depictions of Buddhist hell as a kind of definition of pain, addressing some of the analytical questions regarding pain raised in the introduction and not yet fully reconciled.

Classical Japanese Buddhist writings and scroll paintings mostly depict human pain as being suffered in the fires of hell, where flames consume the poor souls dispatched there by Enmaō, the king of the world of the dead. As we learned from Elaine Scarry in the introduction, because pain is not *of* or *for* anything, crafters of such didactic scrolls always described pain by using *as if* or *as though* expressions. Genshin (942–1017), a monk from the Enryakuji Temple, wrote in 985 that the pain associated with hell felt as if demons were chopping one's body to pieces or one was being devoured by hungry beasts or one was being relentlessly stung by insects or one was being crushed by massive boulders. For Japanese who lived in the medieval age of *mappō* (a Buddhist "Latter Age of the Law"), pain—as an image deployed to lure people into following Buddhist precepts—was the feeling of being burned, ripped open, injured, crushed, or otherwise subjected to horrific punishment.[16] This image of Buddhist hell made sense because Buddhism, as its Four Noble Truths instruct, teaches that life is suffering. We live knowing that the only truth is death. That is, the dominant theology in Japan—Buddhism—focused on pain and suffering: the theological prism through which many Japanese view their own lives is all about the pain of this ephemeral world. Pain, in other words, defines life. To read the diaries of such classic literary figures as Murasaki Shikibu is to be immediately devoured by her pervasive melancholy. Though at times beautiful, her diary is, quite literally, painful to read. For instance, on witnessing two ducks on a pond, she mused: "I too am floating in a sad uncertain world."[17] But according to genre conventions, the diary is supposed to be written in this manner, because articulating the "pathos of life"—*mono no aware*—had been transformed into a potent aesthetic. Pain can be beautiful, too.[18]

Pain's "inexpressibility" has not stopped people from trying to express it. Medieval scroll paintings such as the *Jigokuzōshi* (Illustrated Stories of Hell) and the *Gakizōshi* (Illustrated Stories of Hungry Ghosts) depict people being horribly tortured. For these poor souls, the pain is as if "a red-hot iron dog is always gnawing the legs of these damned" or as if "a steel eaglet with a burning beak is pecking at the heads of the damned and sucking their brains." The "pain is unbearable," explains the *Jigokuzōshi*, "and [the damned] do not cease in their terrible screaming." Whether people are scorched in a burning river, dunked in a pit of filth, forced to weigh measures of red-hot coals, crushed in a mortar, or torn apart by a "terrible rooster full of fire," the *Jigokuzōshi* always uses elements from the mundane world to create its picture of an imaginary realm.[19]

The realm of the hungry ghosts as portrayed in the *Gakizōshi* is equally as nasty but also utilizes elements from the everyday world of experience. The work constitutes, as does the metaphysics of the *Jigokuzōshi*, a kind of medieval Japanese science. William LaFleur writes that "in the medieval period the concepts of hungry ghosts had been part of the best 'science' of the day."[20] Hungry ghosts inhabit humanlike bodies—bodies they can never escape—and the anatomical features of their carefully depicted bodies suggest real human beings in extreme stages of emaciation: gaunt faces, protein-deprived reddening hair, and abdomens protruding from gasses caused by the decomposition of the stomach lining. Japan's times of famine, such as the Kyōhō famine of 1732 and Hachinohe's "wild boar famine" of 1749, offered plenty of emaciated models to draw on for these depictions. The simple fact that hungry ghosts spent their time scrounging for feces and other unsavory excretions from the human body conformed to empirical experience, given that feces vanished from streets relatively quickly. In other words, Buddhist science explained why hungry ghosts appeared the way they did and why feces became discolored and then, after they broke down, disappeared. Hungry ghosts inhabited the realm today reserved for microorganisms, while their depiction in the *Gakizōshi* constituted medieval Japanese science: a depiction of the empirically given. To understand and depict pain, Japanese used their imaginations to grope through the world of given objects, and this included the suffering of others.

Yet, I ask the reader to consider this simple question: what is the difference between the Buddhist representations of being scorched in a burning river, dunked in a pit of filth, forced to weigh measures of red-hot coals, crushed in a mortar, or torn apart by a "terrible rooster full of fire" and the industrial reality of cadmium or mercury poisoning or coal-mining accidents? Let us not mince words: being burned, crushed, and forced to haul (if not measure) coal was part of the coal miner's job description. Surely, Japanese coal miners must have perceived themselves as living the empirical embodiment of pain, the modern manifestation of images that had heretofore been confined to the pages of the medieval *Jigokuzōshi*. This is particularly true during what coal miners called *daihijō*, or "calamities," inside these engineered subterranean spaces.

THE HŌJŌ COLLIERY

If one moment in Japan's coal-mining history proved particularly hellish, it was the coal-dust and methane-gas explosion at the Hōjō colliery in 1914. In an instant, the flames of hell—or at least subterranean flames—burned to death hundreds of souls laboring underground: the blast killed 687 people and 17 horses, and orphaned 94 children.[21] But the explosion also offered a singular glimpse of Buddhist compassion: immediately after the explosion, a one-inch-high statue of Kannon, the Buddhist Goddess of

Mercy, reportedly formed miraculously at the site of one of the cage towers. Buddhism provided the context for imaginaries of the subterranean, as well as its redemptive possibilities.

The Hōjō colliery was born in the context of the late Meiji industrial boom. Mitsubishi formally opened the Hōjō mine, located in Tagawa Province, in 1908. It was the seventh mine opened in an elaborate network of mines in the area known as the Mitsubishi Chikuhō Coalfield. To extract coal from the Chikuhō field, the Hōjō mine deployed technologies of verticality that thrust deep below the surface to harvest this important mineral. Verticality was the key to Meiji mining in the Chikuhō region. The New Mine (Shinnyū Tankō Kyūtatekō) pioneered deep-shaft mining in Japan. Built in 1885, it had a depth of about 98 feet (30 meters). Other mines of about the same depth were the Ōnoura shaft dug in 1886 and the Meiji shaft (Meiji Tankō Tatekō) dug in 1887. The 1890s witnessed the construction of deeper mines: engineers constructed the 151-foot-deep (46 meters) Uruno mine and the 230-foot-deep (70 meters) Shinnyū Tankō Daiichi Kō Tatekō mine. But the Hōjō mine, begun in 1905 and completed in 1908, was among the deeper mines of its day, at the time reaching nearly 295 feet (90 meters) toward the fiery hell that lay waiting in the innermost bowels of Earth. I say "fiery hell" because there is a direct relationship between the technologies of verticality—thrusting deeper into subterranean environments— and technological risk and human pain associated with mines. In the early Meiji years, runaway carts, cave-ins, explosions, fires, and shaft floods had been relatively rare; after the 1890s and the construction of deeper shafts, such incidents, particularly coal-dust and gas explosions, became a veritable hallmark of Japan's coal industry (tables 12–14).[22]

The Hōjō mine area was over 1,235 acres (five million square meters), of which Mitsubishi had commandeered over 16,000 square meters from local farmers. The main coal seam was discovered in 1897, before Mitsubishi arrived. Prior to the official opening of the mine, engineers created the infrastructure. In 1904, for example, engineers laid a railway from nearby Kanada Station; a steel bridge quickly spanned the Hikosan River, a tributary of the Onga River. The mine also featured Asia's first electricity-powered mine-shaft "cage," which lowered miners straight into Earth in about thirty seconds. This is about four times the speed of an average department store elevator: miners had to hold on tight.[23]

The imperial body that was late Meiji Japan thirsted for calories, and the Chikuhō region readily supplied them. Like the Ashio copper mine,

TABLE 12 Changes in Coal-Mining Accident Rates, 1899–1912

					Accident casualties				
Year	Coal production (t)	Efficiency (t/employee/month)	Employees	No. of accidents	Deaths	Serious injuries	Minor injuries	Subtotal	Total
1899	6,755,572	9.23	60,964	45	265	27	25	52	317
1900	7,488,893	8.85	70,508	125	43	78	80	158	201
1901	9,017,506	9.99	75,230	246	180	191	78	269	449
1902	9,701,682	10.25	78,894	375	135	172	219	391	526
1903	10,088,845	9.90	84,941	388	215	279	180	459	674
1904	10,723,796	10.12	88,330	725	189	224	512	736	925
1905	11,542,397	12.10	79,505	2,556	256	190	2,334	2,524	2,780
1906	12,980,103	10.15	106,589	5,022	560	298	4,654	4,952	5,512
1907	13,803,969	8.93	128,772	7,388	468	531	7,012	7,543	8,011
1908	14,825,363	9.73	126,999	8,257	245	431	7,884	8,315	8,560
1909	15,048,113	8.22	152,515	8,188	535	410	7,712	8,122	8,657
1910	15,681,324	9.51	137,467	7,170	307	439	6,549	6,988	7,295
1911	17,632,710	10.11	145,412	13,394	503	847	12,308	13,155	13,658
1912	19,639,755	10.73	152,521	181,635	878	1,389	17,046	18,435	19,313
Total	174,930,028	—	—	235,514	4,779	5,506	66,593	72,099	76,878
Average	12,495,002	9.79	106,332	341	341	393	4,757	5,150	5,491

Source: Kusano Masaki, "Meiji kōki kara Taishō shoki ni okeru Chikuhō sekitan kōgyō to tankō saigai: Taishō sannen Mitsubishi Hōjō tankō tanjin gasu bakuhatsu jiko no bunseki o chūshin to shite" (Chikuhō Coal Industry Disasters from the Late Meiji to the Taisho Periods: An Analysis of the 1914 Mitsubishi Hōjō Coal-Dust and Gas Explosion), Fukuoka ken chiikishi kenkyū 22 (2005): 52.

Note: t = metric ton (or 1.1023 U.S. tons).

TABLE 13 Specific Types of Coal-Mining Accidents in Fukuoka Prefecture, 1900–1903

Year		Cave-ins	Chemical explosions	Flooding	Suffocation	Cart related	Gas/ coal dust	Other	Total
1900	Accidents	24	1	1	1	6	27	17	77
	Deaths	10	—	2	—	3	7	6	28
	Injuries	19	1	—	2	3	56	13	94
1901	Accidents	70	4	11	1	10	35	13	144
	Deaths	12	—	95	2	2	5	6	123
	Injuries	69	7	5	—	8	68	31	188
1902	Accidents	87	6	2	1	21	30	18	165
	Deaths	31	—	1	1	4	21	8	66
	Injuries	82	6	2	—	25	35	28	178
1903	Accidents	97	5	3	3	45	38	36	227
	Deaths	32	—	7	7	4	111	6	165
	Injuries	88	6	2	2	58	105	41	300
Total	Accidents	278	16	17	17	82	130	84	613
	Deaths	85	—	105	105	13	144	26	381
	Injuries	258	20	9	9	94	264	113	760

Source: Kusano Masaki, "Meiji kōki kara Taishō shoki ni okeru Chikuhō sekitan kōgyō to tankō saigai: Taishō sannen Mitsubishi Hōjō tankō tanjin gasu bakuhatsu jiko no bunseki o chūshin to shite" (Chikuhō Coal Industry Disasters from the Late Meiji to the Taisho Periods: An Analysis of the 1914 Mitsubishi Hōjō Coal-Dust and Gas Explosion), *Fukuoka ken chiikishi kenkyū* 22 (2005): 53.

TABLE 14 Major Accidents in the Chikuhō Region, 1899–1917

Date	Coal mine	Deaths	Cause
June 1899	Hōkoku Mine	210	Gas/coal dust
January 1903	Futase Mine, Uruno Shaft	64	Shaft fire
April 1903	Ōmine Mine, Great Shaft	65	Shaft fire
July 1907	Hōkoku Mine	365	Gas/coal dust
November 1909	Ōnoura Mine	256	Gas/coal dust
June 1911	Tadakuma Mine	73	Gas/coal dust
February 1913	Futase Mine, Central Shaft	101	Gas/coal dust
December 1914	Hōjō Mine	665 (or 687)	Gas/coal dust
December 1917	Ōnoura Mine	365	Gas/coal dust

Source: Kusano Masaki, "Meiji kōki kara Taishō shoki ni okeru Chikuhō sekitan kōgyō to tankō saigai: Taishō sannen Mitsubishi Hōjō tankō tanjin gasu bakuhatsu jiko no bunseki o chūshin to shite" (Chikuhō Coal Industry Disasters from the Late-Meiji to the Taisho Periods: An Analysis of the 1914 Mitsubishi Hōjō Coal-Dust and Gas Explosion), Fukuoka ken chiikishi kenkyū 22 (2005): 53.

the Kamioka zinc and lead mines, and the Minamata chemical plant, the Chikuhō Coalfield proved a valuable piece of real estate to Japan's industrialization and empire-building projects. When the Hōjō mine opened in 1908, it produced about 120,000 tons of coal. With the completion of the Jōfū ventilation shaft in 1910, production increased to 200,000 tons. By 1913, production at Hōjō had increased to 230,000 tons. That same year, the Chikuhō Coalfield produced some 10 million tons of high-grade, high-calorie coal, both bituminous and anthracite varieties, which was about half of Japan's total production. To labor at the mines, in 1910 about 1,600 miners called the tiny village of Hōjō home (fig. 6.3).[24]

Despite the promising economic figures of 1913, the next year witnessed tough times for the Chikuhō region. In January, Sakurajima, the island volcano just off the coast of Kagoshima, experienced a major eruption and spewed ash as far north as Hōjō, 156 miles away (about 250 kilometers). This was not Sakurajima's first major eruption in historic times (eruptions also occurred in 1475–76 and 1779), but in the minds of many it portended a tumultuous year. Sakurajima's eruption coincided with the eruption of a political scandal that eventually brought down Yamamoto Gonbei's (1852–1933) cabinet. (In January 1914, the Siemens Incident occurred, which involved ties between Siemens Corporation and the Japanese Imperial Navy. By March, Yamamoto's government had collapsed as a result of the unsavory affair.) Then, in August 1914, Japan entered World War I as an ally of Great Britain and the United States (which entered the war in 1917).[25] Yet the most explosive news for Hōjō Village was yet to come.

On 16 December 1914 the *Fukuoka Daily* reported the horrific news: a massive methane-gas explosion—what miners called *daihijō*, or a "calamity"—had occurred at the Hōjō colliery in the morning of the previous day, and it took until midafternoon of that day to suppress the fires. The newspaper reported that 686 miners and 6 horses were known to have been in the mine at the time of the blast. Improbably, eyewitnesses (including investigators) told of hearing miners cry out from the molten depths of the shafts, as if the denizens of hell were torturing them. Kimura Seisaburō (b. 1897) had just fallen asleep at the time of the explosion, which occurred around 9:40 a.m. It was about 10:00 before he had thrown on some clothes and reached the mine-shaft entrance. The explosion had completely sealed the upper ventilation shaft with rock, clay, and loam. The lower shaft remained open, but he heard the old ventilation machines moaning and groaning under the intense pressure. Dejima Naonobu (b. 1902), only twelve years

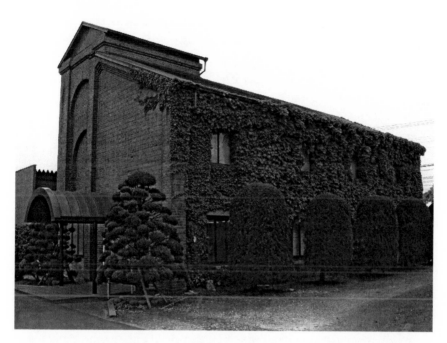

FIG. 6.3 Now owned by Kyushu Hitachi Makuseru, which makes electrical goods, this redbrick office building is about all that remains of the old Hōjō coal mine on the surface, though subterranean shafts, mostly filled with groundwater, still remain but are completely sealed off. Photograph by author.

old at the time, remembered hearing voices crying out from the lower shaft of the mine. Eyewitness Nakamura Jirōkichi (b. 1887) recalled that the blast sealed the upper shaft and that dark smoke belched from the lower one. The blast had been exceptionally powerful. Brick buildings separated from the upper ventilation tower by some thirty feet were destroyed: their destruction sent bricks flying in all directions. Nakamura remembered that bricks even crashed through the glass of the distant Mitsubishi office building.[26]

By 4:00 p.m. on 15 December 1914, the day of the explosion, relief workers had begun removing the charred remains of human and nonhuman bodies from the mine. It proved a slow, gruesome, and incremental process. Initially, relief workers recovered 1 body; by 9:00 a.m. 19 December, 110 bodies; by 4:00 p.m. 20 December, 156 bodies; by 4:00 p.m. 21 December, 192 bodies; and so on. Relief workers lined up the bodies that they had hauled from the mine like cordwood in front of the Seimon Gate. Ikemoto Kiyozō, a relief worker, remembered hauling eight bodies at a time to the cage and then transporting them to the surface. Because the bodies had been "baked like sweet potatoes," they had to be soaked in water at the Seimon Gate to help with identification and stem the odor of charred flesh. Sometimes only limbs or chunks of flesh were discovered. In the end, about 200 bodies would never be identified.[27]

Descriptions of scorched bodies, "baked like sweet potatoes," being hauled from the deepest bowels of Earth by relief workers bring us to an important intersection with my earlier discussion of the inexpressibility of pain. When ancient and medieval Japanese tried to express the horrors of physical pain, they depicted scorched and dismembered bodies burning in subterranean fires. Only now, Japanese mining families in the Chikuhō region, witnessing mangled bodies stacked in front of the Seimon Gate at Hōjō, were experiencing directly this painful hell: industrial mining had realized it. The Hōjō explosion, with all its technological and natural hybrid intricacies, realized some of the earliest Japanese imaginings of pain and suffering.

Indicative of the complexity of any system accident, Mitsubishi industry histories pointed to a number of events that could cause a mine explosion. In a document entitled "Investigative Report on the Hōjō Colliery Explosion" (Hōjō tankō bakuhatsu chōsa hōkoku), investigators explained the complexity of discovering the ultimate causation of any coal mine explosion. In coal mining, the ingredients for a catastrophic event are always in place: you just need ignition:

> For fire to touch off methane gas and even coal dust, there needs to be a source of ignition. The July 28, 1915 report offered a detailed investigation of twelve possible sources of ignition: portable open fire, portable combustion tool, safety lamp left open, the destruction of a safety lamp, ignition caused by electrical equipment, ignition caused by steam pipe, ignition caused by blasting, ignition caused by friction, natural ignition, ignition caused by falling metal items, ignition caused by coal-mining tools, and ignition caused by gunpowder.[28]

What is striking about the Mitsubishi report is that, considering the diversity of ignition sources for coal mine explosions—all of them essential to the enterprise itself—there were not more explosions on the scale of the Hōjō calamity. Later, though, some explosions deserving of our attention occurred within the Japanese Empire.

The Explosion at the Honkeiko (Benxihu) Colliery (1942)

Although the Hōjō calamity was the largest mine explosion to occur on Japanese soil, it was not, as mentioned earlier, the largest explosion at a mine under Japanese control. That dubious distinction is held by the Honkeiko colliery, which was operated by a Japanese firm, the Manchuria Coal Mining Company. The mine went up in flames on 26 April 1942 and killed 1,527 miners. At that time, the only other mining disaster that even approached the Honkeiko incident in scale was the 10 March 1906 explosion at the French mine at the Courrieres, Pas de Calais, which killed 1,110 miners. Both the Guandong (Kwantung) Army and the Japanese civilian government quickly acted to suppress information regarding the Honkeiko explosion, but Allied Occupation investigators pieced together a basic description of the incident immediately after the Pacific War. This report serves as our guide.

The seeds of Japan's tangled involvement in Manchuria paralleled the rise of Japanese industrialization and empire building in the Meiji years. In 1895, Japan went to war with China in order to meddle in Korean affairs, but in doing so it attracted the attention of the equally meddlesome Russians, who had interests in the Liaodong Peninsula and other locations near Korea. One stinging manifestation of this was the so-called Triple Intervention, when Russia, Germany, and France maneuvered to deprive Japan of the spoils of war during the negotiations at Shimonoseki that same year. Eventually, Japan went to war with Russia over disputed colonial spheres of influence in 1905 and defeated the Czarist Empire in what turned out to be an excruciatingly costly conflict for both sides. This time the United States hosted treaty negotiations at Portsmouth, New Hampshire, and Western diplomats managed to snub their Japanese counterparts on almost everything except for their demand to lease the South Manchuria Railway, which they received. Leasing the railway eventually metastasized into the Pacific War. This critical industrial artery came down from Siberia and branched into Manchuria to connect to important ports on Liaodong and elsewhere. It became Japan's diplomatic, economic, and industrial lifeline in the region.[29] In the Manchurian Incident of 1931, zealous officers in the Guandong Army blamed Chinese bandits for bombs that they had secretly placed and detonated on the tracks and used the incident as an excuse for a full-blown military occupation of the region called Manzhouguo.[30] In

1932, the Japanese erected a puppet state in the region, which they called Manshūkoku. After the Marco Polo Bridge Incident of 1937, Japan launched total war with China.[31]

When Guandong officers and Japanese civilian politicians articulated their motivation for occupying Manchuria, access to badly needed natural resources was always among the principal reasons provided. In 1922, "in response to many requests for accurate and concise information" by Americans regarding business opportunities in Manchuria, the South Manchuria Railway Company published a small book on the region's natural resources, and high-calorie coalfields were among the most valuable. The book gushed that under the auspices of Japanese colonial rule, "nowhere else in the world today is there presented so amazing a transition from primitive agricultural life to twentieth century industry and scientific organization."[32] But the link between coal and colonialism was anything but new. Indeed, coal development had also followed Japanese colonization of Hokkaido after the Meiji Restoration. In 1871, geologist Benjamin Lyman (1835–1920), with thirteen Japanese students, surveyed Hokkaido for two years and discovered the Ishikari coalfield.[33] Eight years later the Japanese opened the Horonai mine to exploit this field. Despite formidable transportation difficulties (the mine was located in an inland mountain range), the Meiji government operated the mine (as it did all others until their privatization), and it, along with the Miike and Takashima mines on Kyushu, produced about half of Japan's coal between 1874 and 1886.

Hokkaido collieries experienced much the same history as their counterparts on Kyushu. In 1889, Hokutan—initially, Hokkaidō Tankō Tetsudō Kaisha (Hokkaido Coal Mine Railway Company, 1889); later, Hokkaidō Tankō Kisen Kabushikigaisha (Hokkaido Coal Mine Steamship Company Limited, 1906)—controlled most Hokkaido collieries, overseeing about 90 percent of Hokkaido's coal output. In the early twentieth century, large *zaibatsu* firms began acquiring the mines (just as they acquired the Hōjō and other mines in the Chikuhō region): Mitsui acquired the Hokutan mines in 1913, while Mitsubishi took over the productive Yūbari mines in 1916. In 1883 the Horonai mine began using prisoners from the Sorachi prison to labor in the mine's deep subterranean shafts.[34] Korean labor also became ubiquitous at Horonai, Yūbari, and other mines: in 1928, 1,505 Koreans labored throughout Hokkaido.[35] But as production expanded at Hokkaido collieries, so too did the level of risk and potential for accidents. At Yūbari, between 1892 and 1985 twenty-two accidents killed 1,884 people, with the largest incidents occurring in 1912 and 1914 (the latter the same year as the Hōjō explosion).[36]

Similar to how Japan had thirsted for Hokkaido coal in the late nineteenth and early twentieth centuries, so too did it thirst for Manchurian coal by the mid-twentieth century. In 1931 (the same year as the Manchurian Incident), the Manchurian Coal Mining Company was established. In 1938, one year after the outbreak of war with China, this mining company was placed under the control of the Manchurian Industrial Development Corporation, and by 1942 miners had extracted 5,500,000 metric tons of coal from Manchurian collieries. Japanese worked as managers at the mines (usually serving four-year terms) while conscripted Chinese and Koreans performed most of the subterranean labor. This was the vertical organization of mine labor, which mirrored the vertical technological symmetry of the mine.

The Honkeiko colliery, located on the Benxihu Coalfield, was one site under the management of the corporation. For sixty years the Chinese had been developing the rich Benxihu coal seams, constructing elaborate underground workings, but Japanese management accelerated the pace. By 1941, 4,400 miners labored underground to extract 900,000 metric tons of high-grade coal. Four large surface fans assisted by subterranean booster fans provided ventilation in the shafts. However, engineers and "fire bosses" decided to neither "rock dust" (coal-dust suppression by using water in the shafts) nor take precautions against methane-gas explosions. Despite earlier incidents at the Honkeiko site (revealed during investigations after the 1942 explosion), Japanese operators claimed that the mine was nongassy and that the coal dust was nonexplosive.

Whether motivated by a disregard for Chinese workers (in the first chapter I discussed Japan's bacteriological warfare program against China) or dubious cost-cutting measures, Japanese operators could not have been more mistaken about the explosive potential of the hybrid mine complex. The Honkeiko explosion occurred on the morning of 26 April 1942. The calamity at Honkeiko was caused by a series of dubious human decisions rather than solely by the inherent risk associated with the complex nature of the site. Clearly, Japanese engineers could have taken more precautions against methane-gas and coal-dust explosions. But their decisions drove the Honkeiko's hybrid technological system, where the organic interfaced seamlessly with the mechanical, providing the perfect cascade of events that led to the explosion. That morning, strong winds associated with a typhoon caused recurring power shortages and outages because of the improper installation of the high-tension power lines leading to the Honkeiko complex. When the supervisor ordered repairs made, engineers disconnected the high-tension lines, which stopped the four large ventilation fans on the surface. The high-tension lines came online again after about one hour. When engineers threw the switch, an explosion immediately occurred at the Ryutan "incline" in the Honkeiko mine: the blast was so powerful that it instantly killed a man standing at the shaft opening and crumbled a fairly sturdy building. Mine supervisors quickly mounted a rescue, but the inability of miners to use the twenty functioning oxygen masks stymied efforts. Apparently, one ghostlike miner emerged from the mine immediately after the explosion, and supervisors let him wander home, despite the fact that he had knowledge that hundreds of men were trapped alive in the mine's inner bowels. Eventually, engineers fired up the ventilation fans and began normal rescue procedures. It took ten days to recover the bodies and another twenty days to make the Honkeiko colliery operational: thirty days of lost production. All told, 1,527 miners lost their lives underground, many of them from suffocation rather than the blast or fire.

From what Allied investigators pieced together, here is what happened. When the supervisor ordered repairs of the high-tension wires, he cut power and in doing so turned off the four ventilation fans. Importantly, he did not tell the Chinese mine operators beneath the surface. With the fans off, methane gas began to accumulate in the shafts. Underground and groping in the pitch-black darkness, miners began to wonder what had caused the loss of power, which halted the conveyance systems and other electrically driven parts of the mine. As operators fiddled with electric switches to inspect them, believing the switches to be defective, two wires from the conveyor switch shorted, and when surface operators suddenly turned on the power after the repairs, the exposed wires ignited the methane gas that had accumulated in the shafts. In a chain reaction, the methane flames traveled some fifteen meters to the top gallery of the mine, where they ignited coal dust that had become suspended in the main haulage area and elsewhere. The fire then spread throughout the mine following its fuel—coal dust, for which no countermeasures had been taken. The fires sucked the oxygen out of the shafts, suffocating the trapped miners who had not been burned alive.[37]

The Honkeiko disaster could be labeled a systems accident. Indeed,

Charles Perrow has argued that collisions involving large ships, for example, even if the result of a captain's poor decision, constitute systems accidents because the "error-inducing character of the system lies in the social organization of the personnel aboard ship" and the economic factors that motivate them. A specific kind of maritime social system, the tradition of a "preeminently centralized human system" onboard ships several football fields in length, makes the accidents possible, even if one identifiable decision is to blame.[38] We could extrapolate that Japan's culture of imperialism—mainly, the striking disregard for Chinese and Korean lives within the empire; ethnographic hierarchies; and the lackadaisical nature of Japanese military command on the battlefield in China, which led to such horrors as the Rape of Nanjing in 1937[39]—makes the Honkeiko explosion a systems accident. We might ask: what do you expect from callous mine operators who probably went to school with children who spoke of "brave Japanese" and "cowardly Chinks" in the aftermath of the Sino-Japanese War? Popular ditties in Japan included one with the memorably bigoted lines "Evil Chinamen drop like flies, swatted by our Murata rifles and struck by our swords."[40] Given the imperial, ethnonationalistic social system within which Honkeiko supervisors operated and made decisions, it is not surprising they made the reckless decisions they did. That operators cut power in the Honkeiko complex without warning subterranean workers, who were, as noted earlier, mainly Chinese and Korean, is utterly unsurprising and part of a brutal colonial system. The technologies of the mine—and their accompanying risks—were embedded in the social imperatives of Japanese colonial rule.

Once ignited, the methane-gas explosion started a cascade of coal-dust explosions that were emblematic of the "error-inducing" hybrid nature of the mine: human ideas and decisions, electrical circuitry, economic imperatives, dust clouds, and decaying organic matter (in the form of methane gas) do not mix. Industrialized societies rely on the controlled release of the explosive power of coal; the uncontrolled release of that energy is deadly. Mining is risky business.

The Explosion at the Hōjō Colliery (1914)

Nobody knew the risks of coal mining better than Meguro Suenojō. In April 1915, Meguro, a mine inspector for Fukuoka Prefecture, wrote the definitive investigative report on the Hōjō explosion for the British jour-nal *The Colliery Guardian*. Indeed, given its erudition and forensic detail, it serves as a model for mining-disaster reports. His report serves as our guide, because he saw the Hōjō explosion as a systems accident. He began by describing the elaborate, bulky mechanical systems of this prosthetic bolted onto Chikuhō's shale, sandstone, and volcanic surfaces.

The technological prosthetic looked like this: two shafts, fifty-five meters apart, worked three groups of coal seams, which ranged in thick-ness from the Gosuke seam (about a fifth of a meter) to the Nanaheda seam (nearly two and a half meters). The Hōjō mine worked the Nanaheda and Tagawa seams most extensively, which together possessed the formidable power of 7,353 calories per ton. The two shafts from which miners worked these seams stretched to over 270 meters deep (on average 894 feet deep and 16 feet in diameter). Two twenty-three-meter steel head-frames anchored these technological complexes at the surface, each hoisting cages in excess of one and a half tons from the bowels of the mine.

Once the lift lowered miners the several hundred meters inside the mine, several "inclines" (*oroshi*) penetrated hundreds of meters deeper into Earth's crust in various directions. To clear these inclines of water, two sets of Riedler's steam pumps extracted two and a half cubic meters of water per minute. For fresh air, giant Rateau fans pushed 4,000 cubic meters of air into the up-cast shaft (a ventilation shaft out of which already-circulated air passes), which had the effect of drawing air into the intake shafts. In 1914, the year of the Hōjō explosion, on average 700 tons of coal were extracted every day by about 1,600 miners, along with horses that dragged coal tubs, working the main seams.[41]

Lest the reader lose sight of the connections among coal mines, nations, and the technological risk they create and the pain they inflict, these inclines sported such names as "Tōgō *oroshi*," a reference to Admiral Tōgō Heihachirō (1849–1912), who, during the Russo-Japanese War, famously defeated the Russian fleet at Port Arthur in 1904 and then sank the Russian Baltic fleet at the Battle of Tsushima in 1905. There was also the "Nogi *kata*" (or Nogi "side"), named after General Nogi Maresuke (1849–1912), also a Russo-Japanese War hero, who famously committed suicide the year the Meiji emperor died. Both remain among the most revered military heroes in Japanese history, and these are high honors in a country that boasts cen-turies of military heroes. The point is that the connections between mining and war, particularly the Russo-Japanese War, which evoked a nearly frenzied patriotic response in Japan, operated in the symbolic arena as well as the material one. The Russo-Japanese War also sparked increased production at the Kamioka lead and zinc mines in Toyama Prefecture: environmental pollution is one of the many footprints of war.

As we have seen, the Hōjō explosion occurred on Tuesday, 15 December 1914. The concrete that lined the shaft mouths, as well as steel plates covering the up-cast of the shaft mouths, completely blew off; the cage, which had been resting at the mouth of a shaft, was shot like a bullet out of a rifle barrel seventeen meters into the air, where it smashed into the upper steel head-frame. Surface overseers gathered their wits quickly and, before repairing the cage, managed to lower a telephone and electric lamp into the down-shaft: although they heard nothing over the phone, the voices of severely injured miners emanated, along with smoke, dust, and powdery debris, from the shaft. By 3:00 p.m., engineers had managed to lower the cage and rescue twelve men, who had been mauled badly by the blast. Meguro descended into the shaft with other engineers and operators. "At the bottom a pitiable sight awaited us," he wrote, "Men cried for help, and dead bodies lay here and there." The rescue team tried to proceed deeper into the mine, but several in the party fell into a "comatose state" because of the high levels of "afterdamp" (carbon dioxide, carbon monoxide, and nitrogen gases left in the aftermath of a mine explosion).

Sharp metal fragments, rock, and other debris in the mine shaft prohibited the cage from reaching the bottom, which severely hindered the rescue efforts. Meguro summoned a doctor into the shaft to care for the wounded, but he, too, succumbed to the afterdamp and passed out. When rescuers entered the Nogi *oroshi,* they discovered that over one meter of water had accumulated on the shaft floor, because the water pumps had been broken. They also discovered scores of suffocated dead bodies. When Meguro wrote his investigative article, rescuers had recovered 482 corpses and 22 wounded men (of whom 2 died shortly thereafter); another 183 bodies lay submerged in the water that had filled the shafts. During the recovery efforts, afterdamp exposure killed four rescue workers. It was grim recovery work.

With 1,306 acres aboveground and 36 acres of tunnels, shafts, and inclines, discovering the precise cause—that is, the ignition point—of the Hōjō explosion involved skilled forensic work. Meguro traced the composition of the coke and melted bituminous matter back to the site of the initial blast. What made this difficult was that secondary, chain-reaction explosions occurred when the initial explosion shook coal dust loose from the ribs and walls of the shafts. It formed clouds and then ignited in a cascading series of "explosive waves." The successive explosive waves increased seven to ten times in magnitude, because the blasts raised the temperature of the air in the mine to 1000°–2500° centigrade; subsequently, when the explosion subsided, the cooling air created a powerful vacuum. All of this left specific trace patterns of coke and other burned matter, which led the forensic engineer to the ignition site. It was complicated science, but Meguro was a skilled engineer and, as his investigation revealed, up to the task.

Meguro determined that the ignition point of the explosion was in the southeastern corner of the mine, at the "7½ *oroshi*," which juts out over ten meters from the "16th *kata*." Here the coal was extremely carbonized; bituminous matter had been melted by the high temperatures of the blast and dangled "like thread" from the roof of the shaft. The explosion had blasted the coal tub and brattice (a ventilation partition) to bits. From this ignition point, violent explosive waves then cascaded through the different shafts and inclines in a chain reaction, causing severe damage and leaving "considerably mutilated" bodies in their path. Those souls caught in the explosive waves burned to death; most others underground suffocated as the flame sucked out all the oxygen from the shafts and inclines.

What was the source of the ignition? Meguro mulled over several sources. A few years earlier, the Hōjō mine had experienced an incident of spontaneous combustion, when coal particularized at a fault in the mine and, after increasing in temperature, began to smolder and emit smoke. Miners surrounded the smoldering coal dust with sand and packed the surrounding gallery with shale, stone, plaster, and clay in order to isolate the flame. When Meguro investigated this site, he discovered it unchanged and still successfully isolated, and so spontaneous combustion was considered unlikely. He considered other possible causes, but eventually ruled out sparks from falling stones, electrical sparks (such as at the Honkeiko colliery), and blasting. Meguro focused on "safety lamps." Specifically, safety lamp "No. 193," which belonged to a miner named "Y. Negoro." What caught Meguro's attention was that the lamp was in perfect condition on the outside, but that traces of coke dust adhered inside the gauze net (which, in a safety lamp, is designed to let oxygen in but not such combustible materials as coal dust or methane gas). Normally, the "7½ *oroshi*" was a relatively safe place to work because of proper ventilation, but on this inauspicious day, somebody opened a door that allowed the air current within the mine to circulate differently, which caused gas to accumulate at the site of ignition (fig. 6.4).[42] Later, coal mines integrated into their technological systems doors that closed automatically; but in 1914, to ensure that miners did not leave doors open, foremen made regular rounds to double-check. They missed this one. Moreover, the upper ventilation tower was known to be working poorly, which also contributed to improper air circulation (and hence further methane-gas accumulation) within the shafts and inclines.[43]

Orii Seigo (b. 1931), who has written extensively on the Hōjō mine, reminds us that methane gas is moody when in a mine shaft: in a methane-oxygen mixture that contains between 5 and 11 percent oxygen, methane is highly explosive, but in a mixture of less than 5 percent oxygen, methane just burns. Coal dust is even moodier: if there are between 30 and 100 grams of coal dust per square meter, it is highly volatile, but if it has a moisture content of above 30 percent, it is less volatile. Think of it this way: you can put a lit match to a chunk of coal or a gallon of gasoline and it just burns; but particularized coal dust or gasoline mist, when intermixed with ambient oxygen, is highly explosive. Controlling this explosion is what energizes modern industrial machines.[44] This is what is meant by an explosive wave: the initial explosion shook coal dust from the shaft walls, floor, and ceiling, and while it was still suspended in the air, it was ignited by the lamp-ignited

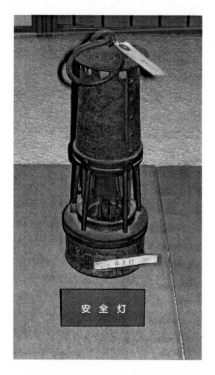

FIG. 6.4 A safety lamp similar to the one that caused the explosion at the Hōjō coal mine. Photograph courtesy of the Tagawa Coal Mining Museum (Sekitan Hakubutsukan), Tagawa, Japan.

methane gas. This caused the cascading wave that traveled throughout the entire mine: in each gallery, shaft, or incline the flame traveled, the burst of the encroaching explosion shook more dust free, which provided fresh fuel for the flame.[45] This chain reaction was possible because Mitsubishi had apparently not taken adequate steps to suppress coal dust by spraying water and dispersing sand.

The morning of the explosion, the clerk in charge of inspecting safety lamps had checked out 687 of them. Mine operators realized that safety lamps constituted a risky, vulnerable spot in the Hōjō mine system, because each miner took one into this dusty, methane-saturated subterranean realm. Mainly, clerks distributed Thomas safety lamps to miners at Hōjō. The reason was simple: an extremely powerful magnet held the lamp together so that, if it went out, miners needed to go to a *hibanjo* (three such fireproof rooms crafted from bamboo were located in the Hōjō mine) to get a new, properly ignited one (fig. 6.5). That is, miners could not reignite their own lamps, because it posed too serious a risk of igniting coal dust or methane gas. These were hand-held lamps that weighed about one kilogram and provided illumination for up to fourteen hours. Safety lamps were ingenious contraptions: what prevented the flame inside the safety lamp from igniting ambient coal dust and methane gas was layer on layer of fine mesh: about 144 openings per square centimeter. Safety lamp "No. 193" had been assembled improperly or was defective and ignited.[46]

Reading through the investigative writings of Meguro Suenojō and Orii Seigo, I became deeply impressed by their erudition. But, despite their explanation of what caused the explosion, I could not help but wonder: who was this poor "Y. Negoro," the man who had haplessly ignited one of the most devastating coal mine explosions in world history. He did not recklessly light a cigarette or accidentally spark a blast cap; rather, he was carrying a carefully checked safety lamp that was a critical tool in his work. It was part of the mining system. To answer that question, I traveled to Kyushu University, in Fukuoka, where I was graciously given complete access to the original official report on the accident by Professor Miwa Munehiro. Following the explosion, Fukuoka Prefecture had organized the investigation.[47] In the report, along with maps of the mine and other information, I came across the haunting death certificates for all the miners who had died in the Hōjō calamity. What I discovered jarred me: "Y. Negoro" was a Hiroshima native by the name of Negoro Yōjirō, who had labored at

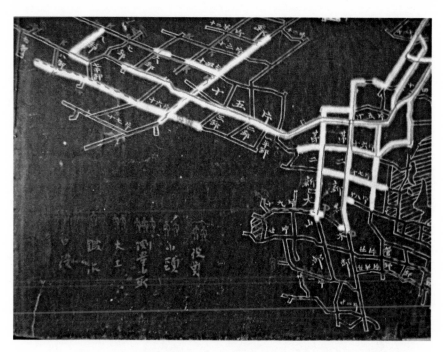

FIG. 6.5 A map of the complex subterranean environment of the Hōjō coal mine indicating where bodies were discovered after the explosion. Photograph courtesy of Kyushu University, Fukuoka, Japan.

the mine with his wife, Shizu, and his eldest daughter, Hatsuyo. Not only had Yōjirō died in the blast (indeed, he had inadvertently ignited it), but his wife and daughter had died as well, his wife by his side in the "7½ *oroshi*."

I found this jarring because it reminded me of the families of Minamata fishers who, in my earlier characterization, constituted patri-ecolocalities or micro-biogeographies, the core ecological units wiped out by industrial pollution. Now here, deep inside the subterranean environs of the Hōjō complex, a family from Hiroshima shouldered the burden of the technological risk associated with fueling the Japanese nation and empire. The nation needed calories to industrialize and wage war; families died in the coal mines to provide them (fig. 6.6). That is, not only did the Confucian *ie*, or family/household, suffer the brunt of parathion poisoning, mercury poisoning, and cadmium poisoning, but it suffered from the inherent technological risks associated with Japan's industrial economy. The Meiji state likened itself to a *kazoku kokka*, or "family state," but the reality was that

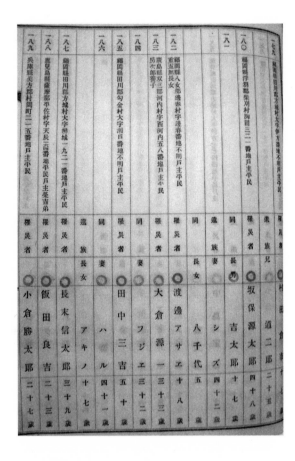

FIG. 6.6 A page from the official Fukuoka prefectural report on the Hōjō coal mine explosion. Red circles, identifying the "victims" (*risaisha*), cover the page. Husband-and-wife teams died, such as Nagamatsu Shintarō and his wife, Haru, who left behind their seventeen-year-old daughter, Akino. Such cruel circumstances proved the rule, not the exception. Photograph courtesy of Kyushu University, Fukuoka, Japan.

it was not a family at all. The Meiji state's frenzied modernization either placed families at serious risk or poisoned them, mainly to patronize the industrialists who owned it.

During the 1950s, the Japanese industrial economy began transforming from coal fueled to petroleum fueled. In time, coal mining in such cities as Tagawa became part of Japan's industrial heritage, and its relics, such as safety lamps and pneumatic drills, were relegated to folksy museums. But these museums disguised the fact that Japan still needed fossil fuels to energize its industrial economy, and like other industrialized nations, it focused its national energy policy on oil. Soon, uncontrolled groundwater filled Hōjō's once-populated shafts and inclines; corporate lodges, once homes to families, were dismantled. Meanwhile, oil-filled supertankers headed for the Japanese archipelago: Japan still thirsted for energy. Japan imported oil from the Middle East and elsewhere, and colossal refining facilities popped up in once-pristine coastal areas to add value to the black, imported crude. Of course, we do not have time to discuss the political and economic intricacies of this energy conversion (historians such as Laura Hein already have), but it is worth briefly exploring the technological risks and environmental dangers associated with refining petroleum, because refining poses the same types of problems as mining. Processing petroleum is no cleaner, though it is probably less dangerous, than producing coal: the most infamous example of the environmental risks of petroleum refining is "Yokkaichi asthma," which I discussed briefly in the introduction.

In previous chapters, we have explored the economic rhythms of coastal fishing communities near Minamata and silkworm farmers in the Shimotsuke Plain, downstream from the Ashio copper mine, and the manner in which industrial pollution poisoned bodies, exterminated families, and destroyed livelihoods. Long an important market center, Yokkaichi, south of Nagoya on the Ise Bay coast, epitomized both the fishing and the silkworm-farming worlds. Folks in Yokkaichi relied on the harvest from Ise Bay for protein: they hauled mackerel, sea bream, and octopus from the bay. In turn, farmers tapped into the eighteenth-century cash-crop industry to tend silkworm nurseries for Japan's booming commercial economy. Not surprisingly, under the Tokugawa shoguns, Yokkaichi was one of fifty-three post stations along the Tōkaidō (Eastern Sea Circuit). Domain lords from southwestern Japan traveled through Yokkaichi on their way to the capital of Edo and patronized its shops and inns. Because Yokkaichi was near the Grand Shrine of Ise, it often served as a stopover for dignitaries and pilgrims traveling to the shrine. Utagawa Hiroshige's (also known as Andō Hiroshige; 1797–1858) wood-block print of Yokkaichi from "fifty-three stages of the Tōkaidō" depicts two travelers walking on elevated platforms suspended over the coastal marsh, braving strong winds. One of them is chasing his hat, which the wind has blown off his head; a single pine tree, growing in the midst of the wetlands, is twisted and contorted from the relentless, punishing winds.

A wealthy Yokkaichi landowner by the name of Inaba San'emon (1837–1915) first conceived of transforming the windswept wetlands of Yokkaichi into a deepwater port. In the summer of 1899, the Yokkaichi port opened and served as a major center for textile exports. Like the stories of chemical insecticides, the Ashio and Kamioka mines, the Minamata nitrogen fixation facilities, and the Hōjō colliery, in the early twentieth century

Yokkaichi's story became entangled in *zaibatsu* capital and Japan's empire-building projects. In 1937, Ishihara Industries, a "new *zaibatsu*" forged during Japan's militarization, reclaimed the Shiohama marshes and built an oil refinery in Yokkaichi. One year later, after the Japanese government brutally exercised eminent domain, the Imperial Navy constructed another oil refinery and an oil storage facility at the site. During the final years of the Pacific War, the bright lights of Yokkaichi's oil refineries proved an irresistible target for American B-29 bombardiers, and in June 1945 the city and its industrial sites were leveled. The point is that the Yokkaichi oil refineries had much in common with the other sites investigated in this book: namely, war fed them.

Immediately after the Allied Occupation, in 1955 the Japanese government again eyed Yokkaichi as a potential industrial site, this time for a massive petrochemical complex. In 1956, construction of the petrochemical complex began in the Shiohama District (reclaimed marshes covered with the bombed-out rubble of earlier oil refineries), and the complex was ready for operation a mere three years later. A joint project of Showa Oil and Shell, the complex was referred to by industrial planners as a *konbinato*, a phonetic Japanese pronunciation of the Russian word *kombinat*, used to describe Soviet-era industrial centers. The idea was simple: the philosophy of the *kombinat* was to cluster petrochemical-related industries near one another so as to increase industrial efficiency. Nearly always on the coast, these sprawling industrial sites enjoyed ease of shipping and railway access and they could conveniently dump waste into the ocean. By 1958, supertankers regularly stopped at Yokkaichi's Showa Oil Refinery, where the refinery transformed the crude oil into gasoline, kerosene, and naphtha. The naphtha was taken to the Mitsubishi Petrochemical Plant, where it was processed into ethylene and other materials used in the manufacture of plastics and other synthetics.

Across the Suzuka River from Yokkaichi colossal petrochemical facilities, the residents of Isozu, the modest fishing village described in the introduction, became sickened from harsh chemical odors and jarring industrial noise, particularly after the Showa Oil Refinery went on a twenty-four-hour production schedule to meet the nation's demands for fuel and plastic. In 1960, some of Isozu's residents appealed to Yokkaichi officials, who essentially shrugged them off. This should come as no surprise: as discussed in the previous chapter, throughout Japanese history coastal communities have been situated outside the traditional palaces of Japanese political power. However, when children at the nearby Mihama Primary School were instructed by their teachers to "breathe as little as possible" because of toxic emissions from the petrochemical plants, some people took notice. In August 1960, the Yokkaichi City Pollution Countermeasures Council was established and determined that ambient sulfur dioxide levels in Isozu were six times higher than in other locations around Yokkaichi. As discussed in chapter 3 in my investigation of the smelters at the Ashio copper mine, sulfur dioxide poisons human and nonhuman bodies. Predictably, Isozu residents began suffering from a new form of asthma, caused by the high levels of sulfur dioxide in the air: nearly half their children had the disease. Isozu became totally engulfed in toxins. Often, the amount of ambient sulfur dioxide exceeded 0.1 μg/g (or micrograms of constituent per gram of tissue; or parts per million); sometimes it increased to 0.5 or even 1.0 μg/g. The disease became known as "Yokkaichi asthma."

Reminiscent of fisheries near Minamata, Isozu fisheries completely collapsed. In the spring of 1960, Tokyo's central fish market, Tsukiji, refused Isozu's catch because it reeked.[48] Fish caught as far as five miles (eight kilometers) from the mouth of the Suzuka River proved inedible. Typical of the response at Ashio and Minamata, the government offered a "settlement" of ¥100 million to be distributed among local fishing unions. Like the tricked fish they hauled onto their small boats, the unions took the bait hook, line, and sinker, even without any assurances of measures to clean up the petrochemical complex. But the situation only grew worse. In June 1963, local fishers moved against the Mie electric power plant, convinced, erroneously, that the yellowish muck coming out of its pipes had caused the collapse of the Suzuka fisheries. Like Tokugawa peasants centuries earlier who sought to "smash and break" the property of wealthier peasants, hundreds of young fishermen took to their vessels, planning to stuff huge sandbags into the electric plant pipes.[49] In response, the Mie electric company cranked up the effluent emissions to prevent them from doing so. A violent clash looked inevitable, until a local patriarch intervened and defused the situation. In 1965, the government offered even more compensation to disgruntled fisher families; but it must have tasted bittersweet to local Isozu residents who made for the "pollution-free room" at the Shiohama Hospital every time the sulfur dioxide levels reached intolerable levels in their homes. Sometimes the pollution-free room and its air-purifying machines helped, and sometimes they did not. In April 1964, Furukawa Yoshirō became the first casualty of Yokkaichi asthma. Then, two other known Yokkaichi asthma sufferers committed suicide in the shadows of the towering *kombinat*, sacrifices to Japan's industrial order.[50]

As this chapter has demonstrated, the key ingredients for baking environmental disasters in Japan, particularly those related to energy production, were as follows. Start with lots of underprivileged and politically powerless people, add a liberal sprinkling of *zaibatsu* capital, a healthy dash of spineless politicians, and slowly heat in the fires of global empire-building projects and war. Voilà: nearly seven hundred dead at the Hōjō mine in one explosion and countless others struggling to breathe in the sulfur-dioxide-saturated air around Yokkaichi. Certainly, such economists as Werner Sombart knew this recipe well, though to him it offered the delicious promise of an industrial society. Sombart, as we learned earlier, crooned in the pages of *Krieg und Kapitalismus* (1913) over the need for better cooperation between the "warlord and capitalist," because war, or the preparation for war, fueled industrial development. But as I hope I have shown, he could just as well have titled his book "War and Environmental Collapse," because the same drivers that caused high-speed industrial growth and increased energy demands also saturated the Japanese archipelago with deadly pollution.

In some respects, it is all a matter of vantage point: the modernization that has proved a celebrated hallmark of Japan's long nineteenth century, when the country transformed from a political hodgepodge of domains ruled by half-bald men sporting sharp swords to a centralized military and industrial powerhouse, had disastrous consequences for Earth and the many humble Japanese families who call it home.

CONCLUSION

" I used to wear it as fairy dust when I was a little girl," she said staring into her beer, as if she were talking to it now and not to me. "It's weightless like dried leaves, you know," she explained. "It was everywhere when I was growing up, near the schools and playgrounds; on the baseball diamonds, tracks, and in gardens."

It was the spring of 2007 and I was in a gritty bar in Libby, Montana, where I was visiting with six Japanese researchers who were part of an asbestos research group, a talented crew organized by the eminent Japanese scholar of environmental problems, Miyamoto Ken'ichi, and led by his student Mori Hiroyuki. Sometime earlier, they had visited New York, New Jersey, and Korea, investigating the international ecoepidemiological dimensions and social costs of asbestos-related health problems. They sought answers regarding how to measure asbestos risk, recognize health problems, clean up communities, and discover synthetic substitutes, as well as legal strategies to hold companies and governments accountable when negligent. It was late, though, and they were sleeping after their long flight from Japan (and then the long drive from Bozeman). I was out on the town gauging the local milieu. I thrive in small towns like this one, particularly after a long drive (fig. C.1).

The woman continued: "When we were little, my friends and I would run and jump into piles of vermiculite near the loading dock and it would almost float away. It's really pretty, you know, with sparkling greens, purples, and reds. That's why it made pretty fairy dust. It's still everywhere." She then placed her beer on the bar and her face formed a slightly gaunt, more serious expression: "I've been checked for asbestosis and the doctors say I'm fine. I've smoked my whole life, though. You've got to die of something, so I figure . . ." She stopped there and, after finishing my beer, I left the bar. As I walked home that night, I could not shake the image of a pretty little Libby girl smearing asbestos-contaminated vermiculite over her body, marveling at its sparkling, magical colors. Fairy dust, she had called it.

I came to learn from the Japanese researchers that asbestos-contaminated vermiculite is anything but fairy dust. A bright young Osaka lawyer named Kobayashi Kuniko, three scholars from Ritsumeikan University, a

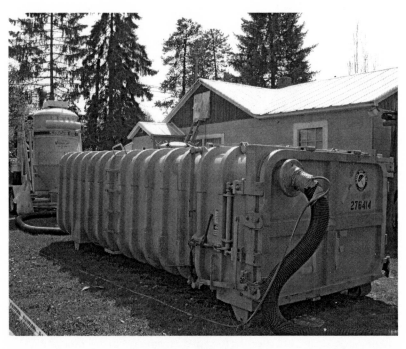

FIG. C.1 In the spring of 2007, the Environmental Protection Agency identified this home in Libby, Montana, as one that needed to be cleaned up because vermiculite was found in the attic and throughout the yard and garden. The entire community of Libby is saturated with vermiculite. Photograph by author.

law professor from Hokkaido University, and a leading community epidemiologist from Nara Medical University—they had all come seeking answers in Libby. Kurumatani Norio, the epidemiologist, was a slender, quiet man but relentlessly inquisitive about everything medical. When talking with Dr. Brad Black, of the Center for Asbestos Related Disease (CARD), about diagnosing the differences between fibrosis and other forms of asbestosis, he proved insistently interested in evidential detail. Translating his questions regarding Libby's unusual set of pleural abnormalities, which differ from the more common forms of asbestosis, such as interstitial fibrosis, was no easy task. I knew little about asbestos before the journey, other than that I wanted nothing to do with it. But here I was in Libby, a small town once bathed in it.[1]

Libby is haunted by a relatively unusual type of asbestos. The majority of Libby's asbestos (which occurs naturally with vermiculite) is called winchite, which contains amphibole (i.e., comprised of silica, calcium, iron, magnesium) asbestos such as actinolite and tremolite (fig. C.2). Some of these are known as crocidolite, or "blue asbestos," which is different and decidedly more deadly than chrysolite, or "white asbestos," for three basic reasons: crocidolite is needle shaped, persists longer in the body, and has chemically toxicological qualities. While in Libby, Mike Cirian, the Environmental Protection Agency's chief engineer, took us on a tour of the W. R. Grace mine in a pressure-controlled, carefully sealed, and air-filtered vehicle. We drove around the mine site for an hour, sweating from the hot sun that baked the mine's moonscape environs and gazing out the window at massive asbestos boulders and outcropping vermiculite seams. Obviously, air-conditioning was out of the question: air in the Libby area can kill. On leaving the mine site, the vehicle went through a thorough decontamination wash, as do all vehicles, including dump trucks that have unloaded asbestos-contaminated soil from around Libby's homes. We also visited sites being decontaminated by the EPA. We saw massive vacuum hoses snaking out of attics and entire yards being dug up with backhoes; men in white hazmat suits and respirators walked in and out of these very modest, plastic-sealed residences.

I knew nothing about the ecoepidemiology of asbestos before talking with Kurumatani about his research on asbestos-related deaths in Amagasaki City (Hyogo Prefecture), caused by the production of giant cement pipes, building columns, and aqueducts at the Kubota-owned Kanzaki factory. In the manufacturing process, laborers mixed bagged asbestos, mostly

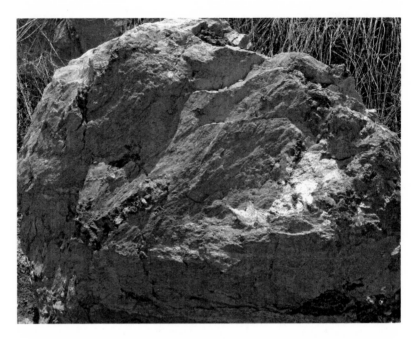

FIG. C.2 Asbestos boulder at the W. R. Grace vermiculite mine in Libby, Montana. This picture was taken from an airtight, pressure-controlled vehicle that was decontaminated on departing the mine site. Photograph by author.

imported from South Africa, with the cement, which gave the pipes better structural integrity. Kubota documents revealed that between 1957 and 1975, the deadly "blue asbestos" was used in the production process, and this is when problems began. In a June 2005 press release, Kubota acknowledged that seventy-five deaths from asbestos-related illnesses had occurred in workers from the Kanzaki factory, and forty-five of those had been from mesothelioma (an often-malignant tumor of mesothelial tissue affecting the pleura or peritoneum). The news was shocking, but not half as shocking as what Kurumatani discovered in his investigation. In a one-mile (1,500-meter) radius of the Kanzaki factory, eighty-five people had died from "environmental exposure" to asbestos (i.e., deaths had occurred not only from the "occupational exposure" or "household exposure" admitted by Kubota). In carefully staged simulations, Kurumatani determined that 0.5 percent of the asbestos had leaked from the plant into the surrounding air, mostly from flues that transported and mixed the asbestos inside the factory. Most of those who died from environmental exposure were women, because they stayed at home or in their neighborhoods during the day, breathing the contaminated ambient air while their husbands were at jobs elsewhere. In epidemiological terms, women had a higher SMR (standard mortality ratio): much like the social construction of industrial disease in the Jinzū River basin, disease was the product of gendered household relations, but this time in a more industrialized, urban setting.

My learning of asbestos-related disease in Amagasaki serves as the ending of this book, and if I had the gumption, it could just as easily serve as the beginning of another one. In essence, there are two possible endings to a book such as this: a guardedly optimistic conclusion and a decidedly pessimistic one. Let me explain. Most of the major environmental pollution cases discussed in this book—organophosphate insecticide saturations, pollution from Ashio tailings and smelter effluents, Kamioka "it hurts, it hurts disease," methylmercury poisoning at Minamata (and in Niigata Prefecture), and Yokkaichi asthma—found their way into the Japanese courts and were, for all intents and purposes, resolved, though not always to everybody's satisfaction. Usually, these environmental pollution cases made their way into the courts because of citizen action, often by disadvantaged victims, which speaks reasonably well of Japan's postwar democratic institutions.[2] The Japanese government also paved the way with important legislative action in 1967 and thereafter. These trends give reason to be guardedly optimistic.

Today, Japan boasts some of the toughest laws in the developed world regarding air pollution and is a model for recycling, fuel efficiency standards, and many other environmentally friendly practices. Some even hail Japan as undergoing "ecological modernization" as a nation. One scholar writes that, since the 1970s, Japan has "made good progress in disengaging its economy from the environment, particularly in terms of energy and resource use, [which has been] associated with structural changes in the economy from mass production-based to value-based industries." (Oddly, this "ecological modernization" theory sounds similar to that modernization ditty crooned by Fukuzawa Yukichi and Maruyama Masao decades earlier: modernity, no matter its form, always preaches triumph over, or "disengagement" from, nature.) Of course, it is impossible to disengage economies or anything else we do from the physical environment—that, I hope, has been the principal lesson of this book—but the development of more sustainable industries in Japan surely must be interpreted as a good sign.[3] Most likely, what is meant by a disengagement from the environment is a disengagement from Japan's environment, which has meant exploiting resources abroad and exporting dirty industries. Pigs fall into this category. In chapter 1, we explored how piggeries located near Japanese cities may have contributed, along with entomological factors (related to mosquitoes), to Japanese B encephalitis outbreaks in the early twentieth century. But Japan's hog industry has been exported to Taiwan, resulting in environmental degradation in that country.[4] Today, given the global nature of environmental problems (global warming, to name just one), it is at best a stopgap measure to focus on "greening" within national boundaries, but it has, to be sure, translated into less Japanese pain as a result of toxins in the archipelago.

Sadly, however, few of these environmental pollution court cases actually remedied the core causes of pollution catastrophes in Japan as identified in this book: reliance on agricultural chemicals, technological hubris, unbridled industrialization, unsustainable habits, modern philosophies that speak of humans as able to "liberate" themselves from nature, discrimination toward the diseased, poor weighing of capitalism's environmental costs, and the overengineering of the Japanese archipelago, including the manipulated nature of many of Japan's landscapes and organisms. Some speak of Japan's moving away from a natural-resource-based economy toward a postindustrial economy, but given that modern societies still need energy and resources, it is hard to decipher precisely what these people are talking about. Even Sony or Nintendo game consoles, designed to entertain the bored postmodern youth of affluent societies and celebrated as part of the postindustrial information-age economy, need copper circuitry, columbite-tantalite (or coltan: a heat-resistant powder that holds an electrical charge) parts, and petrochemical plastics, and just because Japan has exported mining these minerals and manufacturing some of these materials (and their accompanying environmental or political horrors) to other countries does not mean that they do not derive from some physical environment on Earth. Mining coltan, for example, partially supports Rwandan- and Ugandan-supported militias and, thereby, fuels civil war in the African Congo.[5] There is, obviously, less room for optimism on this front. But let us look more closely at some of Japan's early environmental successes.

In 1967, the Japanese government passed the Basic Law for Pollution Control (Kōgai taisaku kihon hō). Though only a skeletal legal framework, the Basic Law sought to "combat environmental pollution" and, in doing so, ensure the "protection of the people's health and the conservation of their living environment." The Basic Law also helped define several key terms in Japan's industrial-pollution vernacular. It defined *kōgai* (literally, "public damage"), for example, which is the term normally used to describe environmental pollution in Japan, as "any situation in which human health and the living environment are damaged by air pollution, water pollution, soil pollution, noise, vibration, ground subsidence, and offensive odors, which arise over a considerable area as a result of industrial or other human activities." Obviously, Japan's nineteenth- and early-twentieth-century experiences with chemical pesticides, mining and smelting pollution, mercury and cadmium poisoning, coal mining, and petrochemical atmospheric emissions defined the key elements that came to constitute *kōgai*. That is, *kōgai* was the product of the history of Japan's toxic archipelago as narrated in this book.[6]

More interesting is the definition of "living environment," which, as articulated in the Basic Law, sadly excluded the disfigured orca calves mentioned in the preface. But it did provide the moral authority to protect the human environment. That is, unlike the "nature" or "wilderness" celebrated in the American tradition, which, as William Cronon argues, represents a place where we humans are not, in Japan the "living environment" comprises those landscapes and organisms most closely associated with human habitation. It is the place where we, and our allied organisms, are present. Though the philosophy behind it differed from the American tradition, the Basic Law did, in some respects, open the door for a more sustainable manner of living. As Cronon has argued of American notions of nature and wilderness, "The place where we are is the place where nature is not. If this is so—if by definition wilderness leaves no place for human beings, save perhaps as contemplative sojourners enjoying their leisurely reverie in God's natural cathedral—then also by definition it can offer no solution to the environmental and other problems that confront us.... We thereby leave ourselves little hope of discovering what an ethical, sustainable, and honorable human place in nature might actually look like."[7]

By contrast, the Basic Law defined the "living environment" as "property closely related to life, and animals and plants closely related to human life and the environment in which such animals and plants live." With the Basic Law, Japan could never be accused of laying the groundwork for the establishment of a Yellowstone National Park or Lee Metcalf Wilderness. Indeed, the Basic Law, with its focus on the "living environment," fails to teach what Donald Worster identifies in the wilderness movement as "moral restraint." He writes that wilderness areas, not the Basic Law's "living environment," exist not only as a "place where evolution can continue on its own terms, where we humans can take refuge from our technological creations, but also as a place where we can learn the virtue of restraint: this far we drive, plow, mine, cut, and no farther."[8] The Basic Law had little language about "moral restraint," but Japanese did begin moving toward a definition of nature that possessed (in Cronon's words) "an ethical, sustainable, and honorable human place in nature."[9] As anthropologists of Japan have observed, Japanese images of nature have long contained strong anthropogenic or anthropocentric elements; in the Japanese language the term "nature" (*shizen*) suggests a process (i.e., "naturally occurring") far more than just a place (i.e., "God's natural cathedral"). Nature is found in a properly functioning vending machine, a carefully manicured Japanese garden, a well-trimmed bonsai tree, and decorous human behavior. "In a sense," write Pamela Asquith and Arne Kalland, "nature is everything around us, whether a mountain or a heap of garbage, a river or a teapot."[10] This, in effect, is the "living environment" reflected in the Basic Law.

The language in the Basic Law had a direct bearing on how Japanese courts tackled what are often referred to as the "big four" pollution cases, which were given considerable attention in this book. Without exception, it is fair to say that the courts favored the victims, though with certain limitations. The "big four" were Niigata methylmercury poisoning (1971), Yokkaichi asthma (1972), Toyama "it hurts, it hurts disease" (1972), and Minamata methylmercury poisoning (1973). Corresponding to these court decisions were the 1970 Pollution Diet (during which fourteen pieces of environmental legislation passed, with the support of the prime minister) and the 1971 establishment of the Environment Agency, which was elevated to the Ministry of Environment (Kankyō Shō) in January 2001. Obtuse language in the Basic Law regarding "harmonizing" pollution control with economic development was also stricken at this time.[11] Paralleling developments in the United States, the early 1970s represented a high point for environmentalism in Japan. Indeed, increasingly "friable" (capable of being crumbled, pulverized, or reduced to powder) asbestos in schools and elsewhere aside, it leaves one optimistic, if guardedly so.

ENVIRONMENTAL PROBLEMS

Considerable environmental problems, such as asbestos ecoepidemics, do remain, however, ones that share a resemblance to the colossal environmental pollution episodes explored in this book. They suggest that, although legal measures were taken to rectify certain high-profile pollution episodes, many of the fundamental historical or ecological lessons were not learned. Today, there is less methylmercury in the Japanese environment than when the Chisso facility was at peak production, but industry and its state supporters have created an entirely new generation of environmental problems, some less threatening than the first, others far more so. The Kubota Kanzaki factory and its "blue asbestos" serve as an excellent example of the latter. In some instances, researchers are only now beginning to understand the human and nonhuman health consequences of classic chemicals that have been saturating agricultural landscapes for decades, such as organochlorine insecticides and plastics factory emissions. This is because the modern fantasy still enchants the Japanese and other industrialized nations: we still desire, almost demand, liberation from nature, to bolster the eroding notion of human exceptionalism. We fix environmental pollution within the Promethean mind-set that technologies will ultimately liberate us and that industrial life is still entirely possible, if only painted a tad greener. We can still engineer Earth and its organisms, only differently from a generation before. We can still transcend, just more fully this time.

But transcendence, disengagement, or liberation (it does not matter what word is used) from nature is a fantasy. Along with asbestos, endocrine-disrupting chemicals provide a frightening example of toxins that will disengage themselves from neither the landscape nor the organisms embedded in it—including us.[12] The potential threat of endocrine disruptors remained poorly understood until the 1990s, but since that time researchers have identified several new environmental toxins, as well as some classic ones, that possess the ability to disrupt hormonal functions and interfere with sexual formation in organisms.[13] Some of these toxins derive from those chemical insecticides explored in chapter 2, while others come from the plastics-manufacturing process discussed in chapter 5. Because of their ability to disrupt sexual formation, endocrine-disrupting chemicals threaten our future in an entirely new fashion.[14] Recently, researchers have discovered new contaminants, such as TCPMe (tris[4-chlorophenyl]methane) and TCPMOH (tris[4-chlorophenyl]methanol), in the adipose tissue (tissue that contains stored cellular lipid fat), liver, and bile from Japanese bodies in higher concentrations than in earlier tests, suggesting their growing persistence and bioaccumulation. These new chemicals, along with classic organochlorines, such as PCBs (polychlorinated biphenyls), DDT (dichloro-diphenyl-trichloroethane), HCB (hexachlorobenzene), and CHL (chlordane compounds), exist in higher amounts in Japanese bodies than in the bodies of those who inhabit most other industrialized countries. The bodies of Japanese, for example, have a PCB level of 1,200 ng/g lipid weight, while in the United States and Canada the level is around 280 (although Americans and Canadians are saturated with far higher levels of DDT). In Japan, the HCB level is 48 ng/g lipid weight; in the United States and Canada it is 8.7.[15] Just like their toxic archipelago, porous Japanese bodies, too, have become industrialized with powerful endocrine-disrupting chemicals that may threaten reproductive health. Given the degree to which these chemicals trespass in human bodies, we really are becoming *Homo sapiens industrialis*.

Take DBP (dibutyl phthalate), a phthalate ester used in the production of polyvinyl chloride resins, or plastics of the type discussed in chapter 5. When genetically male tadpoles of the frog species *Rana rugosa* were exposed to the chemical, they experienced partial or complete gonadal "ovarian structure." In a word, the chemical produces hermaphroditic or female frogs by disrupting the "pathways of testicular differentiation in genetically male animals."[16] It remains to be seen how Japanese society, still dominated by patriarchal values, will respond to environmental toxins that, in principle anyway, can turn little boys (carriers of family names and worshipers of tutelary deities within families) into little girls or hermaphrodites. Certainly, Confucius (551–479 BCE) and his wise disciples would have been horrified. Perhaps an early indication of Japanese governmental interest in the problem was a massive 1998 study, titled "Strategic Program on Environmental Endocrine Disruptors," of the threat posed to the Japanese environment by certain chemicals. The report found discernible amounts of endocrine-disrupting chemicals in a variety of Japanese wildlife, ranging from frogs and raccoon dogs (*Canis procyonoides*) to bears and whales. In whale bodies, scientists detected fourteen kinds of endocrine-disrupting chemicals; in Japanese brown bear (*Ursus arctos*) populations, seven kinds. In some species, scientists observed "histological changes" (such as deformed frogs from Kita Kyūshū City), though it is impossible to determine whether these were caused by endocrine-disrupting toxins or something else.[17] Endocrine disruptors are frightening because we have saturated Earth with them for decades, even though the health consequences are poorly understood.

When I visited Chikuhō coal country in the spring of 2006, I traveled through Kita Kyūshū City, where these frogs chirp, swim, and mutate. It is one of the most densely industrialized cities I have ever seen. The smells and clanking noises render the city like the inside of a giant machine: I always feel as if I might just spontaneously mutate, too. Once on the local train, massive industrial factories quickly gave way to rural engineered landscapes, and I marveled at the new mining industry that had sprouted up around the region's rice paddies and water-filled coal mines: limestone mines for Japan's cement and construction industry (fig. C.3). Between Kita Kyūshū City and the town of Hōjō, miners had decapitated entire mountains to satisfy what Gavan McCormack has labeled the Japanese "pathology" of the "construction state."[18] Since the 1970s, the Ministry of Construction (Kensetsu Shō; now the Ministry of Land, Infrastructure, and Transport, or Kokudo Kōtsū Shō) has been closely tied to political power. Most remarkable were plans to engineer Japan's rivers and waterways with cement. Dams, for example, were constructed throughout the archipelago: between 1956 and 1988, 1,035 dams were constructed in Japan. By 1994 the Nagara River—the only free-flowing river left on the main island of Honshū—was dammed, despite the respectable efforts of the Society against the Nagara River Estuary Dam.[19] Coastal land reclamation also proceeded at an astonishing pace, with 95 percent of Osaka Bay's coastline reclaimed for industrial purposes. Hakata Bay underwent reclamation as well, which destroyed precious habitat for birds migrating between Siberia and Australia and New Zealand (an estimated 60,000 of them per day in the autumn and winter).[20] With all this damming and reclaiming and construction, this book could easily have been titled "The Engineered Archipelago." Engineered landscapes, as I have argued, provide the ecological pathways for certain kinds of pollutants (such as cadmium or endocrine disruptors or asbestos) to interface with naturally occurring systems and, ultimately, human bodies.

Cement makes this engineering possible. Alex Kerr writes that, all told, the River Bureau (Kasen Kyoku, part of the Ministry of Land, Infrastructure, and Transport) has "dammed or diverted all but three of Japan's 113 major rivers." Often, what this means is forcing rivers into concrete chutes, destroying their ecologically vibrant banks and beds. By 1993, engineers had lined 55 percent of Japan's coastlines with cement slabs and concrete tetrapods (fig. C.4). This requires massive quantities of concrete and, therefore, decapitated mountains in the Chikuhō region and elsewhere. "In 1994," writes Kerr, "concrete production in Japan totaled 91.6 million tons, compared with 77.9 million tons in the United States. This means

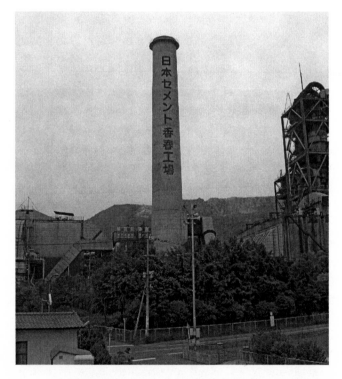

FIG. C.3 A decapitated mountain stands in the background of this cement factory, owned by Nihon Semento, located between Kita Kyūshū City and Tagawa, in north-central Kyushu. Photograph by author.

that Japan lays about thirty times as much per square foot as the United States."[21] Japan's forests have not been spared the engineered fate of its concrete-covered rivers and coastlines. In the postwar years, the Ministry of Agriculture, Forestry, and Fisheries (Nōrin Suisan Shō) has sought to clear-cut Japanese forests and replant them with a monocrop of commercial cedar (*Cryptomeria japonica*). By 1997, the ministry could boast that 43 percent of Japan's woodlands had been replanted with a monoculture of cedar.[22] Cedar pollen allergies are one unanticipated, ecoepidemiological health consequence that has resulted from Japan's overly engineered forests: 10 percent of the Japanese population suffers from the affliction. Other air pollution problems persist: researchers have discovered high dioxin levels near Osaka and Tokorozawa, outside Tokyo, to name just two locations. Thus, engineering continues apace on the archipelago. I could go on, but I need to conclude this book.

Let me end on a hopeful note. No, I do not think that we, as a species, can remedy these problems immediately, perhaps not at all. No, I do not think that industrialized nations will adopt economic systems that adequately

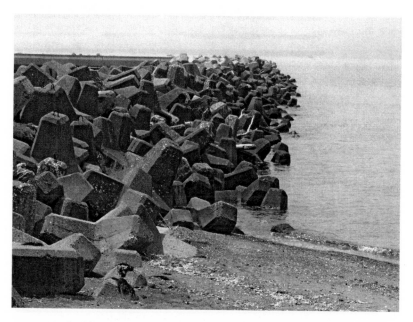

FIG. C.4 Much of the Japanese coast is lined with tetrapods, part of a broader engineering strategy that involves massive amounts of cement. Photograph by author.

measure the social and environmental costs of capitalism. No, I do not think that Earth's carrying capacity can be doubled, let alone tripled, even with better forms of scientific agriculture. Who would want to live there anyway? No, I do not think that we will reverse global warming, nor do I think that we will find new, cleaner technologies that will allow industrialized nations to continue their wild consumer habits. No, I do not think that large carnivores such as tigers can be saved; neither can wolves. Majestic species such as these require naturally occurring space in which to hunt, roar and howl, and raise their young, which is disappearing from what David Quammen has called our "planet of weeds." Tigers and wolves are the "shy creatures that can't tolerate edges," but edges are all we will have left on engineered Earth: the edges between one engineered system and another. What will be left are black rats and house sparrows, those creatures that "play by our rules."[23] This is a grim future, but I do think that, as we experience our environmental collapse, we will witness moments of sublime beauty, which gives me some consolation.

For me, the W. Eugene Smith photograph of mercury-poisoned Uemura Tomoko and her mother bathing together in a small bathtub is absolutely sublime. Also sublime are cedars poking through the ruins of the Kodaki mine site at Ashio, where macaques cradle newborns. But also sublime is a mother orca cradling her deformed calf as they are crushed together against Japan's shores. These moments of selfless compassion and transcendent beauty give me hope: even as the environment collapses under the feet of *Homo sapiens industrialis*, it will expose moments of profound beauty.

NOTES

Prologue

1   Kōnōdo no PCB ya suigin kenshutsu: Shiretoko de shinda shachi (High Levels of PCB and Mercury Found in the Orcas That Died at Shiretoko), *Chūnichi Web Press*, 9 March 2005, http://www.chunichi.co.jp/oo/detail/20050309/fls_detail_062.shtml. For more on PCB poisoning and its physiological affects, see Kentaro Higuchi, ed., *PCB Poisoning and Pollution* (Tokyo: Kodansha; New York: Academic Press, 1976).

2   To narrate environmental "declension" means to emphasize the decline or deterioration of environmental health in one's research. I claim my "declensionist" status while being sympathetic with Gunther Peck's argument that "declensionism may work best when at its bleakest, but it also risks dissuading people from working to protect environments they care about." See Gunther Peck, "The Nature of Labor: Fault Lines and Common Ground in Environmental and Labor History," *Environmental History* 11, no. 2 (April 2006): 232.

3   *Shachi jūnitō ryūhyō de ugokezu Rausu no kaigan* (Twelve Orcas Lodged in Ice Floe along Rausu Coast), *Yomiuri On-Line* (Hokkaidō *hatsu*), 8 February 2005, http://hokkaido.yomiuri.co.jp/shiretoko/shiretoko_article/20050208-1_article.htm; *Ryūhyō no shachi ittō okitsu e Shiretoko jūittō suijaku shinuka* (Of the Orcas Lodged in the Ice Floe: One Heads to Open Sea and Eleven Weaken and Probably Will Die), *Kyodo News On-Line*, 8 February 2005, http://news.livedoor.com/webapp/journal/cid_979065/detail; Koichi Haraguchi, Yousuke Hisamichi, Sachie Moriki, and Tetsuya Endo, "Organohalogen Contaminants and Metabolites in Killer Whale (*Orcinus orca*) and Melon-Headed Whale (*Peponocephala electra*) from Japanese Coastal Water," *Organohalogen Compounds* 68 (2006): 185–54.

1   This theme of death as an expression of sincerity was explored by Ivan Morris in *The Nobility of Failure: Tragic Heroes in the History of Japan* (New York: Holt, Rinehart and Winston, 1975). Some accounts of Minamoto no Yoshitsune's (1159–89) ritualized disembowelment, such as in the fifteenth-century *Gikeiki* (The Chronicle of Yoshitsune), described him as dramatically ripping out his own intestines: "Seizing the sword, Yoshitsune plunged it into his body below the left breast, thrusting it in so far that the blade almost emerged through his back. Then he cut deeply into his stomach and, tearing the wound wide open in three directions, pulled out his intestines" (100). However, as Eiko Ikegami has demonstrated, by the Tokugawa period (1600–1868), "A trend toward a tamer form of seppuku was unmistakable. The former glamorization of violence was clearly fading." Often, instead of disemboweling himself, the samurai motioned toward his short sword or fan, which was a signal to the executioner to slice off his head. See Eiko Ikegami, *The Taming of the Samurai: Honorific Individualism and the Making of Modern Japan* (Cambridge, MA: Harvard University Press, 1995), 257.

2   Bitō Masahide, "The Akō Incident, 1701–1703," *Monumenta Nipponica* 58, no. 3 (Summer 2003): 152. See also Ikegami, *Taming of the Samurai*, 223–240. Four other *Monumenta Nipponica* articles make up the "Three Hundred Years of Chūshingura" series. They are Henry D. Smith II, "The Capacity of Chūshingura," *Monumenta Nipponica* 58, no. 1 (Spring 2003): 1–37; James McMullen, "Confucian Perspectives on the Akō Revenge: Law and Moral Agency," *Monumenta Nipponica* 58, no. 3 (Autumn 2003): 293–311; Federico Marcon and Henry D. Smith II, "A Chūshingura Palimpsest: Young Motoori Norinaga Hears the Story of the Akō Rōnin from a Buddhist Priest," *Monumenta Nipponica* 58, no. 4 (Winter 2003): 439–61; and Hyōdō Hiromi and Henry D. Smith II, "Singing Tales of the Gishi: Naniwabushi and the Forty-Seven Rōnin in Late Meiji Japan," *Monumenta Nipponica* 64, no. 4 (Winter 2007): 459–508.

3   Ikegami, *Taming of the Samurai*, 238. See also Masao Maruyama, *Studies in the Intellectual History of Tokugawa Japan*, trans. Mikiso Hane (Princeton, NJ: Princeton University Press, 1974), 71–72.

4   Norie Huddle and Michael Reich, with Nahum Stiskin, *Islands of Dreams: Environmental Crisis in Japan*, foreword by Paul R. Ehrlich and afterword by Ralph Nader (New York and Tokyo: Autumn Press, 1975), 75–77.

5   Kawana Hideyuki, *Dokyumento Nihon no kōgai: Kōgai no gekka* (Documentation of Japan's Industrial Pollution: Intensification of Industrial Pollution) (Tokyo: Ryokufu Shuppan, 1987), vol. 1, 257–58.

6   On hemophiliac beagles, see Stephen Pemberton, "Canine Technologies, Model Patients: The Historical Production of Hemophiliac Dogs in American Biomedicine," in *Industrializing Organisms: Introducing Evolutionary History*, ed. Susan R. Schrepfer and Philip Scranton, Hagley Center Studies in the History of Business and Technology (New York and London: Routledge, 2004). On science and suf-

fering at Hiroshima, see M. Susan Lindee, *Suffering Made Real: American Science and the Survivors at Hiroshima* (Chicago: University of Chicago Press, 1994).

7   Julia Adeney Thomas, "'To Become as One Dead': Nature and the Political Subject in Modern Japan," in *The Moral Authority of Nature*, ed. Lorraine Daston and Fernando Vidal (Chicago: University of Chicago Press, 2004), 310, 311. For more on concepts of nature in modern Japanese thought, see Julia Adeney Thomas, *Reconfiguring Modernity: Concepts of Nature in Japanese Political Ideology* (Berkeley and Los Angeles: University of California Press, 2001).

8   Michael Pollan, *The Omnivore's Dilemma: A Natural History of Four Meals* (New York: Penguin Press, 2006), 10, 115.

9   The controversial notion that scholars and environmentalists often view themselves outside real "nature" or, more precisely, that they define "wilderness" as a human-less space was tackled by William Cronon in his provocative essay "The Trouble with Wilderness; or, Getting Back to the Wrong Nature," in *Uncommon Ground: Rethinking the Human Place in Nature*, ed. William Cronon (New York: W. W. Norton, 1996), 69–90. In that essay, Cronon writes, "If we allow ourselves to believe that nature, to be true, must also be wild, then our very presence in nature represents its fall. The place where we are is the place where nature is not. If this is so—if by definition wilderness leaves no place for human beings, save perhaps as contemplative sojourners enjoying their leisurely reverie in God's natural cathedral—then also by definition it can offer no solution to the environmental and other problems that confront us. . . . We thereby leave ourselves little hope of discovering what an ethical, sustainable, honorable human place in nature might actually look like" (80–81).

10   David Quammen, *Monster of God: The Man-Eating Predator in the Jungles of History and the Mind* (New York: W. W. Norton, 2003), 13.

11   Alistair Graham and Peter Beard, *Eyelids of Morning: The Mingled Destinies of Crocodiles and Men* (1973; reprint, San Francisco: Chronicle Books, 1990), 11.

12   Linda Nash, *Inescapable Ecologies: A History of Environment, Disease, and Knowledge* (Berkeley and Los Angeles: University of California Press, 2006), 210.

13   That industrial toxins allow scientists to see concrete connections among industrial sites, food webs, and human bodies reminds one of the development of radioecology. In the postwar years, radiotracers allowed ecologists to trace, and thereby see, interrelationships within ecosystems as they never had before. Ironically, radioactivity in the environment contributed to the development of the ecological sciences. See Stephen Bocking, "Ecosystems, Ecologists, and the Atom: Environmental Research at Oak Ridge National Laboratory," *Journal of the History of Biology* 28 (1995): 1–47.

14   Fukuzawa Yukichi, *An Outline of a Theory of Civilization*, trans. David A. Dilworth and G. Cameron Hurst (Tokyo: Sophia University, 1973), 13–15. On Fukuzawa's thoughts on nature, see Thomas, *Reconfiguring Modernity*, 60–83.

15   Daniel V. Botsman, *Punishment and Power in the Making of Modern Japan* (Princeton, NJ: Princeton University Press, 2004).

16 Mary Elizabeth Berry, "Public Peace and Private Attachment: The Goals and Conduct of Power in Early Modern Japan," *Journal of Japanese Studies* 12, no. 2 (Summer 1986): 237–71.

17 Carol Gluck, *Japan's Modern Myths: Ideology in the Late Meiji Period* (Princeton, NJ: Princeton University Press, 1985), 121.

18 Gregory Clancey, *Earthquake Nation: The Cultural Politics of Japanese Seismicity, 1868–1930* (Berkeley and Los Angeles: University of California Press, 2006), 128–34.

19 John W. Dower, *Embracing Defeat: Japan in the Wake of World War II* (New York: W. W. Norton / New Press, 1999), 33–64.

20 Benedict Anderson, *Imagined Communities: Reflections on the Origin and Spread of Nationalism*, rev. ed. (London and New York: Verso, 1991).

21 See Susan L. Burns, *Before the Nation: Kokugaku and the Imagining of Community in Early Modern Japan* (Durham, NC: Duke University Press, 2003), 2.

22 Elaine Scarry, *The Body in Pain: The Making and Unmaking of the World* (Oxford: Oxford University Press, 1985), 4, 162.

23 Ibid., 16.

24 Koyama Hitoshi, ed., *Senzen Shōwaki Osaka no kōgai mondai shiryō* (Sources for Prewar Showa Period Pollution Problems in Osaka) (Suita: Kansai Daigaku Keizai Seiji Kenkyujō, 1973), 1–24; Oda Yasunori, *Kindai Nihon no kōgai mondai: Shiteki keisei katei no kenkyū* (Modern Japan's Pollution Problems) (Kyoto: Sekai Shisōsha, 1983), 177–202.

25 John Lewis Gaddis has called this more inclusive approach to viewing history an "ecological," as opposed to "reductionist," perception of reality. See John Lewis Gaddis, *The Landscape of History: How Historians Map the Past* (Oxford: Oxford University Press, 2002), 54, 75.

26 This reasoning is reminiscent of actor-network theory, where "nature" is viewed as an actor in hybrid environments and social networks. In these hybrid environments, human and nonhuman agents interact to shape historical events. See Bruno Latour, *Reassembling the Social: An Introduction to Actor-Network Theory* (Oxford: Oxford University Press, 2005). The difference, as I see it, is that "nature," such as insects or even chemicals and heavy metals, is not dependent on networks for real agency. Rather, networks shape how humans, the constructors of these elaborate networks of meaning and power, understand how natural agency functions.

27 For an excellent treatment of forms of biomagnification, see Sandra Steingraber, *Having Faith: An Ecologist's Journey to Motherhood* (Cambridge: Perseus Publishing, 2001).

28 Charles Perrow, *Normal Accidents: Living with High-Risk Technologies* (New York: Basic Books, 1984; reprint, Princeton, NJ: Princeton University Press, 1999), 14, 233, 295, 296.

29 For more precise definitions of biological sentinels, see William H. van der Schalie, Hank S. Gardner Jr., John A. Bantle, Chris T. De Rosa, Robert A. Finch, John S. Reif, Roy H. Reuter, Lorraine C. Backer, Joanna Burger, Leroy C. Folmar,

and William S. Stokes, "Animals as Sentinels of Human Health," *Environmental Health Perspectives* 107, no. 4 (April 1999): 309–15.

30 Anne Fadiman, *The Spirit Catches You and You Fall Down: A Hmong Child, Her American Doctors, and the Collision of Two Cultures* (New York: Farrar, Straus and Giroux, 1997), 12–13.

Chapter 1: The Agency of Insects

1 Gregg Mitman, "In Search of Health: Landscape and Disease in American Environmental History," *Environmental History* 10, no. 2 (April 2005): 193. For more on arthropod agency in history, as well as the entomologists who study these insects, see Paul S. Sutter, "Nature's Agents or Agents of Empire? Entomological Workers and Environmental Change during the Construction of the Panama Canal," *Isis* 98, no. 4 (December 2007): 724–54.

2 Charles S. Elton, *The Ecology of Invasions by Animals and Plants* (London: Methuen, 1958; reprint, Chicago: University of Chicago Press, 2000), 52–54.

3 John W. Dower, *War without Mercy: Race and Power in the Pacific War* (New York: Pantheon, 1987).

4 Aldrin and dieldrin are closely related chemicals that fall under the cyclodiene classification of chlorinated hydrocarbons. Once sprayed in the environment, both chemicals bioaccumulate and biomagnify in a manner that kills or inhibits the reproductive success of many nonhuman species, especially avian species.

5 Tachibana Narisue, *Kokon chomonjū* (Notable Tales Old and New), in *Shinchō Nihon koten shūsei* (Shinchō Collection of Classical Japanese Literature), vol. 76, ed. Nishio Kōichi and Kobayashi Yasuharu (Tokyo: Shinchōsha, 1986), vol. 2, 372. For a description of this collection, see Yoshiko K. Dykstra, "Notable Tales Old and New: Tachibana Narisue's *Kokon chomonjū*," *Monumenta Nipponica* 47, no. 4 (Winter 1992): 469–93.

6 Murasaki Shikibu, *The Tale of Genji*, trans. and with an introduction by Edward G. Seidensticker (New York: Alfred A. Knopf, 1997), 671.

7 *Chūryō manroku*, cited in Kasai Masaaki, *Mushi to Nihon bunka* (Insects and Japanese Culture) (Tokyo: Daigyōsha, 1997), 132–33.

8 Kitagawa Morisada, *Ruijū kinsei fūzokushi* (Record of Various Modern Customs), ed. Muromatsu Iwao (Tokyo: Bunchōsha Shoin, 1928), 167.

9 Curtis P. Clausen, J. L. King, and Cho Teranishi, "The Parasites of *Popillia japonica* in Japan and Chosen (Korea), and Their Introduction into the United States," *United States Department of Agriculture Department Bulletin* 1429 (January 1927): 1–55.

10 On the nature of Japan's relative "seclusion" (*sakoku*) and diplomacy during the Tokugawa period, see Ronald P. Toby, *State and Diplomacy in Early Modern Japan: Asia in the Development of the Tokugawa Bakufu* (Princeton, NJ: Princeton University Press, 1984; reprint, Stanford, CA: Stanford University Press, 1991).

11 Edmund P. Russell, "Evolutionary History: Prospectus for a New Field," *Envi-*

ronmental History 8, no. 2 (April 2003): 205–6. See also Edmund P. Russell, "Introduction: The Garden in the Machine; Toward an Evolutionary History of Technology," in *Industrializing Organisms: Introducing Evolutionary History*, ed. Susan R. Schrepfer and Philip Scranton, Hagley Perspectives on Business and Culture, vol. 5 (New York and London: Routledge, 2004).

12 A standard treatment of Heian Japanese aesthetics and cultural sensibilities is Ivan Morris, *The World of the Shining Prince: Court Life in Ancient Japan* (New York: Kodansha International, 1964).

13 Marian R. Goldsmith, Toru Shimada, and Hiroaki Abe, "The Genetics and Genomics of the Silkworm, *Bombyx mori*," *Annual Review of Entomology* 50 (January 2005): 71–100.

14 Kasai, *Mushi to Nihon bunka*, 72–73.

15 *Kojiki* (Record of Ancient Matters), trans. with an introduction and notes by Donald L. Philippi (Tokyo: University of Tokyo Press, 1968), 87.

16 Ibid., 313.

17 Thomas C. Smith, *Native Sources of Japanese Industrialization, 1750–1920* (Berkeley and Los Angeles: University of California Press, 1988), 189–90.

18 Stephen Vlastos, *Peasant Protests and Uprisings in Tokugawa Japan* (Berkeley and Los Angeles: University of California Press, 1986), 94–95.

19 See Tessa Morris-Suzuki, "Sericulture and the Origins of Japanese Industrialization," *Technology and Culture* 33, no. 1 (January 1992): 105–6. In Yonezawa Domain, samurai participated in the sericulture industry to earn extra money. See Mark Ravina, *Land and Lordship in Early Modern Japan* (Stanford, CA: Stanford University Press, 1999), 101–13.

20 Kären Wigen, *The Making of a Japanese Periphery, 1750–1920* (Berkeley and Los Angeles: University of California Press, 1995), 251–52.

21 T. Smith, *Native Sources of Japanese Industrialization*, 205.

22 Brett L. Walker, "Commercial Growth and Environmental Change in Early Modern Japan: Hachinohe's Wild Boar Famine of 1749." *Journal of Asian Studies* 60, no. 2 (Spring 2001): 329–51.

23 Michael Pollan has discussed the theme of coevolution in relation to certain desirable plants in *The Botany of Desire: A Plant's-Eye View of the World* (New York: Random House, 2002).

24 Simon Partner, *Toshié: A Story of Village Life in Twentieth-Century Japan* (Berkeley and Los Angeles: University of California Press, 2004), 17–20.

25 For excellent images of women involved in the sericulture industry, see James T. Ulak, "Utamaro's Views of Sericulture," *Art Institute of Chicago Museum Studies* 18, no. 1 (1992): 70–85.

26 Anne Walthall, *The Weak Body of a Useless Woman: Matsuo Taseko and the Meiji Restoration* (Chicago: University of Chicago Press, 1998), 95.

27 Vlastos, *Peasant Protests*, 99, 101. Kanō Tanboku's *Yōsan hiroku* was translated into French and influenced the European silk industry; see Tsuneo Satō, "Tokugawa Villages and Agriculture," in *Tokugawa Japan: The Social and Economic Anteced-*

ents of Modern Japan, ed. Chie Nakane and Shinzaburō Ōishi, trans. ed. Conrad Totman (Tokyo: University of Tokyo Press, 1990), 79.

28   An excellent treatment of an early modern Japanese rural lending institution is Ronald P. Toby, "Both a Borrower and a Lender Be: From Village Moneylender to Rural Banker in the Tempō Era," *Monumenta Nipponica* 46, no. 4 (Winter 1991): 483–512. In the context of Japan's "household system," it fell on the shoulders of peasant women to care for silkworms and thereby increase the wealth of their husbands' households. See Walthall, *Weak Body of a Useless Woman*.

29   For example, Lady Nijō lamented the death of her lover, the emperor, with a poem that referred to the seasonal (and hence representative of transience) calls of insects and deer. See *The Confessions of Lady Nijō*, trans. Karen Brazell (Stanford, CA: Stanford University Press, 1973).

30   David B. Lurie, "Orientomology: The Insect Literature of Lafcadio Hearn (1850–1904)," in *JAPANimals: History and Culture in Japan's Animal Life*, ed. Gregory M. Pflugfelder and Brett L. Walker (Ann Arbor: Center for Japanese Studies, University of Michigan, 2005), 245–62.

31   Lafcadio Hearn, *Kwaidan: Stories and Studies of Strange Things* (Boston: Houghton, Mifflin, 1904; reprint, Rutland, VT: Charles E. Tuttle, 1971), 184, 207–12.

32   In 1900, Japanese built 1,396 slaughterhouses throughout their country. At these slaughterhouses, between 1893 and 1902, employees dispatched over 1.7 million cattle to fuel the workers and soldiers of modern Japan. Pigs were an important industrialized organism as well. See Department of Agriculture and Commerce, ed., *Japan in the Beginning of the 20th Century* (Tokyo: Shoin, 1904), 184–200.

33   "The Livestock Industry of Japan," Report no. 30, General Headquarters, Supreme Commander for the Allied Powers, Natural Resources Section, APO 500, 18 April 1944.

34   Dower, *Embracing Defeat*, 133.

35   Daniel Barenblatt, *A Plague upon Humanity: The Hidden History of Japan's Biological Warfare Program* (New York: Perennial, 2004), 9–10.

36   "Japanese Use the Chinese as 'Guinea Pigs' to Test Germ Warfare," *Rocky Mountain Medical Journal* 39, no. 8 (August 1942): 571–72; *Materials on the Trial of Former Servicemen of the Japanese Army Charged with Manufacturing and Employing Bacteriological Weapons* (Moscow: Foreign Languages Publishing House, 1950); John W. Powell, "A Hidden Chapter in History," *Bulletin of the Atomic Scientists* 37, no. 8 (October 1981): 49–50.

37   Edmund P. Russell, "'Speaking of Annihilation': Mobilization for War against Human and Insect Enemies, 1914–1945," *Journal of American History* 82, no. 4 (March 1996): 1505–6, 1508, 1511, 1522–27. On the dehumanization of the enemy, both in the United States and in Japan, see Dower, *War without Mercy*.

38   Vlastos, *Peasant Protests*, 99. The classic treatment of the *gōnō* is Thomas C. Smith, *The Agrarian Origins of Modern Japan* (Stanford, CA: Stanford University Press, 1959; reprint, New York: Atheneum, 1966). See also Edward E. Pratt, *Japan's Proto-industrial Elite: The Economic Foundations of the Gōnō* (Cambridge, MA: Harvard University Asia Center, Harvard University Press, 1999), 131–44.

39 Vlastos, *Peasant Protests*, 92–141.

40 Clive Ponting, *A Green History of the World: The Environment and the Collapse of Great Civilizations* (New York: Penguin Books, 1991), 196.

41 Mike Davis, *Late Victorian Holocausts: El Niño Famines and the Making of the Third World* (London and New York: Verso, 2001), 9.

42 Herman Ooms has described Tokugawa governance as colonial in nature in *Tokugawa Village Practice: Class, Status, Power, Law* (Berkeley and Los Angeles: University of California Press, 1996).

43 Ellen Gardner Nakamura, *Practical Pursuits: Takano Chōei, Takahashi Keisaku, and Western Medicine in Nineteenth-Century Japan* (Cambridge, MA: Harvard University Asia Center, Harvard University Press, 2005), 56–57.

44 Brett L. Walker, *The Lost Wolves of Japan*, foreword by William Cronon (Seattle: University of Washington Press, 2005).

45 Brett L. Walker, *The Conquest of Ainu Lands: Ecology and Culture in Japanese Expansion, 1590–1800* (Berkeley and Los Angeles: University of California Press, 2001).

46 Walker, "Commercial Growth."

47 Toshinobu Yasunaga, *Ando Shoeki: Social and Ecological Philosopher of Eighteenth-Century Japan* (New York and Tokyo: Weatherhill, 1992), 27–30.

48 Ibid., 34, 58, 79, 85.

49 Ibid., 36.

50 Ibid., 68.

51 Ibid., 76, 82, 83.

52 Ibid., 123, 351, 361.

53 Richard White, "'Are You an Environmentalist or Do You Work for a Living?' Work and Nature," in *Uncommon Ground: Rethinking the Human Place in Nature*, ed. William Cronon (New York: W. W. Norton, 1996), 171–72.

54 Yasunaga, *Ando Shoeki*, 228, 231.

55 See E. Herbert Norman, *Andō Shōeki and the Anatomy of Japanese Feudalism* (1949; reprint, Washington, DC: University Publications of America, 1979).

56 Yasunaga, *Ando Shoeki*, 139, 141, 159.

57 Ibid., 162.

Chapter 2: The Agency of Chemicals

1 "Kyōhō" refers to a Japanese imperial reign name and era, which in this case lasted from 1716 to 1735.

2 J. H. Mun, Y. H. Song, K. L. Heong, and G. K. Roderick, "Genetic Variation among Asian Populations of Rice Planthoppers, *Nilaparvata lugens* and *Sogatella furcifera* (Hemiptera: Delphacidae): Mitochondrial DNA Sequences," *Bulletin of Entomological Research* 89 (1999): 245–53.

3 Joshua Blu Buhs, *The Fire Ant Wars: Nature, Science, and Public Policy in Twentieth-Century America* (Chicago: University of Chicago Press, 2004), 31–32.

4 *The Ten Foot Square Hut and Tales of the Heike*, trans. A. L. Sadler (Sydney: Angus and Robertson, 1928), 123–24.

5 Robert Borgen, *Sugawara no Michizane and the Early Heian Court* (Honolulu: University of Hawai'i Press, 1986), 278–325.

6 On whaling in Japan, see Arne Kalland and Brian Moeran, *Japanese Whaling: End of an Era?* (London: Curzon Press, 1992).

7 Jeffrey A. Lockwood, *Locust: The Devastating Rise and Mysterious Disappearance of the Insect That Shaped the American Frontier* (New York: Basic Books, 2004).

8 Ōkura Nagatsune, *Jokōroku* (Record of Insect Control), in *Nihon nōsho zenshū* (Complete Works of Japanese Agricultural Writings), vol. 15, ed. Shadan Hōjin Nōsangyoson Bunka Kyōkai (Tokyo: Nōsangyoson Bunka Kyōkai, 1977), 12–118.

9 Kikuchi Isao, *Kinsei no kikin* (Early Modern Japan's Famines) (Tokyo: Yoshikawa Kōbunkan, 1997), 82–89.

10 Conrad Totman, *Early Modern Japan* (Berkeley and Los Angeles: University of California Press, 1993), 236–38.

11 John Briggs and F. David Peat, *Seven Life Lessons of Chaos: Timeless Wisdom from the Science of Change* (New York: HarperCollins, 1999).

12 Carolyn Merchant, *The Death of Nature: Women, Ecology, and the Scientific Revolution* (San Francisco: Harper and Row, 1980; reprint, New York: Harper and Row, 1983).

13 The Meiji Japanese adoption and adaptation of Euro-American science is covered in James R. Bartholomew, *The Formation of Science in Japan* (New Haven, CT: Yale University Press, 1989).

14 On the role of foreign experts in refashioning Hokkaido and agricultural practices there, see Hokkaido Prefectural Government, ed., *Foreign Pioneers: A Short History of the Contribution of Foreigners to the Development of Hokkaido* (Sapporo: Hokkaido Prefectural Government, 1968). See also Fumiko Fujita, *American Pioneers and the Japanese Frontier: American Experts in Nineteenth-Century Japan* (Westport, CT: Greenwood Press, 1994); John M. Maki, *William Smith Clark: A Yankee in Hokkaido* (Sapporo: Hokkaido University Press, 1996).

15 James Whorton, *Before "Silent Spring": Pesticides and Public Health in Pre-DDT America* (Princeton, NJ: Princeton University Press, 1974), 8–9, 12, 15–16, 20, 22, 64–65.

16 Scarry, *Body in Pain*.

17 Matsunaka Shōichi, *Nihon ni okeru nōyaku no rekishi* (Japan's Agricultural Chemical History) (Tokyo: Gakkai Shuppan Sentā, 2002), 9–11. For more specific information on plant disease, insects, and insecticides from the Meiji period through the 1950s, see Tennensha Jiten Henshūbu, ed., *Byōchū nōyaku jiten* (Dictionary of Agricultural Chemicals for Disease and Insects) (Tokyo: Tennensha, 1955).

18 David Vogel, "Consumer Protection and Protectionism in Japan," *Journal of Japanese Studies* 18, no. 1 (Winter 1992): 131–32.

19 See, e.g., Watanabe Yūji, *Kurashi ni hisomu kagaku dokubutsu jiten* (A Dictionary of Chemical Poisons That Lurk in Our Daily Lives) (Tokyo: Ie no Kōkyōkai, 2002), 74; Nakaminami Gen, *Nōyaku genron* (The Principles of Agricultural Chemicals)

(Tokyo: Hokuto Shuppan, 2001), 23–25; Miura Yoshiaki, *Kagaku osen to ningen no rekishi* (Chemical Contamination and Human History) (Tokyo: Tsukiji Shokan, 1999), 73–74; Yasuhara Akio, *Shinobi yoru kagaku busshitsu osen: Chikyū tanjō, seitaikei, gendai bunmei ni okeru kagaku busshitsu osen no keifu* (Exposing Chemical Contamination: The Birth of Earth, Ecological Structure, and the Genealogy of Chemical Contamination in the Context of Modern Civilization) (Tokyo: Gōdō Shuppan, 1999), 143–45; Andō Mitsuru, *Yokuwakaru nōyaku osen: Jintai to kankyō o mushibamu gōsei kagaku busshitsu* (Agricultural Chemical Contamination: The Synthetic Chemical Compounds That Ruin Human Bodies and the Environment) (Tokyo: Gōdō Shuppan, 1990), 21–25.

20 Linda Nash, "The Fruits of Ill-Health: Pesticides and Workers' Bodies in Post-World War II California," *Osiris* 19 (2004): 205, 208. See also Linda Nash, "Finishing Nature: Harmonizing Bodies and Environments in Late-Nineteenth-Century California," *Environmental History* 8 (January 2003): 25–52.

21 Curtis D. Klaassen, ed., *Casarett and Doull's Toxicology: The Basic Science of Poisons*, 5th ed. (New York: McGraw-Hill, Health Professions Division, 1996), 655.

22 Uemura Shinsaku, Kawamura Hiroshi, Tsuji Machiko, Tomita Shigeyuki, and Maeda Shizuo, *Nōyaku dokusei no jiten* (Dictionary of Toxic Agricultural Chemicals) (Tokyo: Sanseidō, 2002), 146–47.

23 Tatsuji Namba, "Oxime Therapy for Poisoning by Alkylphosphate-Insecticides," *Proceedings of the 13th Annual International Congress on Occupational Health, July 25–29, 1960* (1961): 757.

24 Takashi Tanimura, "Embryotoxicity of Acute Exposure to Methyl Parathion in Rats and Mice," *Archives of Environmental Health* 15 (November 1967): 609–13.

25 Namba, "Oxime Therapy."

26 Gerald Markowitz and David Rosner, *Deceit and Denial: The Deadly Politics of Industrial Pollution* (Berkeley and Los Angeles: University of California Press, 2002).

27 Kankyō Hōrei Kenkyūkai, ed., *Kankyō kōgai nenkan* (Yearbook of Environmental Pollution) (Tokyo: Gakuyō Shobō, 1973), 137.

28 Shimokawa Kōshi, ed., *Kankyōshi nenpyō: Shōwa-Heisei hen* (Environmental History Chronology: Shōwa and Heisei Periods) (Tokyo: Kawade Shobō Shinsha, 2004), vol. 2, 193.

29 Sumitomo Kagaku Kōgyō Kabushikigaisha, ed., *Sumitomo Kagaku Kōgyō Kabushikigaisha shi* (A History of Sumitomo Chemical) (Osaka: Sumitomo Kagaku Kōgyō Kabushikigaisha, 1981), 305–9.

30 L. T. Kok, "Toxicity of Insecticides Used for Asiatic Rice Borer Control to Tropical Fish in Rice Paddies," in *The Careless Technology: Ecology and International Development*, ed. M. Taghi Farvar and John P. Milton (Garden City, NY: Natural History Press, 1972), 489–91.

31 Klaassen, *Casarett and Doull's Toxicology*, 673.

32 Yoshitomo Takahashi, Hideto Hirasawa, and Keiko Koyama, "Restriction of Suicide Methods: A Japanese Perspective," *Archives of Suicide Research* 4 (1998): 103–4.

33 Sumitomo Kagaku Kōgyō Kabushikigaisha, *Sumitomo Kagaku Kōgyō Kabushiki-gaisha shi*, 543–44.

34 Shimokawa, *Kankyōshi nenpyō*, 283.

35 G. H. L. Rothschild, "The Biology and Ecology of Rice-Stem Borers in Sarawak (Malaysian Borneo)," *Journal of Applied Ecology* 8, no. 2 (August 1971): 287–322.

36 Syunro Utida, "On Fluctuations in Population Density of the Rice Stem Borer Chilo suppressalis," *Ecology* 39, no. 4 (October 1958): 587–99.

37 Sumitomo Kagaku Kōgyō Kabushikigaisha, *Sumitomo Kagaku Kōgyō Kabushiki-gaisha shi*, 543–44.

38 Pete Daniel, *Toxic Drift: Pesticides and Health in the Post-World War II South* (Baton Rouge: Louisiana State University Press in association with Smithsonian Institution, 2005).

39 Jonathan Weiner explores some insect resistances in *The Beak of the Finch* (New York: Knopf, 1994), 253–55.

Chapter 3: Copper Mining and Ecological Collapse

1   Herman Ooms, *Tokugawa Ideology: Early Constructs, 1570-1680* (Princeton, NJ: Princeton University Press, 1985), 57–59.

2   For more on deer populations at Nikkō, see John Knight, *Waiting for Wolves in Japan: An Anthropological Study of People-Wildlife Relations* (Oxford: Oxford University Press, 2003), 156.

3   Timothy J. LeCain, "'The Heavens and the Earth': Controlling Terrestrial and Subterrestrial Environments in Twentieth Century Western Mining," paper presented at the Third Annual Michael P. Malone Conference, "Spaces of Struggle: Power and the Transformation of Nature," Big Sky, MT, 28 September–2 October 2005.

4   Richard White, *The Organic Machine: The Remaking of the Columbia River* (New York: Hill and Wang, a Division of Farrar, Straus and Giroux, 1995), ix–xi, 37, 38, 61.

5   Kobata Atsushi, *Nihon dōkōgyōshi no kenkyū* (Research on Japan's Copper Mining Industry) (Kyoto: Shibunkaku Shuppan, 1993), 145.

6   Kate Wildman Nakai, *Shogunal Politics: Arai Hakuseki and the Premises of Tokugawa Rule* (Cambridge, MA: Council on East Asian Studies, Harvard University Press, 1988), 97, 106–7.

7   Mary Elizabeth Berry, *Hideyoshi* (Cambridge, MA: Harvard University Press, 1982), 87–93.

8   A. Kobata, "The Production and Uses of Gold and Silver in Sixteenth- and Seventeenth-Century Japan," *Economic History Review*, n.s., 18, no. 2 (1965): 245–66.

9   Wigen, *Making of a Japanese Periphery*, 82.

10 Kenneth Pomeranz, *The Great Divergence: China, Europe, and the Making of the Modern World Economy* (Princeton, NJ: Princeton University Press, 2000), 159.

11 A. Kobata, "Production and Uses of Gold and Silver," 252.

12 George Elison, *Deus Destroyed: The Image of Christianity in Early Modern Japan* (Cambridge, MA: Harvard University Press, 1988), 90–91. On the later persecution of Christians, see Nam-lin Hur, *Death and Social Order in Tokugawa Japan: Buddhism, Anti-Christianity, and the* Danka *System* (Cambridge, MA: Harvard University Asia Center, Harvard University Press, 2007), 37–106.

13 Robert Lero Innes, "The Door Ajar: Japan's Foreign Trade in the Seventeenth Century" (Ph.D. diss., University of Michigan, 1980), 50.

14 Ibid., 21–66.

15 A. Kobata, "Production and Uses of Gold and Silver," 248, 256.

16 Laura Hostetler, *Qing Colonial Enterprise: Ethnography and Cartography in Early Modern China* (Princeton, NJ: Princeton University Press, 2001), 120–21.

17 Bartholomew, *Formation of Science in Japan*, 23–24.

18 C. N. Bromehead, "Ancient Mining Processes as Illustrated by a Japanese Scroll," *Antiquity* 16, no. 63 (September 1942): 193–94, 196, 207.

19 Nagahara Keiji and Kozo Yamamura, "Shaping the Process of Unification: Technological Progress in Sixteenth- and Seventeenth-Century Japan," *Journal of Japanese Studies* 14, no. 1 (Winter 1998): 77–83.

20 Tessa Morris-Suzuki, *The Technological Transformation of Japan: From the Seventeenth to the Twenty-First Century* (Cambridge: Cambridge University Press, 1994), 43–47.

21 Masuda Tsuna, *"Kodō zuroku": Illustrated Book on the Smelting of Copper* (Norwalk, CT: Burndy Library, 1983), 28–54, 70, 74, 80, 84.

22 H. D. Harootunian, *Things Seen and Unseen: Discourse and Ideology in Tokugawa Nativism* (Chicago: University of Chicago Press, 1988), 23, 212; Emiko Ohnuki-Tierney, *Rice as Self: Japanese Identities through Time* (Princeton, NJ: Princeton University Press, 1993), 86–88.

23 Vlastos, *Peasant Protests*.

24 Nimura Kazuo, *The Ashio Riot of 1907: A Social History of Mining in Japan*, ed. Andrew Gordon and trans. Terry Boardman and Andrew Gordon (Durham, NC: Duke University Press, 1997), 15, 30, 38, 99, 102, 109, 134–35, 174.

25 For more on viewing agriculturalists as industrial engineers, see David Igler, *Industrial Cowboys: Miller and Lux and the Transformation of the Far West, 1850–1920* (Berkeley and Los Angeles: University of California Press, 2005).

26 For a discussion of high modernist thought and practice, see James C. Scott, *Seeing like a State: How Certain Schemes to Improve the Human Condition Have Failed* (New Haven, CT: Yale University Press, 1998).

27 Fukuzawa Yukichi, *The Autobiography of Yukichi Fukuzawa*, trans. Eiichi Kiyooka (New York: Columbia University Press, 1966).

28 Muzaffer M. Erselcuk, "Electricity in Japan," *Far Eastern Quarterly* 6 (May 1947): 283–93.

29 On "factory girls," see Mikiso Hane, *Peasants, Rebels, and Outcastes: The Underside of Modern Japan* (New York: Pantheon Books, 1982), 173–204; E. Patricia Tsurumi, *Factory Girls: Women in the Thread Mills of Meiji Japan* (Princeton, NJ: Princeton University Press, 1990).

30   Morris-Suzuki, *Technological Transformation of Japan*, 73.

31   Ibid., 72.

32   Nakano Makiko, *Makiko's Diary: A Merchant Wife in 1910 Kyoto*, trans. and intro. by Kazuko Smith (Stanford, CA: Stanford University Press, 1995), 67.

33   Morris-Suzuki, *Technological Transformation of Japan*, 130.

34   Andrew Gordon, ed., *Postwar Japan as History* (Berkeley and Los Angeles: University of California Press, 1993).

35   Hirose Takeshi, *Kōgai no genten o kōsei ni: Nyūmon Ashio kōdoku jiken* (The Coming of Age of the Cause of Industrial Pollution: Introduction to the Ashio Copper Pollution Incident) (Utsunomiya: Zuisōsha, 2001), 51.

36   Nimura, *Ashio Riot of 1907*, 19, 24–25, 168. See also F. G. Notehelfer, "Japan's First Pollution Incident," *Journal of Japanese Studies* 1, no. 2 (1975): 356.

37   Nash, "Finishing Nature," 42.

38   Robert P. Stolz, "'Yanakagaku': Pollution and Environmental Protest in Modern Japan" (Ph.D. diss., University of Chicago, 2006), 54.

39   Uchimizu Mamoru, *Shiryō Ashio kōdoku jiken* (Sources on the Ashio Copper-Poisoning Incident) (Tokyo: Aki Shobō, 1971), 277–78.

40   Notehelfer, "Japan's First Pollution Incident," 360–61. See also Kichiro Shoji and Masuro Sugai, "The Ashio Copper Mine Pollution Case: The Origins of Environmental Destruction," in *Industrial Pollution in Japan*, ed. Jun Ui (Tokyo: United Nations University Press, 1992), 18–21.

41   Komatsu Hiroshi, *Tanaka Shōzō no kindai* (Tanaka Shōzō's Modernity) (Tokyo: Gendai Kikakushitsu, 2001), 262–63.

42   Kenneth E. Wilkening, *Acid Rain Science and Politics in Japan: A History of Knowledge and Action toward Sustainability* (Cambridge, MA: MIT Press, 2004), 34–35. On Ashio, see 63–68.

43   Klaassen, *Casarett and Doull's Toxicology*, 867–70.

44   Shoji and Sugai, "Ashio Copper Mine Pollution Case," 40–41.

45   Ibid.

46   Kichiro Shoji and Masuro Sugai, "The Arsenic Milk Poisoning Incident," in *Industrial Pollution in Japan*, ed. Jun Ui (Tokyo: United Nations University Press, 1992), 77.

47   Klaassen, *Casarett and Doull's Toxicology*, 696–97.

48   Notehelfer, "Japan's First Pollution Incident," 361–63.

49   Kenneth Strong, *Ox against the Storm: A Biography of Tanaka Shozo—Japan's Conservationist Pioneer* (Tenterden, Kent, UK: Paul Norbury Publications, 1977; reprint, Richmond, Surrey, UK: Japan Library, 1995), 2, 5, 6, 25–28. For an extremely comprehensive look at Tanaka's life and thought, as well as a helpful introduction to the pollution problems at Ashio, see Komatsu, *Tanaka Shōzō no kindai*. For an essay on Tanaka's ideas about humans' ties to nature, see Timothy S. George, "Tanaka Shōzō's Vision of an Alternative Constitutional Modernity for Japan," in *Public Spheres, Private Lives in Modern Japan, 1600–1950: Essays in Honor of Albert M. Craig*, ed. Gail Lee Bernstein, Andrew Gordon, and Kate Wildman Nakai (Cambridge, MA: Harvard University Asia Center, 2005).

50 Strong, *Ox against the Storm*, 19.

51 Roger W. Bowen, *Rebellion and Democracy in Meiji Japan: A Study of Commoners in the Popular Rights Movement* (Berkeley and Los Angeles: University of California Press, 1980).

52 Strong, *Ox against the Storm*, 63–64.

53 Ibid., 74.

54 Ibid., 74–75, 76, 78–79.

55 Ibid., 85, 87, 89–90.

56 Ibid., 129–30.

57 On the topic of Christian converts and protest during the Meiji period, see Irwin Scheiner, *Christian Converts and Social Protest in Meiji Japan* (Berkeley and Los Angeles: University of California Press, 1970).

58 Strong, *Ox against the Storm*, 90–98.

59 Ibid., 104–5.

60 Ibid., 104, 106, 113, 115–16, 121.

61 Ibid., 126–27.

62 Ibid., 128.

63 Ibid., 132–34, 136.

64 The theme of "madness" and radical politics is explored in H. D. Harootunian, *Toward Restoration: The Growth of Political Consciousness in Tokugawa Japan* (Berkeley and Los Angeles: University of California Press, 1991).

65 Strong, *Ox against the Storm*, 153.

66 Ibid., 157, 161, 176–77, 191. On "thinking like a mountain" and the birth of Aldo Leopold's conservationism, see Susan L. Flader, *Thinking Like a Mountain: Aldo Leopold and the Evolution of an Ecological Attitude toward Deer, Wolves, and Forests* (Madison: University of Wisconsin Press, 1994).

67 Strong, *Ox against the Storm*, 192.

68 Ibid., 210, 211.

Chapter 4: *Engineering Pain in the Jinzū River Basin*

1   The Mitsui Group became involved with mining only after the Meiji Restoration of 1868. The Mitsui Group was a *zaibatsu*, or economic conglomerate, which directly controlled many subsidiaries, ranging from banking and shipping to mining and trusts. For a sympathetic, corporate outline of Mitsui's diverse mining subsidiaries, ranging from coal at Miike to sulfur at Iwaonobori, see Oland D. Russell, *The House of Mitsui—a Record of Three Centuries: Past History and Present Enterprises* (Tokyo: Mitsui Gomei Kaisha, 1933), 49–59.

2   Richard J. Samuels, *The Business of the Japanese State: Energy Markets in Comparative and Historical Perspective* (Ithaca, NY: Cornell University Press, 1987), 71–73.

3   My discussion of the history and technological advancements at the Kamioka

mines is based on Matsunami Jun'ichi, *Itai itai byō no kioku* ("It Hurts, It Hurts Disease" Remembrance) (Toyama: Katsura Shobō, 2002), 34–36.

4   O. Russell, *House of Mitsui*, 49. For brief mention of Mitsui's 1887 consolidation of the Kamioka complex, see 55.

5   Mark Metzler, *Lever of Empire: The International Gold Standard and the Crisis of Liberalism in Prewar Japan* (Berkeley and Los Angeles: University of California Press, 2006). In 1896, Matsukata Masayoshi, former finance minister, became prime minister. He saw Japan's participation in the international gold standard as critical to future economic success. And silver was not a part of his strategy. For example, reparation payments in the aftermath of the Sino-Japanese War were originally to be in silver, but, on Matsukata's insistence, they were collected in British pounds. The pounds were then used to purchase gold, which was shipped to Japan as part of the transition to the gold standard.

6   U.S. Geological Survey, *Mineral Resources of the United States, 1914* (Washington, DC: Government Printing Office, 1916), 896. To give some indication of the amount of copper and zinc required in modern warfare, in 1914 European nations ordered over 25 million shells from the United States, which required a total of 101 million pounds of copper and nearly 47 million pounds of zinc for the brass cases (896).

7   On the relationship between technologies and empire, see Daniel R. Headrick, *The Tools of Empire: Technology and European Imperialism in the Nineteenth Century* (Oxford: Oxford University Press, 1981); and Michael Adas, *Machines as the Measure of Men: Science, Technology, and Ideologies of Western Dominance* (Ithaca, NY: Cornell University Press, 1990).

8   Michael Lewis, *Becoming Apart: National Power and Local Politics in Toyama, 1868–1945* (Cambridge, MA: Harvard University Asia Center, 2000), 191.

9   For some information on the practices at the Broken Hill mine in Australia, see K. J. Dickinson, *Mining History of the Silver, Lead, Zinc, and Copper Mines of the Broken Hill District to 1939, Excluding the Main Line of Lode* ([Sydney]: Department of Mines, Geological Survey of New South Wales, V. C. N. Blight, Government Printer, 1972).

10   Kurachi Mitsuo, Tonegawa Haruo, and Hata Akio, eds., *Mitsui shihon to itai itai byō* (Mitsui Capital and "It Hurts, It Hurts Disease") (Tokyo: Ōtsuki Shoten, 1979), 103–4.

11   Ibid., 15–23.

12   The history of the diagnosis of "it hurts, it hurts disease" as cadmium poisoning and the disease's relationship to the Kamioka mines is covered in Lars Friberg, Magnus Piscator, Gunnar F. Nordberg, and Tord Kjellström, *Cadmium in the Environment*, 2nd ed. (Cleveland: CRC Press, 1974), 137–60.

13   Noboru Yamagata and Itsuzo Shigematsu, "Cadmium Pollution in Perspective," *Kōei eisei'in kenkyū hōkoku* (Bulletin of the Institute of Public Health) 19, no. 1 (1970): 2–3, 13–17.

14   Masumi Moritsugu and Jun Kobayashi, "Study on Trace Metals in Bio Materials:

II. Cadmium Content in Polished Rice," in *Berichte des Ohara Instituts für Land-wirtschaftliche Biologie, Okayama Universitat*, 12 (1964): 145–58.

15   Michelle Murphy, *Sick Building Syndrome and the Problem with Uncertainty* (Durham, NC: Duke University Press, 2006), 5, 6–16.

16   Gregg Mitman, *Breathing Space: How Allergens Shape Our Lives and Landscapes* (New Haven, CT: Yale University Press, 2007), 134.

17   J. Kobayashi, "Relation between the 'Itai-Itai' Disease and the Pollution of River Water by Cadmium from a Mine," in *Advances in Water Pollution Research: Proceedings of the Fifth International Water Pollution Research Conference* (n.p., 1970), I 25/1–I 25/8.

18   Sharon L. Sievers, *Flowers in Salt: The Beginnings of Feminist Consciousness in Modern Japan* (Stanford, CA: Stanford University Press, 1983), 22–23.

19   Sharon H. Nolte and Sally Ann Hastings, "The Meiji State's Policy toward Women, 1890–1910," in *Recreating Japanese Women, 1600–1945*, ed. Gail Lee Bernstein (Berkeley and Los Angeles: University of California Press, 1991), 152.

20   Sheldon Garon, *Molding Japanese Minds: The State in Everyday Life* (Princeton, NJ: Princeton University Press, 1997), 115.

21   Sievers, *Flowers in Salt*, 111.

22   Nolte and Hastings, "Meiji State's Policy toward Women," 156.

23   On "factory girls," see Hane, *Peasants, Rebels, and Outcastes*, 173–204; E. Tsurumi, *Factory Girls*. On the tuberculosis epidemics that plagued Japan's textile mills, see William Johnston, *The Modern Epidemic: A History of Tuberculosis in Japan* (Cambridge, MA: Harvard University Press, 1995), 70–90.

24   Jun Kobayashi, "Air and Water Pollution by Cadmium, Lead and Zinc Attributed to the Largest Zinc Refinery in Japan," *Trace Substances in Environmental Health: Proceedings of the University of Missouri's Annual Conference on Trace Substances in Environmental Health* 5 (1972): 119.

25   Friberg et al., *Cadmium in the Environment*, 149–52.

26   Kathleen S. Uno, "Women and Changes in the Household Division of Labor," in *Recreating Japanese Women, 1600–1945*, ed. Gail Lee Bernstein (Berkeley and Los Angeles: University of California Press, 1991), 17–18. The diary of Nakano Makiko provides an excellent example of a late Meiji period woman fulfilling these core filial duties. See Nakano, *Makiko's Diary*.

27   Robert J. Smith and Ella Lury Wiswell, *The Women of Suye Mura* (Chicago: University of Chicago Press, 1982).

28   Friberg et al., *Cadmium in the Environment*, 155.

29   On infanticide and fertility in early modern Japan, see Fabian Drixler, "Demographic Discourses and the End of Japan's Low-Fertility Regime, 1660-1900" (Ph.D. diss., Harvard University, 2007).

30   Thomas C. Smith, *Nakahara: Family Farming and Population in a Japanese Village, 1717–1830* (Stanford, CA: Stanford University Press, 1977), 7–8.

31   Akira Hayami, *The Historical Demography of Pre-modern Japan* (Tokyo: University of Tokyo Press, 1997), 42–50.

32   Of course, the problem with using family size or general population as an indica-

tor of fertility rates or number of children birthed (which is the important contributor in cadmium poisoning) is that infant mortality rates were probably high, which means that, as Laurel Cornell hypothetically points out, "If 250 of 1000 infants died before their first birthdays, then women whom we perceive as having three or six children actually had four or eight. In consequence, all reported figures for fertility in Japan prior to 1870 would inevitably be lower than those reported for pretransitional western Europe, even if the underlying levels were exactly the same." In other words, it is hard to know the degree that fertility rates changed between the late Tokugawa and early Meiji periods. See Laurel L. Cornell, "Infanticide in Early Modern Japan? Demography, Culture, and Population Growth," *Journal of Asian Studies* 55, no. 1 (February 1996): 40.

33   T. Smith, *Nakahara*, 123.
34   Emiko Ochiai, "The Reproductive Revolution at the End of the Tokugawa Period," in *Women and Class in Japanese History*, ed. Hitomi Tonomura, Anne Walthall, and Wakita Haruko (Ann Arbor: Center for Japanese Studies, University of Michigan, 1999), 212.
35   Dower, *War without Mercy*.
36   Bunsō Hashikawa, "Japanese Perspectives on Asia: From Dissociation to Coprosperity," in *The Chinese and the Japanese: Essays in Political and Cultural Interactions*, ed. Akira Iriye and Madeleine Chi (Princeton, NJ: Princeton University Press, 1980), 331–32.
37   Dower, *War without Mercy*, 208–9.
38   Julian Gresser, Koichiro Fujikura, and Akio Morishima, eds., *Environmental Law in Japan* (Cambridge, MA: MIT Press, 1981), 56–57.

Chapter 5: Mercury's Offspring

1   Fadiman, *Spirit Catches You and You Fall Down*, 12–13.
2   Ishimure Michiko, *Paradise in the Sea of Sorrow: Our Minamata Disease*, trans. Livia Monnet (Kyoto: Yamaguchi Publishing House, 1990), 133–74. Ishimure altered the names of most of the people in her book. Sakagami's real name is Murano Tamano. For more on Ishimure Michiko, see Akio Mishima, *Bitter Sea: The Human Cost of Minamata Disease*, foreword by Lester R. Brown (Tokyo: Koei Publishing Co., 1992).
3   Cecilia Segawa Seigle, *Yoshiwara: The Glittering World of the Japanese Courtesan* (Honolulu: University of Hawai'i Press, 1993), 84.
4   Ishimure, *Paradise in the Sea of Sorrow*, 133–74.
5   *Kojiki*, trans. Philippi, 148–58. See also Ohnuki-Tierney, *Rice as Self*, 52–53.
6   Pierre François Souyri, *The World Turned Upside Down: Medieval Japanese Society* (New York: Columbia University Press, 2001), 14, 92–94.
7   For more on modern whaling in U.S.-Japanese relations, see John R. Schmidhauser and George O. Totten, *The Whaling Issue in U.S.-Japan Relations* (Boulder, CO: Westview Press, 1978); Kalland and Moeran, *Japanese Whaling*.

8   Dennis Normile, "Japan's Whaling Program Carries Heavy Baggage," *Science* 289 (29 September 2000): 2264–65.

9   C. Scott Baker, G. M. Lento, F. Cipriano, M. L. Dalebout, S. R. Palumbi, Mutsuo Goto, and Seiji Ohsumi, "Scientific Whaling: Source of Illegal Products for Market?" *Science*, n.s., 290, no. 5497 (1 December 2000): 1695–96.

10 Arthur F. McEvoy, *The Fisherman's Problem: Ecology and Law in the California Fisheries, 1850–1980* (Cambridge: Cambridge University Press, 1986), 21, 30.

11 Garret Hardin, "The Tragedy of the Commons: The Population Problem Has No Technical Solution; It Requires a Fundamental Extension of Morality," *Science* 162 (13 December 1968): 1243–48.

12 Today, Japanese fisheries are far flung and no longer restricted to well-defined territories. On Japanese international fisheries, see Yoshiaki Matsuda, "Changes in Tuna Fisheries Negotiations between Japan and the Pacific Island Nations," in *Resources and Environment in Asia's Marine Sector*, ed. James Barney Marsh (Washington, DC, and London: Taylor and Francis New York, 1992), 41–57; Tadashi Yamamoto and Hajime Imanishi, "Use of Shared Stocks in the Northwest Pacific Ocean with Particular Reference to Japan and the USSR," in *Resources and Environment in Asia's Marine Sector*, ed. James Barney Marsh (Washington, DC, and London: Taylor and Francis New York, 1992), 12–40. Japan has played a particularly prominent role in the decline of shark fisheries around the world. See Sunee C. Sonu, *Shark Fisheries, Trade, and Market of Japan* (Washington, DC: U.S. Department of Commerce, National Oceanic and Atmospheric Administration, National Marine Fisheries Service, October 1998).

13 Arne Kalland, *Fishing Villages in Tokugawa Japan* (Honolulu: University of Hawai'i Press, 1995), 35–52, 91–95, 99–115, 163–79, 180–97, 307–16.

14 On the "ecotone," a kind of hybrid space where creatures neither wild nor domesticated dwell, see Mike Davis, *Ecology of Fear: Los Angeles and the Imagination of Disaster* (New York: Metropolitan Books, 1998).

15 Nishimura Hajime and Okamoto Tatsuaki, *Minamatabyō no kagaku* (The Science of Minamata Disease) (Tokyo: Hyōronsha, 2001), 120–21.

16 Ishimure, *Paradise in the Sea of Sorrow*, 76.

17 Nishimura and Okamoto, *Minamatabyō no kagaku*, 120–21. For more on the history of cats in Japan, see Hiraiwa Yonekichi, *Neko no rekishi to kiwa* (Cat's History and Stories) (Tokyo: Tsukiji Shokan, 1992).

18 Ishimure, *Paradise in the Sea of Sorrow*, 73.

19 Barry Commoner, *The Closing Circle: Nature, Man, and Technology* (New York: Alfred A. Knopf, 1971), 163; Jeffrey L. Meikle, *American Plastic: A Cultural History* (New Brunswick, NJ: Rutgers University Press, 1995), 137–38.

20 Ishimure, *Paradise in the Sea of Sorrow*, 73–74.

21 Ibid., 227; Commoner, *Closing Circle*, 228–30.

22 Ishimure, *Paradise in the Sea of Sorrow*, 71, 74.

23 Steingraber, *Having Faith*, 48–49.

24 Shoji Kitamura, "Determination on Mercury Content in the Bodies of Inhabitants, Cats, Fishes and Shells in Minamata District and in the Mud of Minamata

Bay," in *Minamata Disease*, ed. Study Group of Minamata Disease (Kumamoto: Kumamoto University, 1968), 258–65.

25 Katsuro Irukayama, "Animal Experiments with Substances Obtained by Various Treatments of the Poisonous Fish and Shellfish," in *Minamata Disease*, ed. Study Group of Minamata Disease (Kumamoto: Kumamoto University, 1968), 254–56.

26 Nishimura and Okamoto, *Minamatabyō no kagaku*, 152–57.

27 Ibid., 169–77.

28 Gregory T. Cushman, "'The Most Valuable Birds in the World': Science and the Revival of Peru's Guano Industry, 1909–1965," *Environmental History* 10, no. 3 (July 2005): 477–78.

29 Ponting, *Green History of the World*, 218–21.

30 J. R. McNeill, *Something New under the Sun: An Environmental History of the Twentieth-Century World* (New York: W. W. Norton, 2000), 25–26.

31 William M. Tsutsui, "Landscapes in the Dark Valley: Toward an Environmental History of Wartime Japan," *Environmental History* 8, no. 2 (April 2003): 294–311.

32 On the development of the herring fertilizer industry on Hokkaido, see David L. Howell, *Capitalism from Within: Economy, Society, and the State in a Japanese Fishery* (Berkeley and Los Angeles: University of California Press, 1995). For an examination of the Japanese presence on Hokkaido in the seventeenth and eighteenth centuries, see my *Conquest of Ainu Lands*.

33 Jason P. Kaye, Peter M. Groffman, Nancy B. Grimm, Lawrence A. Baker, and Richard V. Pouyat, "A Distinct Urban Biochemistry?" *TRENDS in Ecology and Evolution* 21, no. 4 (April 2006): 192.

34 This famous thesis was outlined in T. Smith, *Agrarian Origins of Modern Japan*.

35 See, e.g., Anne Walthall, "Village Networks: Sōdai and the Sale of Edo Nightsoil," *Monumenta Nipponica* 43, no. 3 (Autumn 1988): 279–303.

36 Ann P. Kinzig and J. Morgan Grove, "Urban-Suburban Ecology," in *Encyclopedia of Biodiversity* (New York: Academic Press, 2001), vol. 5, 733–45.

37 For more on the *mibunsei*, or "status system," see David L. Howell, *Geographies of Identity in Nineteenth-Century Japan* (Berkeley and Los Angeles: University of California Press, 2005).

38 Susan B. Hanley, "Urban Sanitation in Preindustrial Japan," *Journal of Interdisciplinary History* 18, no. 1 (Summer 1987): 1–26.

39 Partner, *Toshié*, 127–28.

40 The Frank-Caro process refers to the German chemist Adolph Frank (1834–1916) and the Polish chemist Nikodem Caro (1871–1935).

41 For a thorough account of the technological developments at Chisso, see Timothy S. George, *Minamata: Pollution and the Struggle for Democracy in Postwar Japan* (Cambridge, MA: Harvard University Asia Center, 2001), 13–41. See also Kazuko Tsurumi, "Man, Nature and Technology: A Case of Minamata," in *Aspects of Endogenous Development in Modern Japan*, ed. Kazuko Tsurumi, Sophia University, Institute of International Relations Research Papers, series A-38, part 3 (Tokyo: Sophia University, 1979), 12–13; Barbara Molony, *Technology and Investment: The Prewar Japanese Chemical Industry* (Cambridge, MA: Harvard Univer-

sity Press, 1990), 17–266; Morris-Suzuki, *Technological Transformation of Japan*, 114–15; Yahagi Tadashi, "Nihon Chisso hiryō (kabu) ni kansuru kenkyū" (Research on Chisso Corporation), *Urawa ronsō* 10 (March 1993): 55–96; Yahagi Tadashi, "Sengo Chisso shi 1945–55" (A History of Postwar Chisso, 1945–55), *Urawa ronsō* 14 (June 1995): 145–78; Yahagi Tadashi, "Chisso shi 1955–60 Minamatabyō" (Chisso History, 1955–60: Minamata Disease), *Urawa ronsō* 17 (January 1997): 23–46; Yahagi Tadashi, "Chisso shi 1960–65 Goi kōjō kensetsu" (Chisso History, 1960–65: Construction of the Goi Factory), *Urawa ronsō* 20 (June 1998): 21–60.

42 Masayoshi Sugimoto and David L. Swain, *Science and Culture in Traditional Japan, A.D. 600–1854* (Cambridge, MA: MIT Press, 1978), 90–91.

43 Meikle, *American Plastic*, 83.

44 W. Eugene Smith and Aileen M. Smith, *Minamata* (New York: Holt, Rinehart and Winston, 1975), 28, 33.

45 Julia Adeney Thomas, "Photography, National Identity, and the 'Cataract of Times': Wartime Images and the Case of Japan," *American Historical Review* 103, no. 5 (December 1998): 1475–1501.

46 Helena María Viramontes, *The Moths and Other Stories* (Houston: Arte Público Press, 1985), 23–28.

47 Bridget Kevane and Juanita Heredia, eds., *Latina Self-Portraits: Interviews with Contemporary Women Writers* (Albuquerque: University of New Mexico Press, 2000), 141–54.

48 Meikle, *American Plastic*, xiv, 3, 63–67.

49 Ibid., 16, 20.

50 Mitman, "In Search of Health," 185.

51 Gregg Mitman, Michelle Murphy, and Christopher Sellers, "Introduction: A Cloud over History," *Osiris*, 2nd ser., 19, Landscapes of Exposure: Knowledge and Illness in Modern Environments (2004): 2.

52 Yuki Terazawa, "Gender, Knowledge, and Power: Reproductive Medicine in Japan, 1690–93" (Ph.D. diss., University of California, Los Angeles, 2001).

53 Margaret M. Lock, *East Asian Medicine in Urban Japan: Varieties of Medical Experience* (Berkeley and Los Angeles: University of California Press, 1980), 23–66.

54 *The Yellow Emperor's Classic of Internal Medicine*, trans. Ilza Veith, foreword by Ken Rose (Berkeley and Los Angeles: University of California Press, 2002), 105, 149.

55 On the geographies of health in the United States, see Gregg Mitman, "Geographies of Hope: Mining the Frontiers of Health in Denver and Beyond, 1870–1965," *Osiris*, 2nd ser., 19, Landscapes of Exposure: Knowledge and Illness in Modern Environments (2004): 93–111. See also Mitman, *Breathing Space*.

56 Terazawa, "Gender, Knowledge, and Power," 21–79, 80–193, 195–291, quotation on 92.

57 Jennifer Robertson, "The Shingaku Woman: Straight from the Heart," in *Recreating Japanese Women, 1600–1945*, ed. Gail Lee Bernstein (Berkeley and Los Angeles: University of California Press, 1991), 94–95.

58 Janet R. Goodwin, Bettina Gramlich-Oka, Elizabeth A. Leicester, Yuki Terazawa,

and Anne Walthall, trans., "Solitary Thoughts: A Translation of Tadano Makuzu's *Hitori Kangae*," *Monumenta Nipponica* 56, no. 1 (Spring 2001): 25.

59 Terazawa, "Gender, Knowledge, and Power," 21–79, 80–193, 195–291, quotations on 100.

60 Nakamura, *Practical Pursuits*, 60–61.

61 *The Gossamer Years: A Diary by a Noblewoman of Heian Japan*, trans. Edward Seidensticker (Tokyo: Charles E. Tuttle, 1964), 42.

62 *Confessions of Lady Nijō*, trans. Brazell, 13–14.

63 Ibid., 39, 45, 50–51.

64 Hitomi Tonomura, "Sexual Violence against Women: Legal and Extralegal Treatment in Premodern Warrior Societies," in *Women and Class in Japanese History*, ed. Hitomi Tonomura, Anne Walthall, and Wakita Haruko (Ann Arbor: Center for Japanese Studies, University of Michigan, 1999), 150.

65 Terazawa, "Gender, Knowledge, and Power," 124–25.

66 Ibid., 109.

67 Ibid., 21–79, 80–193, 195–291. See also Ochiai, "Reproductive Revolution at the End of the Tokugawa Period," 187–215.

68 Steingraber, *Having Faith*.

69 Laurel L. Cornell, "The Deaths of Old Women: Folklore and Differential Morality in Nineteenth-Century Japan," in *Recreating Japanese Women, 1600–1945*, ed. Gail Lee Bernstein (Berkeley and Los Angeles: University of California Press, 1991), 71–87.

70 T. Smith, *Nakahara*, 59–85.

71 Helen Hardacre, *Marketing the Menacing Fetus in Japan* (Berkeley and Los Angeles: University of California Press, 1997).

72 William R. LaFleur, *Liquid Life: Abortion and Buddhism in Japan* (Princeton, NJ: Princeton University Press, 1992).

73 Negishi Yasumori, *Mimibukuro* (Ear Bag), ed. Suzuki Tōzō (Tokyo: Heibonsha, 2000), vol. 1, 295, 344–45.

74 See Ria Koopmans-de Bruijn, "Fabled Liaisons: Serpentine Spouses in Japanese Folktales," in *JAPANimals: History and Culture in Japan's Animal Life*, ed. Gregory M. Pflugfelder and Brett L. Walker (Ann Arbor: Center for Japanese Studies, University of Michigan, 2005), 61–88.

75 *Confessions of Lady Nijō*, trans. Brazell, 206.

76 Negishi, *Mimibukuro*, vol. 1, 295, 344–45.

77 Timon Screech, *The Lens within the Heart: The Western Scientific Gaze and Popular Imagery in Later Edo Japan* (Honolulu: University of Hawai'i Press, 2002), 133–65.

78 Yoshitaka Harada, "Congenital (or Fetal) Minamata Disease," in *Minamata Disease*, ed. Study Group of Minamata Disease (Kumamoto: Kumamoto University, 1968), 93–117, quotations on 116–17.

79 For scholarship on the struggles for recognition and compensation, see Huddle and Reich, with Stiskin, *Islands of Dreams*, 102–32; Frank K. Upham, *Law and Social Change in Postwar Japan* (Cambridge, MA: Harvard University Press,

1989), 28–77; Jun Ui, *Industrial Pollution in Japan* (Tokyo: United Nations University Press, 1992), 103–32; George, *Minamata*. On the pathology of Minamata disease, see Masazumi Harada, with Aileen M. Smith, "Minamata Disease: A Medical Report," in *Minamata*, W. Eugene Smith and Aileen M. Smith, ed. (New York: Holt, Rinehart and Winston, 1975), 180–92; Tadao Tsubaki and Katsuro Irukayama, eds., *Minamata Disease: Methylmercury Poisoning in Minamata and Niigata, Japan* (Tokyo: Kodansha; Amsterdam: Elsevier Scientific Publishing, 1977); Tadao Takeuchi and Komyo Eto, *The Pathology of Minamata Disease: A Tragic Story of Water Pollution* (Fukuoka: Kyushu University Press, 1999).

80   Ishimure, *Paradise in the Sea of Sorrow*, 350–51.

Chapter 6: Hell at the Hōjō Colliery

1   On another large-scale coal mine explosion, one that caused long-term carbon monoxide poisoning, see Masazumi Harada, *Minamata Disease*, trans. Tsushima Sachie and Timothy S. George, trans. ed. Timothy S. George (Kumamoto: Kumamoto Nichinichi Shinbun Culture and Information Center, 2004), 80–81.

2   Werner Sombart, *Krieg und Kapitalismus* (War and Capitalism) (Manchester, NH: Ayer Co. Publishers, 1975).

3   Richard J. Samuels, *"Rich Nation Strong Army": National Security and the Technological Transformation of Japan* (Ithaca, NY: Cornell University Press, 1994), 9, 35–38.

4   Orii Seigo, *Hōjō daihijō* (Calamity at Hōjō) (Tokyo: Asahi Shinbunsha, 1979), 5.

5   Kusano Masaki, "Meiji kōki kara Taishō shoki ni okeru Chikuhō sekitan kōgyō to tankō saigai: Taishō sannen Mitsubishi Hōjō tankō tanjin gasu bakuhatsu jiko no bunseki o chūshin to shite" (Chikuhō Coal Industry Disasters from the Late Meiji to the Taisho Period: An Analysis of the 1914 Mitsubishi Hōjō Coal-Dust and Gas Explosion), *Fukuoka ken chiikishi kenkyū* 22 (2005): 50.

6   Laura E. Hein, *Fueling Growth: The Energy Revolution and Economic Policy in Postwar Japan* (Cambridge, MA: Council on East Asian Studies, Harvard University, 1990), 32.

7   Hane, *Peasants, Rebels, and Outcastes*, 235.

8   Michael Lewis has written about early-twentieth-century riots at coal mines in *Rioters and Citizens: Mass Protest in Imperial Japan* (Berkeley and Los Angeles: University of California Press, 1990).

9   Matthew Allen, *Undermining the Japanese Miracle: Work and Conflict in a Coal Mining Community* (Cambridge: Cambridge University Press, 1994), 12–14, 54–57.

10   Ibid., 54–63, 82.

11   Hane, *Peasants, Rebels, and Outcastes*, 227.

12   Joyce Chapman Lebra, "Women in an All-Male Industry: The Case of Sake Brewer Tatsu'uma Kiyo," in *Recreating Japanese Women, 1600–1945*, ed. Gail Lee Bernstein (Berkeley and Los Angeles: University of California Press, 1991), 132–33.

13   Baroness Shidzué Ishimoto, *Facing Two Ways: The Story of My Life*, intro. Barbara

Molony (New York: Farrar and Rinehart, 1935; reprint, Stanford, CA: Stanford University Press, 1984), 148, 150, 158–59, 160, 161, 163.

14 Yutaka Nishinarita, "The Coal-Mining Industry," in *Technology Change and Female Labour in Japan*, ed. Masanori Nakamura (Tokyo and New York: United Nations University Press, 1994), 60, 62–63, 69, 72.

15 Charles S. Elton described organisms as "connected energy transformers" that came together to create "loop channels in the ecosystem." See his *Ecology of Invasions by Animals and Plants*, 125–26.

16 Allan A. Andrews, *The Teachings Essential for Rebirth: A Study of Genshin's "Ōjō yōshū,"* Monumenta Nipponica Monograph (Tokyo: Sophia University, 1973).

17 Richard Bowring, trans., *The Diary of Lady Murasaki* (New York: Penguin Classic, 1999), 22.

18 Not all forms of Buddhism viewed life so tragically, and neither did the Shinto belief system. For an exploration of the relationship between play and prayer in late Tokugawa society, see Nam-lin Hur, *Prayer and Play in Late Tokugawa Japan: Asakusa Sensōji and Edo Society* (Cambridge, MA: Harvard University Asia Center, 2000).

19 Fernando G. Gutiérrez, "Emakimono Depicting the Pains of the Damned," *Monumenta Nipponica* 22, nos. 3/4 (1967): 281–86.

20 William R. LaFleur, "Hungry Ghosts and Hungry People: Somaticity and Rationality in Medieval Japan," in *Fragments for a History of the Human Body*, parts 1–3, ed. Michael Feher, with Ramona Naddaff and Nadia Tazi (New York: Zone Books, 1989), 273.

21 Ueda Tatsuo, *Hōjō-chō to tankō* (Hōjō Township and Coal Mining) (Hōjō: Hōjō-chō Kyōiku Iinkai and Hōjō-chō Bunkazai Senmon Iinkai, 1994), 175–78.

22 Kusano, "Meiji kōki kara Taishō shoki ni okeru Chikuhō sekitan kōgyō to tankō saigai," 50–51.

23 Orii, *Hōjō daihijō*, 6–8.

24 Ibid., 8.

25 Ibid.

26 Ibid., 36–40.

27 Ibid., 53, 60, 61.

28 The document titled "Hōjō tankō bakuhatsu chōsa hōkoku" (Investigative Report on the Hōjō Colliery Explosion) is cited in Orii, *Hōjō daihijō*, 174.

29 Yoshihisa Tak Matsusaka, *The Making of Japanese Manchuria, 1904–1932*, Harvard East Asian Monographs 196 (Cambridge, MA: Harvard University Press, 2001).

30 Mark R. Peattie, *Ishiwara Kanji and Japan's Confrontation with the West* (Princeton, NJ: Princeton University Press, 1975), 87–139.

31 Much of this ground regarding Japanese imperialism is covered in W. G. Beasely, *Japanese Imperialism, 1894–1945* (Oxford: Clarendon Press, 1987).

32 *Manchuria: Land of Opportunities* (New York: South Manchuria Railway, 1922), v, 30–37.

33 Fujita, *American Pioneers and the Japanese Frontier*, 43–68.

34 Botsman, *Punishment and Power in the Making of Modern Japan*, 184–86.

35 Kuwabara Masato, *Senzenki Hokkaidō no shiteki kenkyū* (Prewar Hokkaido and Historical Research) (Sapporo: Hokkaidō Daigaku Tosho Kankōkai, 1993), 215, 218.

36 Suzanne Culter, *Managing Decline: Japan's Coal Industry Restructuring and Community Response* (Honolulu: University of Hawai'i Press, 1999), 36–37, 113.

37 "The Honkeiko Colliery Disaster (26 April 1942)," Report no. 29 (18 April 1946), General Headquarters, Supreme Commander for the Allied Powers, Natural Resources Section, 1–8.

38 Perrow, *Normal Accidents*, 230–31.

39 "Judgment of the International Military Tribunal for the Far East," in *Documents on the Rape of Nanking*, ed. Timothy Brook (Ann Arbor: University of Michigan Press, 1999), 258–59.

40 Saburō Ienaga, *The Pacific War, 1931–1945: A Critical Perspective on Japan's Role in World War II by a Leading Japanese Scholar* (New York: Pantheon Books, 1978), 6–7.

41 S. Meguro, "Report on the Explosion at the Hojo Colliery, Japan," *Colliery Guardian and Journal of the Coal and Iron Trades* 109, no. 2835 (30 April 1915): 907–9.

42 S. Meguro, "Report on the Explosion at the Hojo Colliery, Japan," *Colliery Guardian and Journal of the Coal and Iron Trades* 109, no. 2836 (7 May 1915): 964–65.

43 Orii, *Hōjō daihijō*, 178–90.

44 Orii Seigo, *Nazo no Hōjō tankō daibakuhatsu* (The Reason for the Great Explosion at the Hōjō Colliery) (Tokyo: Kokudosha, 1981), 138–40.

45 Meguro, "Report on the Explosion at the Hojo Colliery, Japan," *Colliery Guardian and Journal of the Coal and Iron Trades* 109, no. 2836 (7 May 1915): 964–65.

46 Orii, *Hōjō daihijō*, 178–90.

47 For a printed version of the original Fukuoka report, minus the death certificates, see "Hōjō tankō hensai shorui (Documents Regarding the Disaster at the Hōjō Coal Mine)," *Sekitan kenkyū shiryō sōsho* (Resource Series for Coal Research) 26 (March 2005): 3–68.

48 On this giant fish market, see Theodore C. Bestor, *Tsukiji: The Fish Market at the Center of the World* (Berkeley and Los Angeles: University of California Press, 2004).

49 For the classic discussion of the motivations behind Tokugawa peasant rebellions, see Irwin Scheiner, "Benevolent Lords and Honorable Peasants: Rebellion and Peasant Consciousness in Tokugawa Japan," in *Japanese Thought in the Tokugawa Period, 1600–1868: Methods and Metaphors*, ed. Tetsuo Najita and Irwin Scheiner (Chicago: University of Chicago Press, 1978), 39–62. For an assessment of Tokugawa peasant rebellion literature, see Conrad Totman, "Tokugawa Peasants: Win, Lose, or Draw," *Monumenta Nipponica* 41, no. 4 (Winter 1986): 457–76.

50 Huddle and Reich, with Stiskin, *Islands of Dreams*, 51–77. See also Yoshida Katsumi, *Yokkaichi kōgai: Sono kyōkun to 21-seiki e no kadai* (Yokkaichi Industrial Pollution: Its Lessons and Challenges in the 21st Century) (Tokyo: Kashiwa Shobō, 2002); and Ueno Tatsuhiko and Paku Keishuku, eds., *Kankyō kaitei toshi o meza-*

shite: Yokkaichi kōgai kara no teigen (Aiming for an Environmentally Agreeable City: A Proposal from Yokkaichi Industrial Pollution) (Tokyo: Chūō Hōki, 2004).

Conclusion

1   Andrea Peacock, *Libby, Montana: Asbestos and the Deadly Silence of an American Corporation* (Boulder, CO: Johnson Books, 2003); Andrew Schneider and David McCumber, *An Air That Kills: How the Asbestos Poisoning of Libby, Montana, Uncovered a National Scandal* (New York: Berkley Books, 2004).

2   See, e.g., Ellis S. Krauss and Bradford L. Simcock, "Citizens' Movements: The Growth and Impact of Environmental Protest in Japan," in *Political Opposition and Local Politics in Japan*, ed. Kurt Steiner, Ellis S. Krauss, and Scott C. Flanagan (Princeton, NJ: Princeton University Press, 1980), 187–227; Jack G. Lewis, "Civic Protest in Mishima: Citizens' Movements and the Politics of the Environment in Contemporary Japan," in *Political Opposition and Local Politics in Japan*, ed. Kurt Steiner, Ellis S. Krauss, and Scott C. Flanagan (Princeton, NJ: Princeton University Press, 1980), 274–313; Margaret A. McKean, *Environmental Protest and Citizen Politics in Japan* (Berkeley and Los Angeles: University of California Press, 1981); Upham, *Law and Social Change in Postwar Japan*, 28–77; John Knight, "The Forest Grant Movement in Japan," in *Environmental Movements in Asia*, ed. Arne Kalland and Gerard Persoon (Richmond, Surrey, UK: Curzon Press, 1998), 110–30; Anny Wong, "The Anti-tropical Timber Campaign in Japan," in *Environmental Movements in Asia*, ed. Arne Kalland and Gerard Persoon (Richmond, Surrey, UK: Curzon Press, 1998), 131–50; George, *Minamata*.

3   See Brendan F. D. Barrett, "Conclusions," in *Ecological Modernisation and Japan* (London and New York: Routledge, 2005), 172. For my evaluation of "ecological modernization theory" and review of *Ecological Modernisation and Japan*, see *Journal of Japanese Studies* 33, no. 1 (Winter 2007): 294–98.

4   Gavan McCormack, *The Emptiness of Japanese Affluence*, rev. ed., foreword by Norma Field (New York and London: M. E. Sharpe, 2001), 133–34.

5   See www.friendsofthecongo.org.

6   Gresser, Fujikura, and Morishima, *Environmental Law in Japan*, 395–96.

7   Cronon, "The Trouble with Wilderness," 80–81.

8   Donald Worster, "The Wilderness of History," *Wild Earth*, Fall 1997, 12–13.

9   For the Basic Law, see Gresser, Fujikura, and Morishima, *Environmental Law in Japan*, 395–96.

10 Pamela J. Asquith and Arne Kalland, "Japanese Perceptions of Nature: Ideals and Illusions," in *Japanese Images of Nature: Cultural Perspectives* (Richmond, Surrey, UK: Curzon Press, 1997), 15.

11 Wilkening, *Acid Rain Science and Politics in Japan*, 126–31.

12 Iguchi Taisen, Sumi Manabu, and Tanabe Shinsuke, "Endocrine Disruptor Issues in Japan," *Congenital Anomalies* 40, no. 2 (2002): 106–19. Endocrine disruptors

are "an exogenous substance or mixture that alters the function of the endocrine system and consequently causes adverse health effects in an intact organism or its progeny or subpopulations." See "The State of the Science on Endocrine Disruptors," *Environmental Health Perspectives* 106, no. 7 (July 1998): A319.

13 See, e.g., Nancy Langston, "The Retreat from Precaution: Regulating Diethylstilbestrol (DES), Endocrine Disruptors, and Environmental Health," *Environmental History* 13, no. 1 (January 2008): 41–65.

14 See, e.g., Theo Colborn, Dianne Dumanoski, and John Peterson Myers, *Our Stolen Future: Are We Threatening Our Fertility, Intelligence, and Survival?* (New York: Plume, 1997); and Sheldon Krimsky, *Hormonal Chaos: The Scientific and Social Origins of the Environmental Endocrine Hypothesis*, foreword by Lynn Goldman (Baltimore, MD: Johns Hopkins University Press, 2002).

15 Tu Binh Minh, Mafumi Watanabe, Shinsuke Tanabe, Taketo Yamada, Jun'ichi Hata, and Shaw Watanabe, "Specific Accumulation and Elimination Kinetics of Tris(4-Chlorophenyl)Methane, Tris(4-Chlorophenyl)Methanol, and Other Persistent Organochlorines in Humans from Japan," *Environmental Health Perspectives* 109, no. 9 (September 2001): 927, 929, 930.

16 Hiromi Ohtani, Ikuo Miura, and Youko Ichikawa, "Effects of Dibutyl Phthalate as an Environmental Endocrine Disruptor on Gonadal Sex Differentiation of Genetic Males of the Frog *Rana rugosa*," *Environmental Health Perspectives* 108, no. 12 (December 2000): 1189.

17 See "Strategic Program on Environmental Endocrine Disruptors" (SPEED '98), Environmental Agency, Government of Japan (www.env.go.jp/en), 347, 353–54, 355, 360–61. See also Nakata Kotoko, "Endocrine Disruptors and Environmental Impact in Japan," *Cad. Saúde Pública* 18, no. 2 (March–April 2002): 531–48, http://www.scielosp.org/scielo.php?script=sci_arttext&pid=S0102-311X2002000200019&nrm=iso&tlng=pt.

18 McCormack, *Emptiness of Japanese Affluence*, 27.

19 Niikura Toshiko, "Campaigns against Dams in Japan and the Nagara River Estuary Dam," *Organization and Environment* 12, no. 1 (March 1999): 99–104.

20 McCormack, *Emptiness of Japanese Affluence*, 25–77.

21 Alex Kerr, *Dogs and Demons: Tales from the Dark Side of Japan* (New York: Hill and Wang, 2001), 47.

22 Conrad Totman has written extensively on Japan's forestry, particularly in the prewar years. See, e.g., *Green Archipelago: Forestry in Pre-industrial Japan* (Berkeley and Los Angeles: University of California Press, 1989; reprint, Athens: Ohio University Press, 1998); and, more recently, *Japan's Imperial Forest: Goryōrin, 1889–1945* (Folkestone, Kent, UK: Global Oriental, 2007). For material on Japan's role in global deforestation, see Thomas R. Cox, "The North American–Japanese Timber Trade: A Survey of Its Social, Economic, and Environmental Impact," in *World Deforestation in the Twentieth Century*, ed. John F. Richards and Richard P. Tucker, Duke Press Policy Studies (Durham, NC: Duke University Press, 1988).

23 David Quammen, "Planet of Weeds: Tallying the Losses of Earth's Animals and Plants," *Harper's Magazine*, October 1998, 57–69.

WORKS CITED

Adas, Michael. *Machines as the Measure of Men: Science, Technology, and Ideologies of Western Dominance*. Ithaca, NY: Cornell University Press, 1990.

Allen, Matthew. *Undermining the Japanese Miracle: Work and Conflict in a Coal Mining Community*. Cambridge: Cambridge University Press, 1994.

Anderson, Benedict. *Imagined Communities: Reflections on the Origin and Spread of Nationalism*. Rev. ed. London and New York: Verso, 1991.

Andō Mitsuru. *Yokuwakaru nōyaku osen: Jintai to kankyō o mushibamu gōsei kagaku busshitsu* (Agricultural Chemical Contamination: The Synthetic Chemical Compounds That Ruin Human Bodies and the Environment). Tokyo: Gōdō Shuppan, 1990.

Andrews, Allan A. *The Teachings Essential for Rebirth: A Study of Genshin's "Ōjō yōshū."* Monumenta Nipponica Monograph. Tokyo: Sophia University, 1973.

Asquith, Pamela J., and Kalland, Arne. "Japanese Perceptions of Nature: Ideals and Illusions." In *Japanese Images of Nature: Cultural Perspectives*. Richmond, Surrey, UK: Curzon Press, 1997.

Baker, C. Scott, G. M. Lento, F. Cipriano, M. L. Dalebout, S. R. Palumbi, Mutsuo Goto, and Seiji Ohsumi. "Scientific Whaling: Source of Illegal Products for Market?" *Science*, n.s., 290, no. 5497 (1 December 2000): 1695–96.

Barenblatt, Daniel. *A Plague upon Humanity: The Hidden History of Japan's Biological Warfare Program*. New York: Perennial, 2004.

Barrett, Brendan F. D. "Conclusions." In *Ecological Modernisation and Japan*. London and New York: Routledge, 2005.

Bartholomew, James R. *The Formation of Science in Japan*. New Haven, CT: Yale University Press, 1989.

Beasely, W. G. *Japanese Imperialism, 1894–1945.* Oxford: Clarendon Press, 1987.

Berry, Mary Elizabeth. *Hideyoshi.* Cambridge, MA: Harvard University Press, 1982.

———. "Public Peace and Private Attachment: The Goals and Conduct of Power in Early Modern Japan." *Journal of Japanese Studies* 12, no. 2 (Summer 1986): 237–71.

Bestor, Theodore C. *Tsukiji: The Fish Market at the Center of the World.* Berkeley and Los Angeles: University of California Press, 2004.

Bitō Masahide. "The Akō Incident, 1701–1703." *Monumenta Nipponica* 58, no. 3 (Summer 2003): 149–69.

Bocking, Stephen. "Ecosystems, Ecologists, and the Atom: Environmental Research at Oak Ridge National Laboratory." *Journal of the History of Biology* 28 (1995): 1–47.

Borgen, Robert. *Sugawara no Michizane and the Early Heian Court.* Honolulu: University of Hawai'i Press, 1986.

Botsman, Daniel V. *Punishment and Power in the Making of Modern Japan.* Princeton, NJ: Princeton University Press, 2004.

Bowen, Roger W. *Rebellion and Democracy in Meiji Japan: A Study of Commoners in the Popular Rights Movement.* Berkeley and Los Angeles: University of California Press, 1980.

Bowring, Richard, trans. *The Diary of Lady Murasaki.* New York: Penguin Classic, 1999.

Briggs, John, and F. David Peat. *Seven Life Lessons of Chaos: Timeless Wisdom from the Science of Change.* New York: HarperCollins, 1999.

Bromehead, C. N. "Ancient Mining Processes as Illustrated by a Japanese Scroll." *Antiquity* 16, no. 63 (September 1942): 193–207.

Buhs, Joshua Blu. *The Fire Ant Wars: Nature, Science, and Public Policy in Twentieth-Century America.* Chicago: University of Chicago Press, 2004.

Burns, Susan L. *Before the Nation: Kokugaku and the Imagining of Community in Early Modern Japan.* Durham, NC: Duke University Press, 2003.

Clancey, Gregory. *Earthquake Nation: The Cultural Politics of Japanese Seismicity, 1868–1930.* Berkeley and Los Angeles: University of California Press, 2006.

Clausen, Curtis P., J. L. King, and Cho Teranishi. "The Parasites of *Popillia japonica* in Japan and Chosen (Korea), and Their Introduction into the United States." *United States Department of Agriculture Department Bulletin* 1429 (January 1927): 1–55.

Colborn, Theo, Dianne Dumanoski, and John Peterson Myers. *Our Stolen Future: Are We Threatening Our Fertility, Intelligence, and Survival?* New York: Plume, 1997.

Commoner, Barry. *The Closing Circle: Nature, Man, and Technology.* New York: Alfred A. Knopf, 1971.

The Confessions of Lady Nijō. Translated by Karen Brazell. Stanford, CA: Stanford University Press, 1973.

Cornell, Laurel L. "The Deaths of Old Women: Folklore and Differential Morality in Nineteenth-Century Japan." In *Recreating Japanese Women, 1600–1945,* edited by Gail Lee Bernstein. Berkeley and Los Angeles: University of California Press, 1991.

———. "Infanticide in Early Modern Japan? Demography, Culture, and Population Growth." *Journal of Asian Studies* 55, no. 1 (February 1996): 22–50.

Cox, Thomas R. "The North American–Japanese Timber Trade: A Survey of Its Social,

Economic, and Environmental Impact." In *World Deforestation in the Twentieth Century*, edited by John F. Richards and Richard P. Tucker. Duke Press Policy Studies. Durham, NC: Duke University Press, 1988.

Cronon, William. "The Trouble with Wilderness; or, Getting Back to the Wrong Nature." In *Uncommon Ground: Rethinking the Human Place in Nature*, edited by William Cronon. New York: W. W. Norton, 1996.

Culter, Suzanne. *Managing Decline: Japan's Coal Industry Restructuring and Community Response*. Honolulu: University of Hawai'i Press, 1999.

Cushman, Gregory T. "'The Most Valuable Birds in the World': Science and the Revival of Peru's Guano Industry, 1909–1965." *Environmental History* 10, no. 3 (July 2005): 477–78.

Daniel, Pete. *Toxic Drift: Pesticides and Health in the Post-World War II South*. Baton Rouge: Louisiana State University Press in association with Smithsonian Institution, 2005.

Davis, Mike. *Ecology of Fear: Los Angeles and the Imagination of Disaster*. New York: Metropolitan Books, 1998.

———. *Late Victorian Holocausts: El Niño Famines and the Making of the Third World*. London and New York: Verso, 2001.

Department of Agriculture and Commerce, ed. *Japan in the Beginning of the 20th Century*. Tokyo: Shoin, 1904.

Dickinson, K. J. *Mining History of the Silver, Lead, Zinc, and Copper Mines of the Broken Hill District to 1939, Excluding the Main Line of Lode*. [Sydney]: Department of Mines, Geological Survey of New South Wales, V. C. N. Blight, Government Printer, 1972.

Dower, John W. *Embracing Defeat: Japan in the Wake of World War II*. New York: W. W. Norton / The New Press, 1999.

———. *War without Mercy: Race and Power in the Pacific War*. New York: Pantheon, 1987.

Drixler, Fabian. "Demographic Discourses and the End of Japan's Low-Fertility Regime, 1660–1900." Ph.D. diss., Harvard University, 2007.

Dykstra, Yoshiko K. "Notable Tales Old and New: Tachibana Narisue's *Kokon Chomonjū*." *Monumenta Nipponica* 47, no. 4 (Winter 1992): 469–93.

Elison, George. *Deus Destroyed: The Image of Christianity in Early Modern Japan*. Cambridge, MA: Harvard University Press, 1988.

Elton, Charles S. *The Ecology of Invasions by Animals and Plants*. London: Methuen, 1958. Reprint, Chicago: University of Chicago Press, 2000.

Erselcuk, Muzaffer M. "Electricity in Japan." *Far Eastern Quarterly* 6 (May 1947): 283–93.

Fadiman, Anne. *The Spirit Catches You and You Fall Down: A Hmong Child, Her American Doctors, and the Collision of Two Cultures*. New York: Farrar, Straus and Giroux, 1997.

Flader, Susan L. *Thinking like a Mountain: Aldo Leopold and the Evolution of an Ecological Attitude toward Deer, Wolves, and Forests*. Madison: University of Wisconsin Press, 1994.

Friberg, Lars, Magnus Piscator, Gunnar F. Nordberg, and Tord Kjellström. *Cadmium in the Environment*. 2nd ed. Cleveland: CRC Press, 1974.

Fujita, Fumiko. *American Pioneers and the Japanese Frontier: American Experts in Nineteenth-Century Japan*. Westport, CT: Greenwood Press, 1994.

Fukuzawa Yukichi. *The Autobiography of Yukichi Fukuzawa*. Translated by Eiichi Kiyooka. New York: Columbia University Press, 1966.

———. *An Outline of a Theory of Civilization*. Translated by David A. Dilworth and G. Cameron Hurst. Tokyo: Sophia University, 1973.

Gaddis, John Lewis. *The Landscape of History: How Historians Map the Past*. Oxford: Oxford University Press, 2002.

Garon, Sheldon. *Molding Japanese Minds: The State in Everyday Life*. Princeton, NJ: Princeton University Press, 1997.

George, Timothy S. *Minamata: Pollution and the Struggle for Democracy in Postwar Japan*. Cambridge, MA: Harvard University Asia Center, 2001.

———. "Tanaka Shōzō's Vision of an Alternative Constitutional Modernity for Japan." In *Public Spheres, Private Lives in Modern Japan, 1600–1950: Essays in Honor of Albert M. Craig*, edited by Gail Lee Bernstein, Andrew Gordon, and Kate Wildman Nakai. Cambridge, MA: Harvard University Asia Center, 2005.

Gluck, Carol. *Japan's Modern Myths: Ideology in the Late Meiji Period*. Princeton, NJ: Princeton University Press, 1985.

Goldsmith, Marian R., Toru Shimada, and Hiroaki Abe. "The Genetics and Genomics of the Silkworm, *Bombyx mori*." *Annual Review of Entomology* 50 (January 2005): 71–100.

Goodwin, Janet R., Bettina Gramlich-Oka, Elizabeth A. Leicester, Yuki Terazawa, and Anne Walthall, trans. "Solitary Thoughts: A Translation of Tadano Makuzu's *Hitori Kangae*." *Monumenta Nipponica* 56, no. 1 (Spring 2001): 21–38.

Gordon, Andrew, ed. *Postwar Japan as History*. Berkeley and Los Angeles: University of California Press, 1993.

The Gossamer Years: A Diary by a Noblewoman of Heian Japan. Translated by Edward Seidensticker. Tokyo: Charles E. Tuttle, 1964.

Graham, Alistair, and Peter Beard. *Eyelids of Morning: The Mingled Destinies of Crocodiles and Men*. San Francisco, CA: Chronicle Books, 1990.

Gresser, Julian, Koichiro Fujikura, and Akio Morishima, eds. *Environmental Law in Japan*. Cambridge, MA: MIT Press, 1981.

Gutiérrez, Fernando G. "Emakimono Depicting the Pains of the Damned." *Monumenta Nipponica* 22, nos. 3/4 (1967): 278–89.

Hane, Mikiso. *Peasants, Rebels, and Outcastes: The Underside of Modern Japan*. New York: Pantheon Books, 1982.

Hanley, Susan B. "Urban Sanitation in Preindustrial Japan." *Journal of Interdisciplinary History* 18, no. 1 (Summer 1987): 1–26.

Harada, Masazumi. *Minamata Disease*. Translated by Tsushima Sachie and Timothy S. George. Translation edited by Timothy S. George. Kumamoto: Kumamoto Nichi-nichi Shinbun Culture and Information Center, 2004.

Harada, Masazumi, with Aileen M. Smith. "Minamata Disease: A Medical Report." In

Minamata, by W. Eugene Smith and Aileen M. Smith. New York: Holt, Rinehart and Winston, 1975.

Harada, Yoshitaka. "Congenital (or Fetal) Minamata Disease." In *Minamata Disease*, edited by Study Group of Minamata Disease. Kumamoto: Kumamoto University, 1968.

Hardacre, Helen. *Marketing the Menacing Fetus in Japan*. Berkeley and Los Angeles: University of California Press, 1997.

Hardin, Garret. "The Tragedy of the Commons: The Population Problem Has No Technical Solution; It Requires a Fundamental Extension of Morality." *Science* 162 (13 December 1968): 1243–48.

Harootunian, H. D. *Things Seen and Unseen: Discourse and Ideology in Tokugawa Nativism*. Chicago: University of Chicago Press, 1988.

———. *Toward Restoration: The Growth of Political Consciousness in Tokugawa Japan*. Berkeley and Los Angeles: University of California Press, 1991.

Hashikawa, Bunsō. "Japanese Perspectives on Asia: From Dissociation to Coprosperity." In *The Chinese and the Japanese: Essays in Political and Cultural Interactions*, edited by Akira Iriye and Madeleine Chi. Princeton, NJ: Princeton University Press, 1980.

Hayami, Akira. *The Historical Demography of Pre-modern Japan*. Tokyo: University of Tokyo Press, 1997.

Headrick, Daniel R. *The Tools of Empire: Technology and European Imperialism in the Nineteenth Century*. Oxford: Oxford University Press, 1981.

Hearn, Lafcadio. *Kwaidan: Stories and Studies of Strange Things*. Boston: Houghton, Mifflin, 1904. Reprint, Rutland, VT: Charles E. Tuttle, 1971.

Hein, Laura E. *Fueling Growth: The Energy Revolution and Economic Policy in Postwar Japan*. Cambridge, MA: Council on East Asian Studies, Harvard University, 1990.

Hiraiwa Yonekichi. *Neko no rekishi to kiwa* (Cat's History and Stories). Tokyo: Tsukiji Shokan, 1992.

Hirose Takeshi. *Kōgai no genten o kōsei ni: Nyūmon Ashio kōdoku jiken* (The Coming of Age of the Cause of Industrial Pollution: Introduction to the Ashio Copper Pollution Incident). Utsunomiya: Zuisōsha, 2001.

"Hōjō tankō hensai shorui" (Documents Regarding the Disaster at the Hōjō Coal Mine). *Sekitan kenkyū shiryō sōsho* (Resource Series for Coal Research) 26 (March 2005): 3–68.

Hokkaido Prefectural Government, ed. *Foreign Pioneers: A Short History of the Contribution of Foreigners to the Development of Hokkaido*. Sapporo: Hokkaido Prefectural Government, 1968.

"The Honkeiko Colliery Disaster (26 April 1942)." Report no. 29 (18 April 1946), General Headquarters, Supreme Commander for the Allied Powers, Natural Resources Section, 1–8.

Hostetler, Laura. *Qing Colonial Enterprise: Ethnography and Cartography in Early Modern China*. Princeton, NJ: Princeton University Press, 2001.

Howell, David L. *Capitalism from Within: Economy, Society, and the State in a Japanese Fishery*. Berkeley and Los Angeles: University of California Press, 1995.

————. *Geographies of Identity in Nineteenth-Century Japan.* Berkeley and Los Angeles: University of California Press, 2005.

Huddle, Norie, and Michael Reich, with Nahum Stiskin. *Islands of Dreams: Environmental Crisis in Japan.* Foreword by Paul R. Ehrlich. Afterword by Ralph Nader. New York and Tokyo: Autumn Press, 1975.

Hur, Nam-lin. *Death and Social Order in Tokugawa Japan: Buddhism, Anti-Christianity, and the* Danka *System.* Cambridge, MA: Harvard University Asia Center, Harvard University Press, 2007.

————. *Prayer and Play in Late Tokugawa Japan: Asakusa Sensōji and Edo Society.* Cambridge, MA: Harvard University Asia Center, 2000.

Hyōdō Hiromi and Henry D. Smith II. "Singing Tales of the Gishi: Naniwabushi and the Forty-Seven Rōnin in Late Meiji Japan." *Monumenta Nipponica* 64, no. 4 (Winter 2007): 459–508.

Ienaga, Saburō. *The Pacific War, 1931–1945: A Critical Perspective on Japan's Role in World War II by a Leading Japanese Scholar.* New York: Pantheon Books, 1978.

Igler, David. *Industrial Cowboys: Miller and Lux and the Transformation of the Far West, 1850–1920.* Berkeley and Los Angeles: University of California Press, 2005.

Iguchi Taisen, Sumi Manabu, and Tanabe Shinsuke. "Endocrine Disruptor Issues in Japan." *Congenital Anomalies* 40, no. 2 (2002): 106–19.

Ikegami, Eiko. *The Taming of the Samurai: Honorific Individualism and the Making of Modern Japan.* Cambridge, MA: Harvard University Press, 1995.

Innes, Robert Lero. "The Door Ajar: Japan's Foreign Trade in the Seventeenth Century." Ph.D. diss., University of Michigan, 1980.

Irukayama, Katsuro. "Animal Experiments with Substances Obtained by Various Treatments of the Poisonous Fish and Shellfish." In *Minamata Disease,* edited by Study Group of Minamata Disease. Kumamoto: Kumamoto University, 1968.

Ishimoto, Baroness Shidzué. *Facing Two Ways: The Story of My Life.* Introduction by Barbara Molony. New York: Farrar and Rinehart, 1935. Reprint, Stanford, CA: Stanford University Press, 1984.

Ishimure Michiko. *Paradise in the Sea of Sorrow: Our Minamata Disease.* Translated by Livia Monnet. Kyoto: Yamaguchi Publishing House, 1990.

"Japanese Use the Chinese as 'Guinea Pigs' to Test Germ Warfare." *Rocky Mountain Medical Journal* 39, no. 8 (August 1942): 571–72.

Johnston, William. *The Modern Epidemic: A History of Tuberculosis in Japan.* Cambridge, MA: Harvard University Press, 1995.

"Judgment of the International Military Tribunal for the Far East." In *Documents on the Rape of Nanking,* edited by Timothy Brook. Ann Arbor: University of Michigan Press, 1999.

Kalland, Arne. *Fishing Villages in Tokugawa Japan.* Honolulu: University of Hawai'i Press, 1995.

Kalland, Arne, and Brian Moeran. *Japanese Whaling: End of an Era?* London: Curzon Press, 1992.

Kankyō Hōrei Kenkyūkai, ed. *Kankyō kōgai nenkan* (Yearbook of Environmental Pollution). Tokyo: Gakuyō Shobō, 1973.

Kasai Masaaki. *Mushi to Nihon bunka* (Insects and Japanese Culture). Tokyo: Daigyōsha, 1997.

Kawana Hideyuki. *Dokyumento Nihon no kōgai: Kōgai no gekka* (Documentation of Japan's Industrial Pollution: Intensification of Industrial Pollution). Vol 1. Tokyo: Ryokufu Shuppan, 1987.

Kaye, Jason P., Peter M. Groffman, Nancy B. Grimm, Lawrence A. Baker, and Richard V. Pouyat. "A Distinct Urban Biochemistry?" *TRENDS in Ecology and Evolution* 21, no. 4 (April 2006): 192–99.

Kentaro Higuchi, ed. *PCB Poisoning and Pollution*. Tokyo: Kodansha; New York: Academic Press, 1976.

Kerr, Alex. *Dogs and Demons: Tales from the Dark Side of Japan*. New York: Hill and Wang, 2001.

Kevane, Bridget, and Juanita Heredia, eds. *Latina Self-Portraits: Interviews with Contemporary Women Writers*. Albuquerque: University of New Mexico Press, 2000.

Kikuchi Isao. *Kinsei no kikin* (Early Modern Japan's Famines). Tokyo: Yoshikawa Kōbunkan, 1997.

Kinzig, Ann P., and J. Morgan Grove. "Urban-Suburban Ecology." In *Encyclopedia of Biodiversity*, vol. 5, 733–45. New York: Academic Press, 2001.

Kitagawa Morisada. *Ruijū kinsei fūzokushi* (Record of Various Modern Customs), edited by Muromatsu Iwao. Tokyo: Bunchōsha Shoin, 1928.

Kitamura, Shoji. "Determination on Mercury Content in the Bodies of Inhabitants, Cats, Fishes and Shells in Minamata District and in the Mud of Minamata Bay." In *Minamata Disease*, edited by Study Group of Minamata Disease. Kumamoto: Kumamoto University, 1968.

Klaasen, Curtis D., ed. *Casarett and Doull's Toxicology: The Basic Science of Poisons*. 5th ed. New York: McGraw-Hill, Health Professions Division, 1996.

Knight, John. "The Forest Grant Movement in Japan." In *Environmental Movements in Asia*, edited by Arne Kalland and Gerard Persoon. Richmond, Surrey, UK: Curzon Press, 1998.

———. *Waiting for Wolves in Japan: An Anthropological Study of People-Wildlife Relations*. Oxford: Oxford University Press, 2003.

Kobata, A. "The Production and Uses of Gold and Silver in Sixteenth- and Seventeenth-Century Japan." *Economic History Review*, n.s., 18, no. 2 (1965): 245–66.

Kobata Atsushi. *Nihon dōkōgyōshi no kenkyū* (Research on Japan's Copper-Mining Industry). Kyoto: Shibunkaku Shuppan, 1993.

Kobayashi, J. "Relation between the 'Itai-Itai' Disease and the Pollution of River Water by Cadmium from a Mine." In *Advances in Water Pollution Research: Proceedings of the Fifth International Water Pollution Research Conference*, I 25/1–I 25/8. N.p., 1970.

Kobayashi, Jun. "Air and Water Pollution by Cadmium, Lead and Zinc Attributed to the Largest Zinc Refinery in Japan." *Trace Substances in Environmental Health: Proceedings of the University of Missouri's Annual Conference on Trace Substances in Environmental Health* 5 (1972): 117–28.

Koichi Haraguchi, Yousuke Hisamichi, Sachie Moriki, and Tetsuya Endo. "Organohalogen Contaminants and Metabolites in Killer Whale (*Orcinus orca*) and Melon-Headed Whale (*Peponocephala electra*) from Japanese Coastal Water." *Organohalogen Compounds* 68 (2006): 1851–54.

Kojiki (Record of Ancient Matters). Translated with an introduction and notes by Donald L. Philippi. Tokyo: University of Tokyo Press, 1968.

Kok, L. T. "Toxicity of Insecticides Used for Asiatic Rice Borer Control to Tropical Fish in Rice Paddies." In *The Careless Technology: Ecology and International Development*, edited by M. Taghi Farvar and John P. Milton. Garden City, NY: Natural History Press, 1972.

Komatsu Hiroshi. *Tanaka Shōzō no kindai* (Tanaka Shōzō's Modernity). Tokyo: Gendai Kikakushitsu, 2001.

Kōnōdo no PCB ya suigin kenshutsu: Shiretoko de shinda shachi (High Levels of PCB and Mercury Found in the Orcas That Died at Shiretoko). *Chūnichi Web Press*, 9 March 2005. http://www.chunichi.co.jp/00/detail/20050309/fls_detail_062.shtml.

Koyama Hitoshi, ed. *Senzen Shōwaki Osaka no kōgai mondai shiryō* (Sources for Prewar Showa Period Pollution Problems in Osaka). Suita: Kansai Daigaku Keizai Seiji Kenkyūjo, 1973.

Krauss, Ellis S., and Bradford L. Simcock. "Citizens' Movements: The Growth and Impact of Environmental Protest in Japan." In *Political Opposition and Local Politics in Japan*, edited by Kurt Steiner, Ellis S. Krauss, and Scott C. Flanagan. Princeton, NJ: Princeton University Press, 1980.

Krimsky, Sheldon. *Hormonal Chaos: The Scientific and Social Origins of the Environmental Endocrine Hypothesis*. Foreword by Lynn Goldman. Baltimore, MD: Johns Hopkins University Press, 2002.

Kurachi Mitsuo, Tonegawa Haruo, and Hata Akio, eds. *Mitsui shihon to itai itai byō* (Mitsui Capital and "It Hurts, It Hurts Disease"). Tokyo: Ōtsuki Shoten, 1979.

Kusano Masaki. "Meiji kōki kara Taishō shoki ni okeru Chikuhō sekitan kōgyō to tankō saigai: Taishō sannen Mitsubishi Hōjō tankō tanjin gasu bakuhatsu jiko no bunseki o chūshin to shite" (Chikuhō Coal Industry Disasters from the Late Meiji to the Taisho Periods: An Analysis of the 1914 Mitsubishi Hōjō Coal-Dust and Gas Explosion). *Fukuoka ken chiikishi kenkyū* 22 (2005): 49–79.

Kuwabara Masato. *Senzenki Hokkaidō no shiteki kenkyū* (Prewar Hokkaido and Historical Research). Sapporo: Hokkaidō Daigaku Tosho Kankōkai, 1993.

LaFleur, William R. "Hungry Ghosts and Hungry People: Somaticity and Rationality in Medieval Japan." In *Fragments for a History of the Human Body*, parts 1–3, edited by Michael Feher, with Ramona Naddaff and Nadia Tazi. New York: Zone Books, 1989.

———. *Liquid Life: Abortion and Buddhism in Japan*. Princeton, NJ: Princeton University Press, 1992.

Langston, Nancy. "The Retreat from Precaution: Regulating Diethylstilbestrol (DES), Endocrine Disruptors, and Environmental Health." *Environmental History* 13, no. 1 (January 2008): 41–65.

Latour, Bruno. *Reassembling the Social: An Introduction to Actor-Network Theory*. Oxford: Oxford University Press, 2005.

Lebra, Joyce Chapman. "Women in an All-Male Industry: The Case of Sake Brewer Tatsu'uma Kiyo." In *Recreating Japanese Women, 1600–1945*, edited by Gail Lee Bernstein. Berkeley and Los Angeles: University of California Press, 1991.

LeCain, Timothy J. "'The Heavens and the Earth': Controlling Terrestrial and Subterrestrial Environments in Twentieth Century Western Mining." Paper presented at the Third Annual Michael P. Malone Conference, "Spaces of Struggle: Power and the Transformation of Nature," Big Sky, MT, 28 September–2 October 2005.

Lewis, Jack G. "Civic Protest in Mishima: Citizens' Movements and the Politics of the Environment in Contemporary Japan." In *Political Opposition and Local Politics in Japan,* edited by Kurt Steiner, Ellis S. Krauss, and Scott C. Flanagan. Princeton, NJ: Princeton University Press, 1980.

Lewis, Michael. *Becoming Apart: National Power and Local Politics in Toyama, 1868–1945.* Cambridge, MA: Harvard University Asia Center, 2000.

———. *Rioters and Citizens: Mass Protest in Imperial Japan.* Berkeley and Los Angeles: University of California Press, 1990.

Lindee, M. Susan. *Suffering Made Real: American Science and the Survivors at Hiroshima.* Chicago: University of Chicago Press, 1994.

"The Livestock Industry of Japan." Report no. 30, General Headquarters, Supreme Commander for the Allied Powers, Natural Resources Section, APO 500, 18 April 1944.

Lock, Margaret M. *East Asian Medicine in Urban Japan: Varieties of Medical Experience.* Berkeley and Los Angeles: University of California Press, 1980.

Lockwood, Jeffrey A. *Locust: The Devastating Rise and Mysterious Disappearance of the Insect That Shaped the American Frontier.* New York: Basic Books, 2004.

Lurie, David B. "Orientomology: The Insect Literature of Lafcadio Hearn (1850–1904)." In *JAPANimals: History and Culture in Japan's Animal Life,* edited by Gregory M. Pflugfelder and Brett L. Walker. Ann Arbor: Center for Japanese Studies, University of Michigan, 2005.

Maki, John M. *William Smith Clark: A Yankee in Hokkaido.* Sapporo: Hokkaido University Press, 1996.

Manchuria: Land of Opportunities. New York: South Manchuria Railway, 1922.

Marcon, Federico, and Henry D. Smith II. "A Chūshingura Palimpsest: Young Motoori Norinaga Hears the Story of the Akō Rōnin from a Buddhist Priest." *Monumenta Nipponica* 58, no. 4 (Winter 2003): 439–61.

Markowitz, Gerald, and David Rosner. *Deceit and Denial: The Deadly Politics of Industrial Pollution.* Berkeley and Los Angeles: University of California Press, 2002.

Maruyama, Masao. *Studies in the Intellectual History of Tokugawa Japan.* Translated by Mikiso Hane. Princeton, NJ: Princeton University Press, 1974.

Masuda Tsuna. *"Kodō zuroku": Illustrated Book on the Smelting of Copper.* Norwalk, CT: Burndy Library, 1983.

Materials on the Trial of Former Servicemen of the Japanese Army Charged with Manufacturing and Employing Bacteriological Weapons. Moscow: Foreign Languages Publishing House, 1950.

Matsubara Hiromichi. *Nihon nōyakugakushi nenpyō* (A Historical Chronology of the

Development of Agricultural Chemicals). Tokyo: Gakkai Shuppan Sentā, 1984.

Matsuda, Yoshiaki. "Changes in Tuna Fisheries Negotiations between Japan and the Pacific Island Nations." In *Resources and Environment in Asia's Marine Sector,* edited by James Barney Marsh. Washington, DC, and London: Taylor and Francis New York, 1992.

Matsunaka Shōichi. *Nihon ni okeru nōyaku no rekishi* (Japan's Agricultural Chemical History). Tokyo: Gakkai Shuppan Sentā, 2002.

Matsunami Jun'ichi. *Itai itai byō no kioku* ("It Hurts, It Hurts Disease" Remembrance). Toyama: Katsura Shobō, 2002.

Matsusaka, Yoshihisa Tak. *The Making of Japanese Manchuria, 1904–1932.* Harvard East Asian Monographs 196. Cambridge, MA: Harvard University Press, 2001.

McCormack, Gavan. *The Emptiness of Japanese Affluence.* Rev. ed. Foreword by Norma Field. New York and London: M. E. Sharpe, 2001.

McEvoy, Arthur F. *The Fisherman's Problem: Ecology and Law in the California Fisheries, 1850–1980.* Cambridge: Cambridge University Press, 1986.

McKean, Margaret A. *Environmental Protest and Citizen Politics in Japan.* Berkeley and Los Angeles: University of California Press, 1981.

McMullen, James. "Confucian Perspectives on the Akō Revenge: Law and Moral Agency." *Monumenta Nipponica* 58, no. 3 (Autumn 2003): 293–311.

McNeill, J. R. *Something New under the Sun: An Environmental History of the Twentieth-Century World.* New York: W. W. Norton, 2000.

Meguro, S. "Report on the Explosion at the Hojo Colliery, Japan." *Colliery Guardian and Journal of the Coal and Iron Trades* 109, no. 2835 (30 April 1915): 907–9.

———. "Report on the Explosion at the Hojo Colliery, Japan." *Colliery Guardian and Journal of the Coal and Iron Trades* 109, no. 2836 (7 May 1915): 964–65.

Meikle, Jeffrey L. *American Plastic: A Cultural History.* New Brunswick, NJ: Rutgers University Press, 1995.

Merchant, Carolyn. *The Death of Nature: Women, Ecology, and the Scientific Revolution.* San Francisco: Harper and Row, 1980. Reprint, New York: Harper and Row, 1983.

Metzler, Mark. *Lever of Empire: The International Gold Standard and the Crisis of Liberalism in Prewar Japan.* Berkeley and Los Angeles: University of California Press, 2006.

Minh, Tu Binh, Mafumi Watanabe, Shinsuke Tanabe, Taketo Yamada, Jun'ichi Hata, and Shaw Watanabe. "Specific Accumulation and Elimination Kinetics of Tris(4-Chlorophenyl)Methane, Tris(4-Chlorophenyl)Methanol, and Other Persistent Organochlorines in Humans from Japan." *Environmental Health Perspectives* 109, no. 9 (September 2001): 927–35.

Mishima, Akio. *Bitter Sea: The Human Cost of Minamata Disease.* Foreword by Lester R. Brown. Tokyo: Koei Publishing Co., 1992.

Mitman, Gregg. *Breathing Space: How Allergens Shape Our Lives and Landscapes.* New Haven, CT: Yale University Press, 2007.

———. "Geographies of Hope: Mining the Frontiers of Health in Denver and Beyond, 1870–1965." In "Landscapes of Exposure: Knowledge and Illness in Modern Environments," *Osiris,* 2nd ser., 19 (2004): 93–111.

———. "In Search of Health: Landscape and Disease in American Environmental History." *Environmental History* 10, no. 2 (April 2005): 184–210.

Mitman, Gregg, Michelle Murphy, and Christopher Sellers. "Introduction: A Cloud over History." In "Landscapes of Exposure: Knowledge and Illness in Modern Environments," *Osiris*, 2nd ser., 19 (2004): 1–17.

Mitsui Kinzoku Kōgyō Kabushikigaisha Shūshi Iinkai Jimukyoku, ed. *Kamioka kōzan shashinshū* (Photograph collection of the Kamioka mine). Tokyo: Mitsui Kinzoku Kōgyō Kabushikigaisha, 1975.

Miura Yoshiaki. *Kagaku osen to ningen no rekishi* (Chemical Contamination and Human History). Tokyo: Tsukiji Shokan, 1999.

Molony, Barbara. *Technology and Investment: The Prewar Japanese Chemical Industry.* Cambridge, MA: Harvard University Press, 1990.

Moritsugu, Masumi, and Jun Kobayashi. "Study on Trace Metals in Bio Materials: II. Cadmium Content in Polished Rice." *Berichte des Ohara Instituts für Landwirtschaftliche Biologie, Okayama Universitat,* 12 (1964): 145–58.

Morris, Ivan. *The Nobility of Failure: Tragic Heroes in the History of Japan.* New York: Holt, Rinehart and Winston, 1975.

———. *The World of the Shining Prince: Court Life in Ancient Japan.* New York: Kodansha International, 1964.

Morris-Suzuki, Tessa. "Sericulture and the Origins of Japanese Industrialization." *Technology and Culture* 33, no. 1 (January 1992): 101–21.

———. *The Technological Transformation of Japan: From the Seventeenth to the Twenty-First Century.* Cambridge: Cambridge University Press, 1994.

Mun, J. H., Y. H. Song, K. L. Heong, and G. K. Roderick. "Genetic Variation among Asian Populations of Rice Planthoppers, *Nilaparvata lugens* and *Sogatella furcifera* (Hemiptera: Delphacidae): Mitochondrial DNA Sequences." *Bulletin of Entomological Research* 89 (1999): 245–53.

Murasaki Shikibu. *The Tale of Genji.* Translated and with an introduction by Edward G. Seidensticker. New York: Alfred A. Knopf, 1997.

Murphy, Michelle. *Sick Building Syndrome and the Problem with Uncertainty.* Durham, NC: Duke University Press, 2006.

Nagahara Keiji and Kozo Yamamura. "Shaping the Process of Unification: Technological Progress in Sixteenth- and Seventeenth-Century Japan." *Journal of Japanese Studies* 14, no. 1 (Winter 1998): 77–109.

Nakai, Kate Wildman. *Shogunal Politics: Arai Hakuseki and the Premises of Tokugawa Rule.* Cambridge, MA: Council on East Asian Studies, Harvard University Press, 1988.

Nakaminami Gen. *Nōyaku genron* (The Principles of Agricultural Chemicals). Tokyo: Hokuto Shuppan, 2001.

Nakamura, Ellen Gardner. *Practical Pursuits: Takano Chōei, Takahashi Keisaku, and Western Medicine in Nineteenth-Century Japan.* Cambridge, MA: Harvard University Asia Center, Harvard University Press, 2005.

Nakano Makiko. *Makiko's Diary: A Merchant Wife in 1910 Kyoto.* Translated and introduction by Kazuko Smith. Stanford, CA: Stanford University Press, 1995.

Nakata Kotoko. "Endocrine Disruptors and Environmental Impact in Japan." *Cad. Saúde Pública* 18, no. 2 (March–April 2002): 531–48. http://www.scielosp.org/scielo.php?script=sci_arttext&pid=S0102-311X2002000200019&nrm=iso&tlng=pt.

Namba, Tatsuji. "Oxime Therapy for Poisoning by Alkylphosphate-Insecticides." *Proceedings of the 13th Annual International Congress on Occupational Health, July 25–29, 1960* (1961): 757–58.

Nash, Linda. "Finishing Nature: Harmonizing Bodies and Environments in Late-Nineteenth-Century California." *Environmental History* 8 (January 2003): 25–52.

————. "The Fruits of Ill-Health: Pesticides and Workers' Bodies in Post–World War II California." In "Landscapes of Exposure: Knowledge and Illness in Modern Environments," *Osiris*, 2nd ser., 19 (2004): 203–19.

————. *Inescapable Ecologies: A History of Environment, Disease, and Knowledge.* Berkeley and Los Angeles: University of California Press, 2006.

Negishi Yasumori. *Mimibukuro* (Ear Bag). Vol. 1. Edited by Suzuki Tōzō. Tokyo: Heibonsha, 2000.

Niikura Toshiko. "Campaigns against Dams in Japan and the Nagara River Estuary Dam." *Organization and Environment* 12, no. 1 (March 1999): 99–104.

Nimura Kazuo. *The Ashio Riot of 1907: A Social History of Mining in Japan.* Edited by Andrew Gordon. Translated by Terry Boardman and Andrew Gordon. Durham, NC: Duke University Press, 1997.

Nishimura Hajime and Okamoto Tatsuaki. *Minamatabyō no kagaku* (The Science of Minamata Disease). Tokyo: Hyōronsha, 2001.

Nishinarita, Yutaka. "The Coal-Mining Industry." In *Technology Change and Female Labour in Japan*, edited by Masanori Nakamura. Tokyo and New York: United Nations University Press, 1994.

Nolte, Sharon H., and Sally Ann Hastings. "The Meiji State's Policy toward Women, 1890–1910." In *Recreating Japanese Women, 1600–1945*, edited by Gail Lee Bernstein. Berkeley and Los Angeles: University of California Press, 1991.

Norman, E. Herbert. *Andō Shōeki and the Anatomy of Japanese Feudalism.* 1949. Reprint, Washington, DC: University Publications of America, 1979.

Normile, Dennis. "Japan's Whaling Program Carries Heavy Baggage." *Science* 289 (29 September 2000): 2264–65.

Notehelfer, F. G. "Japan's First Pollution Incident." *Journal of Japanese Studies* 1, no. 2 (1975): 351–83.

Ochiai, Emiko. "The Reproductive Revolution at the End of the Tokugawa Period." In *Women and Class in Japanese History*, edited by Hitomi Tonomura, Anne Walthall, and Wakita Haruko. Ann Arbor: Center for Japanese Studies, University of Michigan, 1999.

Oda Yasunori. *Kindai Nihon no kōgai mondai: Shiteki keisei katei no kenkyū* (Modern Japan's Pollution Problems). Kyoto: Sekai Shisōsha, 1983.

Ohnuki-Tierney, Emiko. *Rice as Self: Japanese Identities through Time.* Princeton, NJ: Princeton University Press, 1993.

Ohtani, Hiromi, Ikuo Miura, and Youko Ichikawa. "Effects of Dibutyl Phthalate as an Environmental Endocrine Disruptor on Gonadal Sex Differentiation of Genetic

Males of the Frog *Rana rugosa.*" *Environmental Health Perspectives* 108, no. 12 (December 2000): 1189–93.

Ōkura Nagatsune. *Jokōroku* (Record of Insect Control). In *Nihon nōsho zenshū* (Complete Works of Japanese Agricultural Writings), vol. 15, edited by Shadan Hōjin Nōsangyoson Bunka Kyōkai. Tokyo: Nōsangyoson Bunka Kyōkai, 1977.

Ooms, Herman. *Tokugawa Ideology: Early Constructs, 1570–1680.* Princeton, NJ: Princeton University Press, 1985.

———. *Tokugawa Village Practice: Class, Status, Power, Law.* Berkeley and Los Angeles: University of California Press, 1996.

Orii Seigo. *Hōjō daihijō* (Calamity at Hōjō). Tokyo: Asahi Shinbunsha, 1979.

———. *Nazo no Hōjō tankō daibakuhatsu* (The Reason for the Great Explosion at the Hōjō Colliery). Tokyo: Kokudosha, 1981.

Partner, Simon. *Toshié: A Story of Village Life in Twentieth-Century Japan.* Berkeley and Los Angeles: University of California Press, 2004.

Peacock, Andrea. *Libby, Montana: Asbestos and the Deadly Silence of an American Corporation.* Boulder, CO: Johnson Books, 2003.

Peattie, Mark R. *Ishiwara Kanji and Japan's Confrontation with the West.* Princeton, NJ: Princeton University Press, 1975.

Peck, Gunther. "The Nature of Labor: Fault Lines and Common Ground in Environmental and Labor History." *Environmental History* 11, no. 2 (April 2006): 212–38.

Pemberton, Stephen. "Canine Technologies, Model Patients: The Historical Production of Hemophiliac Dogs in American Biomedicine." In *Industrializing Organisms: Introducing Evolutionary History,* edited by Susan R. Schrepfer and Philip Scranton. Hagley Center Studies in the History of Business and Technology. New York and London: Routledge, 2004.

Perrow, Charles. *Normal Accidents: Living with High-Risk Technologies.* New York: Basic Books, 1984. Reprint, Princeton, NJ: Princeton University Press, 1999.

Pflugfelder, Gregory M., and Brett L. Walker, eds. *JAPANimals: History and Culture in Japan's Animal Life.* Ann Arbor: Center for Japanese Studies, University of Michigan, 2005.

Pollan, Michael. *The Botany of Desire: A Plant's-Eye View of the World.* New York: Random House, 2002.

———. *The Omnivore's Dilemma: A Natural History of Four Meals.* New York: Penguin Press, 2006.

Pomeranz, Kenneth. *The Great Divergence: China, Europe, and the Making of the Modern World Economy.* Princeton, NJ: Princeton University Press, 2000.

Ponting, Clive. *A Green History of the World: The Environment and the Collapse of Great Civilizations.* New York: Penguin Books, 1991.

Powell, John W. "A Hidden Chapter in History." *Bulletin of the Atomic Scientists* 37, no. 8 (October 1981): 43–53.

Pratt, Edward E. *Japan's Proto-industrial Elite: The Economic Foundations of the Gōnō.* Cambridge, MA: Harvard University Asia Center, Harvard University Press, 1999.

Quammen, David. *Monster of God: The Man-Eating Predator in the Jungles of History and the Mind.* New York: W. W. Norton, 2003.

———. "Planet of Weeds: Tallying the Losses of Earth's Animals and Plants." *Harper's Magazine,* October 1998, 57–69.

Ravina, Mark. *Land and Lordship in Early Modern Japan.* Stanford, CA: Stanford University Press, 1999.

Robertson, Jennifer. "The Shingaku Woman: Straight from the Heart." In *Recreating Japanese Women, 1600–1945,* edited by Gail Lee Bernstein. Berkeley and Los Angeles: University of California Press, 1991.

Rothschild, G. H. L. "The Biology and Ecology of Rice-Stem Borers in Sarawak (Malaysian Borneo)." *Journal of Applied Ecology* 8, no. 2 (August 1971): 287–322.

Russell, Edmund P. "Evolutionary History: Prospectus for a New Field." *Environmental History* 8, no. 2 (April 2003): 204–28.

———. "Introduction: The Garden in the Machine; Toward an Evolutionary History of Technology." In *Industrializing Organisms: Introducing Evolutionary History,* edited by Susan R. Schrepfer and Philip Scranton. Hagley Perspectives on Business and Culture, vol. 5. New York and London: Routledge, 2004.

———. "'Speaking of Annihilation': Mobilization for War against Human and Insect Enemies, 1914–1945." *Journal of American History* 82, no. 4 (March 1996): 1505–29.

Russell, Oland D. *The House of Mitsui—a Record of Three Centuries: Past History and Present Enterprises.* Tokyo: Mitsui Gomei Kaisha, 1933.

Ryūhyō no shachi ittō okitsu e Shiretoko jūittō suijaku shinuka (Of the Orcas Lodged in the Ice Floe: One Heads to Open Sea and Eleven Weaken and Probably Will Die). *Kyodo News On-Line,* 8 February 2005. http://news.livedoor.com/webapp/journal/cid_979065/detail.

Samuels, Richard J. *The Business of the Japanese State: Energy Markets in Comparative and Historical Perspective.* Ithaca, NY: Cornell University Press, 1987.

———. *"Rich Nation Strong Army": National Security and the Technological Transformation of Japan.* Ithaca, NY: Cornell University Press, 1994.

Satō, Tsuneo. "Tokugawa Villages and Agriculture." In *Tokugawa Japan: The Social and Economic Antecedents of Modern Japan,* edited by Chie Nakane and Shinzaburō Ōishi. Translation edited by Conrad Totman. Tokyo: University of Tokyo Press, 1990.

Scarry, Elaine. *The Body in Pain: The Making and Unmaking of the World.* Oxford: Oxford University Press, 1985.

Scheiner, Irwin. "Benevolent Lords and Honorable Peasants: Rebellion and Peasant Consciousness in Tokugawa Japan." In *Japanese Thought in the Tokugawa Period, 1600–1868: Methods and Metaphors,* edited by Tetsuo Najita and Irwin Scheiner. Chicago: University of Chicago Press, 1978.

———. *Christian Converts and Social Protest in Meiji Japan.* Berkeley and Los Angeles: University of California Press, 1970.

Schmidhauser, John R., and George O. Totten. *The Whaling Issue in U.S.-Japan Relations.* Boulder, CO: Westview Press, 1978.

Schneider, Andrew, and David McCumber. *An Air That Kills: How the Asbestos Poisoning of Libby, Montana, Uncovered a National Scandal.* New York: Berkley Books, 2004.

Scott, James C. *Seeing like a State: How Certain Schemes to Improve the Human Condition Have Failed.* New Haven, CT: Yale University Press, 1998.

Screech, Timon. *The Lens within the Heart: The Western Scientific Gaze and Popular Imagery in Later Edo Japan.* Honolulu: University of Hawai'i Press, 2002.

Seigle, Cecilia Segawa. *Yoshiwara: The Glittering World of the Japanese Courtesan.* Honolulu: University of Hawai'i Press, 1993.

Shachi jūnitō ryūhyō de ugokezu Rausu no kaigan (Twelve Orcas Lodged in Ice Floe along Rausu Coast). *Yomiuri On-Line* (Hokkaidō *hatsu*), 8 February 2005. http://hokkaido.yomiuri.co.jp/shiretoko/shiretoko_article/20050208-1_article.htm.

Shimokawa Kōshi, ed. *Kankyōshi nenpyō: Shōwa-Heisei hen* (Environmental History Chronology: Shōwa and Heisei Periods). Vol. 2. Tokyo: Kawade Shobō Shinsha, 2004.

Shoji, Kichiro, and Masuro Sugai. "The Arsenic Milk Poisoning Incident." In *Industrial Pollution in Japan,* edited by Jun Ui. Tokyo: United Nations University Press, 1992.

———. "The Ashio Copper Mine Pollution Case: The Origins of Environmental Destruction." In *Industrial Pollution in Japan,* edited by Jun Ui. Tokyo: United Nations University Press, 1992.

Sievers, Sharon L. *Flowers in Salt: The Beginnings of Feminist Consciousness in Modern Japan.* Stanford, CA: Stanford University Press, 1983.

Smith, Henry D., II. "The Capacity of Chūshingura." *Monumenta Nipponica* 58, no. 1 (Spring 2003): 1–37.

Smith, Robert J., and Ella Lury Wiswell. *The Women of Suye Mura.* Chicago: University of Chicago Press, 1982.

Smith, Thomas C. *The Agrarian Origins of Modern Japan.* Stanford, CA: Stanford University Press, 1959. Reprint, New York: Atheneum, 1966.

———. *Nakahara: Family Farming and Population in a Japanese Village, 1717–1830.* Stanford, CA: Stanford University Press, 1977.

———. *Native Sources of Japanese Industrialization, 1750–1920.* Berkeley and Los Angeles: University of California Press, 1988.

Smith, W. Eugene, and Aileen M. Smith. *Minamata.* New York: Holt, Rinehart and Winston, 1975.

Sombart, Werner. *Krieg und Kapitalismus* (War and Capitalism). Manchester, NH: Ayer Co. Publishers, 1975.

Sonu, Sunee C. *Shark Fisheries, Trade, and Market of Japan.* Washington, DC: U.S. Department of Commerce, National Oceanic and Atmospheric Administration, National Marine Fisheries Service, October 1998.

Souyri, Pierre François. *The World Turned Upside Down: Medieval Japanese Society.* New York: Columbia University Press, 2001.

"The State of the Science on Endocrine Disruptors." *Environmental Health Perspectives* 106, no. 7 (July 1998): A319–A320.

Steingraber, Sandra. *Having Faith: An Ecologist's Journey to Motherhood.* Cambridge: Perseus Publishing, 2001.

Stolz, Robert P. "'Yanakagaku': Pollution and Environmental Protest in Modern Japan." Ph.D. diss., University of Chicago, 2006.

"Strategic Program on Environmental Endocrine Disruptors" (SPEED '98). Environmental Agency, Government of Japan. www.env.go.jp/en.

Strong, Kenneth. *Ox against the Storm: A Biography of Tanaka Shozo—Japan's Conservationist Pioneer.* Tenterden, Kent, UK: Paul Norbury Publications, 1977. Reprint, Richmond, Surrey, UK: Japan Library, 1995.

Sugimoto, Masayoshi, and David L. Swain. *Science and Culture in Traditional Japan, A.D. 600–1854.* Cambridge, MA: MIT Press, 1978.

Sumitomo Kagaku Kōgyō Kabushikigaisha, ed. *Sumitomo Kagaku Kōgyō Kabushikigaisha shi* (A History of Sumitomo Chemical). Osaka: Sumitomo Kagaku Kōgyō Kabushikigaisha, 1981.

Sutter, Paul S. "Nature's Agents or Agents of Empire? Entomological Workers and Environmental Change during the Construction of the Panama Canal." *Isis* 98, no. 4 (December 2007): 724–54.

Suzuki Takeshi and Ogata Kazuki. *Nihon no eisei gaichū: Sono seitai to kujo* (Japan's Hygiene and Insect Pests). Tokyo: Shinshichōsha, 1958.

Tachibana Narisue. *Kokon chomonjū* (Notable Tales Old and New). Vol. 2. In *Shinchō Nihon koten shūsei* (Shinchō Collection of Classical Japanese Literature), vol. 76, edited by Nishio Kōichi and Kobayashi Yasuharu. Tokyo: Shinchōsha, 1986.

Takahashi, Yoshitomo, Hideto Hirasawa, and Keiko Koyama. "Restriction of Suicide Methods: A Japanese Perspective." *Archives of Suicide Research* 4 (1998): 101–7.

Takeuchi, Tadao, and Komyo Eto. *The Pathology of Minamata Disease: A Tragic Story of Water Pollution.* Fukuoka: Kyushu University Press, 1999.

Tanimura, Takashi. "Embryotoxicity of Acute Exposure to Methyl Parathion in Rats and Mice." *Archives of Environmental Health* 15 (November 1967): 609–13.

The Ten Foot Square Hut and Tales of the Heike. Translated by A. L. Sadler. Sydney: Angus and Robertson, 1928.

Tennensha Jiten Henshūbu, ed. *Byōchū nōyaku jiten* (Dictionary of Agricultural Chemicals for Disease and Insects). Tokyo: Tennensha, 1955.

Terazawa, Yuki. "Gender, Knowledge, and Power: Reproductive Medicine in Japan, 1690–93." Ph.D. diss., University of California, Los Angeles, 2001.

Thomas, Julia Adeney. "Photography, National Identity, and the 'Cataract of Times': Wartime Images and the Case of Japan." *American Historical Review* 103, no. 5 (December 1998): 1475–1501.

———. *Reconfiguring Modernity: Concepts of Nature in Japanese Political Ideology.* Berkeley and Los Angeles: University of California Press, 2001.

———. "'To Become as One Dead': Nature and the Political Subject in Modern Japan." In *The Moral Authority of Nature*, edited by Lorraine Daston and Fernando Vidal. Chicago: University of Chicago Press, 2004.

Toby, Ronald P. "Both a Borrower and a Lender Be: From Village Moneylender to Rural Banker in the Tempō Era." *Monumenta Nipponica* 46, no. 4 (Winter 1991): 483–512.

———. *State and Diplomacy in Early Modern Japan: Asia in the Development of the Tokugawa Bakufu.* Princeton, NJ: Princeton University Press, 1984. Reprint, Stanford, CA: Stanford University Press, 1991.

Tonomura, Hitomi. "Sexual Violence against Women: Legal and Extralegal Treatment in Premodern Warrior Societies." In *Women and Class in Japanese History*, edited by Hitomi Tonomura, Anne Walthall, and Wakita Haruko. Ann Arbor: Center for Japanese Studies, University of Michigan, 1999.

Totman, Conrad. *Early Modern Japan*. Berkeley and Los Angeles: University of California Press, 1993.

———. *Green Archipelago: Forestry in Pre-industrial Japan*. Berkeley and Los Angeles: University of California Press, 1989. Reprint, Athens: Ohio University Press, 1998.

———. *Japan's Imperial Forest: Goryōrin, 1889–1945*. Folkestone, Kent, UK: Global Oriental, 2007.

———. "Tokugawa Peasants: Win, Lose, or Draw." *Monumenta Nipponica* 41, no. 4 (Winter 1986): 457–76.

Tsubaki, Tadao, and Katsuro Irukayama, eds. *Minamata Disease: Methylmercury Poisoning in Minamata and Niigata, Japan*. Tokyo: Kodansha; Amsterdam: Elsevier Scientific Publishing, 1977.

Tsurumi, E. Patricia. *Factory Girls: Women in the Thread Mills of Meiji Japan*. Princeton, NJ: Princeton University Press, 1990.

Tsurumi, Kazuko. "Man, Nature and Technology: A Case of Minamata." In *Aspects of Endogenous Development in Modern Japan*, edited by Kazuko Tsurumi. Sophia University, Institute of International Relations Research Papers, series A-38, part 3. Tokyo: Sophia University, 1979.

Tsutsui, William M. "Landscapes in the Dark Valley: Toward an Environmental History of Wartime Japan." *Environmental History* 8, no. 2 (April 2003): 294–311.

Uchimizu Mamoru. *Shiryō Ashio kōdoku jiken* (Sources on the Ashio Copper-Poisoning Incident). Tokyo: Aki Shobō, 1971.

Ueda Tatsuo. *Hōjō-chō to tankō* (Hōjō Township and Coal Mining). Hōjō: Hōjō-chō Kyōiku Iinkai and Hōjō-chō Bunkazai Senmon Iinkai, 1994.

Uemura Shinsaku, Kawamura Hiroshi, Tsuji Machiko, Tomita Shigeyuki, and Maeda Shizuo. *Nōyaku dokusei no jiten* (Dictionary of Toxic Agricultural Chemicals). Tokyo: Sanseidō, 2002.

Ueno Tatsuhiko and Paku Keishuku, eds. *Kankyō kaitei toshi o mezashite: Yokkaichi kōgai kara no teigen* (Aiming for an Environmentally Agreeable City: A Proposal from Yokkaichi Industrial Pollution). Tokyo: Chūō Hōki, 2004.

Ui, Jun. *Industrial Pollution in Japan*. Tokyo: United Nations University Press, 1992.

Ulak, James T. "Utamaro's Views of Sericulture." *Art Institute of Chicago Museum Studies* 18, no. 1 (1992): 70–85.

Uno, Kathleen S. "Women and Changes in the Household Division of Labor." In *Recreating Japanese Women, 1600–1945*, edited by Gail Lee Bernstein. Berkeley and Los Angeles: University of California Press, 1991.

Upham, Frank K. *Law and Social Change in Postwar Japan*. Cambridge, MA: Harvard University Press, 1989.

U.S. Geological Survey. *Mineral Resources of the United States, 1914*. Washington, DC: Government Printing Office, 1916.

Utida, Syunro. "On Fluctuations in Population Density of the Rice Stem Borer *Chilo suppressalis*." *Ecology* 39, no. 4 (October 1958): 587–99.

van der Schalie, William H., Hank S. Gardner Jr., John A. Bantle, Chris T. De Rosa, Robert A. Finch, John S. Reif, Roy H. Reuter, Lorraine C. Backer, Joanna Burger, Leroy C. Folmar, and William S. Stokes. "Animals as Sentinels of Human Health." *Environmental Health Perspectives* 107, no. 4 (April 1999): 309–15.

Viramontes, Helena María. *The Moths and Other Stories*. Houston: Arte Público Press, 1985.

Vlastos, Stephen. *Peasant Protests and Uprisings in Tokugawa Japan*. Berkeley and Los Angeles: University of California Press, 1986.

Vogel, David. "Consumer Protection and Protectionism in Japan," *Journal of Japanese Studies* 18, no. 1 (Winter 1992): 119–54.

Walker, Brett L. "Commercial Growth and Environmental Change in Early Modern Japan: Hachinohe's Wild Boar Famine of 1749." *Journal of Asian Studies* 60, no. 2 (Spring 2001): 329–51.

———. *The Conquest of Ainu Lands: Ecology and Culture in Japanese Expansion, 1590–1800*. Berkeley and Los Angeles: University of California Press, 2001.

———. *The Lost Wolves of Japan*. Foreword by William Cronon. Seattle: University of Washington Press, 2005.

———. Review of *Ecological Modernisation and Japan*, by Brendan F. D. Barrett. *Journal of Japanese Studies* 33, no. 1 (Winter 2007): 294–98.

Walthall, Anne. "Village Networks: Sōdai and the Sale of Edo Nightsoil." *Monumenta Nipponica* 43, no. 3 (Autumn 1988): 279–303.

———. *The Weak Body of a Useless Woman: Matsuo Taseko and the Meiji Restoration*. Chicago: University of Chicago Press, 1998.

Watanabe Yūji. *Kurashi ni hisomu kagaku dokubutsu jiten* (A Dictionary of Chemical Poisons That Lurk in Our Daily Lives). Tokyo: Ie no Kōkyōkai, 2002.

Weiner, Jonathan. *The Beak of the Finch*. New York: Knopf, 1994.

White, Richard. "'Are You an Environmentalist or Do You Work for a Living?' Work and Nature." In *Uncommon Ground: Rethinking the Human Place in Nature*, edited by William Cronon. New York: W. W. Norton, 1996.

———. *The Organic Machine: The Remaking of the Columbia River*. New York: Hill and Wang, a Division of Farrar, Straus and Giroux, 1995.

Whorton, James. *Before "Silent Spring": Pesticides and Public Health in Pre-DDT America*. Princeton, NJ: Princeton University Press, 1974.

Wigen, Kären. *The Making of a Japanese Periphery, 1750–1920*. Berkeley and Los Angeles: University of California Press, 1995.

Wilkening, Kenneth E. *Acid Rain Science and Politics in Japan: A History of Knowledge and Action toward Sustainability*. Cambridge, MA: MIT Press, 2004.

Wong, Anny. "The Anti-tropical Timber Campaign in Japan." In *Environmental Movements in Asia*, edited by Arne Kalland and Gerard Persoon. Richmond, Surrey, UK: Curzon Press, 1998.

Worster, Donald. "The Wilderness of History." *Wild Earth*, Fall 1997, 12–13.

Yahagi Tadashi. "Chisso shi 1955–60 Minamatabyō" (Chisso History, 1955–60: Minamata Disease). *Urawa ronsō* 17 (January 1997): 23–46.

———. "Chisso shi 1960–65 Goi kōjō kensetsu" (Chisso History, 1960–65: Construction of the Goi Factory). *Urawa ronsō* 20 (June 1998): 21–60.

———. "Nihon Chisso hiryō (kabu) ni kansuru kenkyū" (Research on Chisso Corporation). *Urawa ronsō* 10 (March 1993): 55–96.

———. "Sengo Chisso shi 1945–55" (A History of Postwar Chisso, 1945–55). *Urawa ronsō* 14 (June 1995): 145–78.

Yamagata, Noboru, and Itsuzo Shigematsu. "Cadmium Pollution in Perspective." *Kōei eisei'in kenkyū hōkoku* (Bulletin of the Institute of Public Health) 19, no. 1 (1970): 1–27.

Yamamoto, Tadashi, and Hajime Imanishi. "Use of Shared Stocks in the Northwest Pacific Ocean with Particular Reference to Japan and the USSR." In *Resources and Environment in Asia's Marine Sector,* edited by James Barney Marsh. Washington, DC, and London: Taylor and Francis New York, 1992.

Yasuhara Akio. *Shinobi yoru kagaku busshitsu osen: Chikyū tanjō, seitaikei, gendai bunmei ni okeru kagaku busshitsu osen no keifu* (Exposing Chemical Contamination: The Birth of Earth, Ecological Structure, and the Genealogy of Chemical Contamination in the Context of Modern Civilization). Tokyo: Gōdō Shuppan, 1999.

Yasunaga, Toshinobu. *Ando Shoeki: Social and Ecological Philosopher of Eighteenth-Century Japan.* New York and Tokyo: Weatherhill, 1992.

The Yellow Emperor's Classic of Internal Medicine. Translated by Ilza Veith. Foreword by Ken Rose. Berkeley and Los Angeles: University of California Press, 2002.

Yoshida Katsumi. *Yokkaichi kōgai: Sono kyōkun to 21-seiki e no kadai* (Yokkaichi Industrial Pollution: Its Lessons and Challenges in the 21st Century). Tokyo: Kashiwa Shobō, 2002.

INDEX

Note: page numbers in *italics* refer to illustrations; those followed by "t" refer to tables.

chaos theory, 54, 59

chemical weapons, 59–60

Chikuhō region, 176, 180, 221, 222. *See also* coal mines

childbirth, 129–31, 166–67

Chilo suppressalis (Asiatic rice borers), 60, 62, 68–69

China: copper and silver trade with, 74–76, 77, 78t; fertilizers from, 154; Honkeiko mine and explosion (1942, Manchuria), 179, 195–96, 197–99; Japanese biological weapons program in, 37; silk and, 29, 30, 32, 74; Sino-Japanese War (1895), 177–78, 195

chisan, chisui ("care for mountains and forests, care for rivers and streams"), 106

Chisso Corporation: announcement and responses to Minamata disease, 173–74; in industrial-natural system, 16–17; lawsuit against, 174; "nitrogen problem" and, 157–58; octyl alchohol facility, 161; production technologies, 158–60; waste diversion by, 148–49. *See also* Minamata disease (methylmercury poisoning)

CHL (chlordane compounds), 220

chlorinated fluorocarbons, 24–25

chlorinated hydrocarbons, 58, 229n4

chokkō (Right Cultivation), 41, 42–43

cholinesterase inhibitors, 60

chrysanthemum-based insecticides, 57, 58

chrysanthemum-petroleum emulsion, 57

chrysolite, 213

Chūjō School of obstetrics, 165

cicadas, 34–35

Cicadula sexnotata (leaf hopper), 47

Cirian, Mike, 213

cisterns in cemeteries, 35–36

"civilization and enlightenment" (*bunmei kaika*), 177

coal mines: accident rates, 189t, 190t, 191t; Buddhist image of hell and hungry ghosts, 184–87; Chikuhō region and, 176; colonialism and, 196; Hōjō colliery, 177, 187–94; Hōjō explosion (1914), 187–88,

192–94, 199–206; Hokkaido collieries, 196–97; Honkeiko mine and explosion, Manchuria (1942), 179, 195–96, 197–99; Meiji modernization and, 88, 177–81; replaced by petroleum, 206–7; riots in, 81; women and families in, 180, 181–84, *183*

Coal Priority Production legislation (1946), 181

coevolution and silkworms, 33, 38

colonialism, 38–39, 196. *See also* Manchuria

coltan, 216

"compulsory purchases," 105

Confucianism and Neo-Confucianism: Andō and, 39, 41, 42; Ashio mine and paternalism of, 100; coal mining and family unit, 182; fishing communities and, 142; "good wife, wise mother" slogan and, 129; *ie* family/household system, 140–41, 144, 184, 205–6; medical notions, 164; sustainability and, 144

Confucius, 220

consequences, unintended. *See* unanticipated consequences

conservationism, modern, 106. *See also* environmentalism

consumerism and the "Plastic Age," 161

copper mines: history of trade and, 74–77, 78t; labor riots, 81–83; Meiji technological advances, 86–89; technological advances and environmental connections, 72–74; Tokugawa technological advances, 77–81; war demands and, 113, 239n6; women and, 81. *See also* Ashio copper mine

Cornell, Laurel, 131, 241n32

court cases, 134, 174, 215, 216, 218

creation mythologies, 30

crickets, 26–27

crocidolite, 213

Cronon, William, 7, 217–18, 227n9

cupellation smelting *(haibuki)*, 79–80

currency system, 75–76, 112, 239n5

cyanamide, 159

Cyclators, 173–74

Cyprinus carpio (carp), 63

Kamimura Tomoko, 160

Kamioka mine complex and Jinzū River Basin, *112*; hybrid causation and technological interfaces, 108–11; industrial disease in Tokugawa and early Meiji periods, 121–22; metals mined at, 112–13; Mitsui Group and Meiji government, 111–12; ore-processing facilities, *116*; oxidation and bioavailability, 110, 121; prisoner and unskilled labor at, 117, 120; situation and historical overview, 111; technologies and productivity, 113–17, 114t, 120–21, 122; warfare and empire building and, 113, 239n6; zinc and cadmium wasted in process, 116t, 118t, 119t. *See also* "it hurts, it hurts disease" (*itai itai byō*, cadmium poisoning)

Kannon (Goddess of Mercy), 187–88

Kanō Tanboku, 34, 38

Kasama Domain, 132

katakuchiiwashi anchovies (*Engraulis japonicus*), 149–50

Katō Shidzue, 182–84

Katsuki Gyūzan, 163–68

Katsuro Irukayama, 148

Kawabe Village (Saitama Prefecture), 105

Kawamata Incident (1900), 103

Kerr, Alex, 222

Kihira Usaburō, 4–5

Kimura Seisaburō, 192

Kira Yoshinaka, 3–4

Kitagawa Morisada, 27

Kita Kyūshū City, 221

Kitamura, Shoji, 148

Kobayashi Jun, 126

Kobayashi Kuniko, 212–13

Kodō zuroku (Illustrated Record of Copper Smelting) (Masuda), 80–81

kōgai ("public damage"), 217

Koizumi Yakumo (Lafcadio Hearn), 35

Kojiki (Records of Ancient Matters), 30, 31, 141

Komatsu Domain, 46–47

konbinato, 208

Korea, silver trade with, 76

Korean prisoners as laborers, 117, 180, 196

Kotoku Shushui, 104

Kubota Kanzaki factory, 213–15, 219

Kumamoto University, 138–39, 168, 171–73

Kurumatani Norio, 213–14

Kyōhō famine, 50–52

labor and work: Andō on Right Cultivation and, 43; in coal mines, 180; copper mine riots, 81–83; copper mines and interconnectedness, 73; Kamioka mines and, 117, 120; prisoners of war as laborers, 117, 120, 180, 196

labor control offices, 180

lactation deficiencies, 91

LaFleur, William, 186

language, pain as destruction of, 14

laws. *See* legal controls, regulations, and bans

lawsuits, 134, 174, 215, 216, 218

lead, 79, 112, 113, 114t

leaf hopper (*Cicadula sexnotata*), 47

legal controls, regulations, and bans: Agricultural Chemical Control Law (1948), 61; Basic Law for Pollution Control (1967), 217–19; pesticides, 66, 67t; status of, 215

Leopold, Aldo, 106

Lewis, Michael, 113

limestone mines, 221

"lime sulfur," 56

"living environment," 217–18

lodge system, 180

logging, 94

"Louseous Japanicas," 24, 132

Lurie, David, 35

Lyman, Benjamin, 196

macaques, 84

machines as organic, 73

Manchuria, 179, 195–96, 197–99

Manchuria Coal Mining Company, 195, 197

Markowitz, Gerald, 61

Maruyama Masao, 7, 8, 42, 215

WEYERHAEUSER ENVIRONMENTAL BOOKS

The Natural History of Puget Sound Country by Arthur R. Kruckeberg

*Forest Dreams, Forest Nightmares: The Paradox of Old Growth
    in the Inland West* by Nancy Langston

Landscapes of Promise: The Oregon Story, 1800–1940 by William G. Robbins

*The Dawn of Conservation Diplomacy: U.S.-Canadian Wildlife Protection Treaties
    in the Progressive Era* by Kurkpatrick Dorsey

Irrigated Eden: The Making of an Agricultural Landscape in the American West
    by Mark Fiege

Making Salmon: An Environmental History of the Northwest Fisheries Crisis
    by Joseph E. Taylor III

George Perkins Marsh, Prophet of Conservation by David Lowenthal

*Driven Wild: How the Fight against Automobiles Launched the Modern Wilderness
    Movement* by Paul S. Sutter

The Rhine: An Eco-Biography, 1815–2000 by Mark Cioc

Where Land and Water Meet: A Western Landscape Transformed
    by Nancy Langston

The Nature of Gold: An Environmental History of the Alaska/Yukon Gold Rush
    by Kathryn Morse

Faith in Nature: Environmentalism as Religious Quest by Thomas R. Dunlap

Landscapes of Conflict: The Oregon Story, 1940–2000 by William G. Robbins

The Lost Wolves of Japan by Brett L. Walker

Wilderness Forever: Howard Zahniser and the Path to the Wilderness Act
    by Mark Harvey

On the Road Again: Montana's Changing Landscape by William Wyckoff

Public Power, Private Dams: The Hells Canyon High Dam Controversy
    by Karl Boyd Brooks

Windshield Wilderness: Cars, Roads, and Nature in Washington's National Parks
    by David Louter

Native Seattle: Histories from the Crossing-Over Place by Coll Thrush

The Country in the City: The Greening of the San Francisco Bay Area
    by Richard A. Walker

Drawing Lines in the Forest: Creating Wilderness Areas in the Pacific Northwest
    by Kevin R. Marsh

Plowed Under: Agriculture and Environment in the Palouse by Andrew P. Duffin

Making Mountains: New York City and the Catskills by David Stradling

The Fishermen's Frontier: People and Salmon in Southeast Alaska
   by David F. Arnold
Shaping the Shoreline: Fisheries and Tourism on the Monterey Coast
   by Connie Y. Chiang
Dreaming of Sheep in Navajo Country by Marsha Weisiger
The Toxic Archipelago: A History of Industrial Disease in Japan by Brett L. Walker

WEYERHAEUSER ENVIRONMENTAL CLASSICS

The Great Columbia Plain: A Historical Geography, 1805–1910 by D. W. Meinig
*Mountain Gloom and Mountain Glory: The Development of the Aesthetics of the
   Infinite* by Marjorie Hope Nicolson
Tutira: The Story of a New Zealand Sheep Station by Herbert Guthrie-Smith
A Symbol of Wilderness: Echo Park and the American Conservation Movement
   by Mark Harvey
Man and Nature: Or, Physical Geography as Modified by Human Action
   by George Perkins Marsh; edited and annotated by David Lowenthal
Conservation in the Progressive Era: Classic Texts edited by David Stradling
DDT, Silent Spring, and the Rise of Environmentalism: Classic Texts
   edited by Thomas R. Dunlap

CYCLE OF FIRE BY STEPHEN J. PYNE

Fire: A Brief History
World Fire: The Culture of Fire on Earth
Vestal Fire: An Environmental History, Told through Fire,
   of Europe and Europe's Encounter with the World
Fire in America: A Cultural History of Wildland and Rural Fire
Burning Bush: A Fire History of Australia
The Ice: A Journey to Antarctica

CPSIA information can be obtained at www.ICGtesting.com
260591BV00002B/2/P